Human Gene Transfer

Transfert de gènes chez l'homme

Colloques **INSERM**
ISSN 0768-3154

Other *Colloques* published as co-editions by John Libbey Eurotext and INSERM

133 Cardiovascular and Respiratory Physiology in the Fetus and Neonate. *Physiologie Cardiovasculaire et Respiratoire du Fœtus et du Nouveau-né.*
Scientific Committee : P. Karlberg,
A. Minkowski, W. Oh and L. Stern;
Managing Editor : M. Monset-Couchard.
ISBN : John Libbey Eurotext 0 86196 125 0
INSERM 2 85598 340 1

134 Porphyrins and Porphyrias. *Porphyrines et Porphyries.*
Edited by Y. Nordmann.
ISBN : John Libbey Eurotext 0 86196 087 4
INSERM 2 85598 281 2

137 Neo-Adjuvant Chemotherapy. *Chimiothérapie Néo-Adjuvante.*
Edited by C. Jacquillat, M. Weil and D. Khayat.
ISBN : John Libbey Eurotext 0 86196 125 0
INSERM 2 85598 340 1

139 Hormones and Cell Regulation (10th European Symposium). *Hormones et Régulation Cellulaire (10ᵉ Symposium Européen).*
Edited by J. Nunez, J.E. Dumont and R.J.B. King.
ISBN : John Libbey Eurotext 0 86196 125 0X
INSERM 2 85598 340 1

147 Modern Trends in Aging Research. *Nouvelles Perspectives de la Recherche sur le Vieillissement.*
Edited by Y. Courtois, B. Faucheux, B. Forette,
D.L. Knook and J.A. Tréton.
ISBN : John Libbey Eurotext 0 86196 126 0X
INSERM 2 85598 340 1

149 Binding Proteins of Steroid Hormones. *Protéines de liaison des Hormones Stéroïdes.*
Edited by M.G. Forest and M. Pugeat.
ISBN : John Libbey Eurotext 0 86196 125 0
INSERM 2 85598 340 1X

151 Control and Management of Parturition. *La Maîtrise de la Parturition.*
Edited by C. Sureau, P. Blot, D. Cabrol, F. Cavaillé and G. Germain.
ISBN : John Libbey Eurotext 0 86196 125 0
INSERM 2 85598 340 1

Suite page 361

Human Gene Transfer

Transfert de gènes chez l'homme

Proceedings of the International Workshop on Human Gene Transfer held at the Château de Montvillargenne, Gouvieux-Chantilly (France), April 11-13, 1991

Sponsored by the Institut National de la Santé et de la Recherche Médicale (INSERM), Fondation de France (Fondation contre la Leucémie), Association Française contre les Myopathies and Société Beckman

Edited by

Odile Cohen-Haguenauer
Michel Boiron

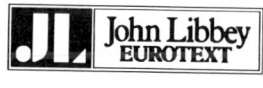

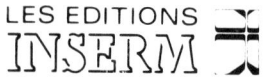

British Library Cataloguing in Publication Data
Human gene transfer
  I. Cohen-Haguenauer, Odile
  II. Boiron, Michel
  616.042

ISBN 0-86196-301-6
ISSN 0768-3154

First published in 1991 by

Editions John Libbey Eurotext
6 rue Blanche, 92120 Montrouge, France. (33) (1) 47 35 85 52
ISBN 0 86196 301 6

John Libbey and Company Ltd
13 Smiths Yard, Summerley Street, London SW18 4HR, England.
(44) (81) 947 27 77

Institut National de la Santé et de la Recherche Médicale
101 rue de Tolbiac, 75654 Paris Cedex 13, France.
(33) (1) 44 23 60 00
ISBN 2 855 98 497 1

ISSN 0768-3154

© 1991 Colloques INSERM/John Libbey Eurotext Ltd,
All rights reserved
Unauthorized publication contravenes applicable laws

Foreword

Outstanding international experts met at Montvillargenne (Chantilly-Gouvieux) near Paris in April 1991 for a three-day study on the subject of Gene Transfer in man.

Presentations and discussions were particularly fascinating. Beside senior scientists, a large number of young researchers and physicians was invited and participated actively in the discussion.

What were our reasons for organizing a workshop on gene transfer into somatic cells ?

- First of all, we wanted to promote contact between scientists and physicians and between young and more experienced people.

- Second, we thought it would be useful to provide an overview of recent progress in the field, in both the scientific and therapeutic domains.

- And third, we thought it important to consider which diseases are, or will be, the most suitable candidates for gene therapy and to discuss the relevance of gene therapy versus other methods of treatment for those that are not good targets. After all, organ transplants, when they are performed for hereditary diseases, can be considered a first attempt at gene therapy since one of their goals is actually to provide a functional gene.

It is important to evaluate gene therapy from every angle with care. It is a sensitive subject which questions Man's relation to himself and to God and, as such, it naturally provokes both high enthusiasm and deep concern.

It is fact, for example, that by the early 70s gene therapy had already acquired most of its theoretical support from knowledge of the mechanisms governing cell transformation by tumor viruses. And yet twenty years elapsed before its first medical application.

On the other hand, the success of gene therapy in Man in the context of ADA deficiency immediately elicited extremely enthusiastic reactions and already appears to be one of the great milestones of human medicine.

We know that much progress has been made in the development of gene transfer techniques and in the evaluation of potential cellular targets. But we also know that many difficulties and obstacles await us in the future. There are problems with the application of bone marrow modification techniques in animals and in Man.

The *in vivo* survival of modified skin fibroblasts grafts is relatively short-lived. Transplantation of genetically modified hepatocytes into the intact liver or ectopic sites must be improved. Direct transfer of DNA into the liver or muscle appears promising but further developments are necessary.

Up until now, researchers have been working to control genetic diseases. The future may paradoxically teach us that non-genetic diseases are the best targets for gene therapy.

In this context, genetically modified cells will be used as mini-factories for the production and distribution of biological substances : thrombolytic factors, "humanized" monoclonal anti-bodies, neurotrophic substances, CD4 molecules, etc.

This could represent an entirely new approach to vascular, infectious, neurological and cancerous diseases.

Pr Michel Boiron

I express my thanks to Odile Cohen-Haguenauer who has been the soul and spirit of the organization of this workshop, to Christèle Baudet for her excellent secretarial assistance and to our sponsors : Fondation contre la Leucémie, Association Française contre les Myopathies, Institut National de la Santé et de la Recherche Médicale, Société Beckman.

Avant-propos

Plusieurs éminents spécialistes internationaux se sont réunis à Montvillargenne (Chantilly-Gouvieux) pour un séminaire de trois jours sur le thème du transfert de gènes chez l'homme.

Les présentations et les discussions qui se sont tenues ont été particulièrement enrichissantes. En effet, à côté de scientifiques confirmés, de nombreux médecins et jeunes chercheurs invités à ce colloque ont activement pris part aux discussions.

Quelles raisons nous ont conduits à organiser un colloque consacré au transfert de gènes dans les cellules somatiques ?
- Nous souhaitions, tout d'abord, promouvoir des contacts entre scientifiques et médecins, et favoriser les échanges entre chercheurs confirmés et plus jeunes.
- Il nous a semblé, en outre, opportun de permettre de faire le point sur les plus récents progrès en ce domaine, tant dans ses aspects thérapeutiques que de recherche fondamentale.

- Enfin, il paraissait justifié de déterminer, parmi les maladies humaines, celles qui pourraient être les candidats les plus appropriés à la thérapie génique et de débattre de la pertinence de cette option thérapeutique par rapport à d'autres.

Puisque les transplantations d'organes dans leurs indications pour des maladies héréditaires viennent compenser l'anomalie d'expression d'un gène, elles peuvent, d'une certaine manière, être considérées comme les premières tentatives de thérapie génique.

Il importe d'envisager avec prudence l'ensemble des aspects de la thérapie génique. Il s'agit, en effet, d'un domaine sensible qui conduit l'homme à s'interroger sur des questions d'ordre existentiel et mystique, suscitant de ce fait à la fois un enthousiasme certain et une interpellation profonde.

En atteste, par exemple, le fait que les bases théoriques de la thérapie génique étaient jetées dès les années 70, dès lors que les mécanismes gouvernant la transformation cellulaire par les virus des tumeurs étaient appréhendés. Cependant, vingt années se sont écoulées avant que les première applications médicales ne voient le jour.

Par ailleurs, l'évolution favorable des premières tentatives de thérapie génique chez l'homme, dans le contexte du déficit en adénosine désaminase, a immédiatement suscité des réactions extrêmement enthousiastes, apparaissant ainsi comme une étape marquante de l'histoire de la médecine.

Comme on le sait, des progrès significatifs ont été réalisés à la fois dans le développement des techniques de transfert génétique et dans l'évaluation des cibles cellulaires potentielles. Néanmoins, de nombreux obstacles et difficultés sont à prévoir. Des problèmes persistent dans l'application des techniques de modification de la moelle osseuse chez les grands animaux non consanguins et chez l'homme.

La persistance de greffons de fibroblastes cutanés manipulés est relativement courte. L'introduction d'hépatocytes génétiquement modifiés dans un foie intact ou à un site ectopique demande à être perfectionnée. Le transfert direct d'ADN dans le foie ou le muscle semble prometteur mais des mises au point restent à effectuer.

Si jusqu'à présent les recherches se sont orientées électivement vers la correction de maladies génétiques, des développements futurs pourraient démontrer que les maladies non héréditaires constituent de meilleures cibles pour la thérapie génique.

Dans ce contexte des cellules manipulées génétiquement pourront être utilisées comme de petites usines destinées à produire et distribuer des substances biologiques telles que : facteurs thrombolytiques, anticorps monoclonaux «humanisés», substances neurotrophiques, molécules CD 4, etc.

L'approche thérapeutique de maladies vasculaires, infectieuses, neurologiques ou des cancers pourrait s'en trouver radicalement modifiée.

Pr Michel Boiron

Je tiens à remercier Odile Cohen-Haguenauer qui a été «l'âme et l'esprit» de l'organisation de ce colloque, Christèle Baudet pour sa parfaite assistance, ainsi que les organismes qui ont permis l'organisation de cette manifestation : Fondation contre la Leucémie, Association Française contre les Myopathies, Institut National de la Santé et de la Recherche Médicale, Société Beckman.

Organizing Committee
Comité d'organisation

Michel Boiron *(Président)*
Pascale Briand
Odile Cohen-Haguenauer
Olivier Danos
Yves Dumez
Alain Fischer
Eliane Gluckman
Jean-Michel Heard

Bertrand Jordan
Claudine Junien
Axel Kahn
Christian Larsen
Yves Najean
Michel Perricaudet
Gérard Schaison
Pierre Tambourin

List of authors and chairmen
Liste des auteurs et présidents de session

Beuzard Yves, INSERM U 91, Hôpital Henri Mondor, 51, avenue du Maréchal de Lattre de Tassigny, 94010 Créteil, France

Blaese R. Michael, Molecular Hematology Branch, Bldg, 10, 7D-18, National Heart, Lung and Blood Institute, NIH, Bethesda, Maryland 20892, États-Unis

Boiron Michel, Centre Hayem, Hôpital Saint-Louis, 1, avenue Claude Vellefaux, 75010 Paris, France

Bordignon Claudio, Istituto Scientifico H.S. Raffaele, Department of Laboratory Medicine, Via Olgettina, 60, 20132 Milano, Italie

Briand Pascale, Institut Cochin de Génétique Moléculaire, INSERM CJF 90-03, 22, rue Méchain, 75674 Paris Cedex 14, France

Broxmeyer Hal E., Walther Oncology Center, Indiana University School of Medicine, 975 W. Walnut Street, Indianapolis, Indiana 46202-5121, États-Unis

Capecchi Mario R., Howard Hughes Medical Institute, Department of Biology, University of Utah, 337, South Biology Bld, Salt Lake City, Utah 84112, États-Unis

Caskey C. Thomas, Institute for Molecular Genetics and Howard Hugues Medical Institute, Baylo College of Medicine, One Baylor Plaza, Houston TX 77030, États-Unis

Cohen-Haguenauer Odile, Service de Médecine Nucléaire, Hôpital Saint-Louis, 1, avenue Claude-Vellefaux, 75010 Paris, France

Crystal Ronald G., Pulmonary Branch, NHLBI, National Institutes of Health, Building 10, Room 6D03, Bethesda, Maryland 20892, États-Unis

Danos Olivier, Laboratoire Rétrovirus et Transfert génétique, Institut Pasteur, 28, rue du Docteur Roux, 75015 Paris, France

Fischer Alain, INSERM U 132, Unité d'Immunologie et d'Hématologie, Département de Pédiatrie, Hôpital Necker, 149, rue de Sèvres, 75743 Paris Cedex 15, France

Geller Alfred I., The Jimmy Fund, Dana Farber Cancer Institute, 44, Binney Street, Boston, MA 02115, États-Unis

Girard Marc, Département de Virologie, Institut Pasteur, 28, rue du Docteur Roux, 75724 Paris Cedex 15, France

Gluckman Eliane, Service de Greffes de Moelle, Trèfle 3, Hôpital Saint-Louis, 1, avenue Claude-Vellefaux, 75475 Paris Cedex 10, France

Goff Stephen P., Departments of Biochemistry and Molecular Biophysics, College of Physicians and Surgeons, Columbia University, 630 W. 168th Street, New York, NY 10032, États-Unis

Gottesman Michael M., Laboratory of Cell Biology, Bld 37, Room 2E18, Department of Health and Human Services, National Institutes of Health, Bethesda, Maryland 20892, États-Unis

Grosveld Frank G., Medical Research Council, National Institute for Medical Research, The Ridgeway, Mill Hill, London NW7 1AA, Royaume-Uni

Guénet Jean-Louis, Génétique des Mammifères, Institut Pasteur, 28, rue du Docteur Roux, 75724 Paris Cedex 15, France

Hofnung Maurice, Unité de Programmation Moléculaire et Toxicologie Génétique, Institut Pasteur, 28, rue du Docteur Roux, 75724 Paris Cedex 15, France

Houssin Didier, Clinique Chirurgicale, Groupe Hospitalier Cochin, 27, rue du Faubourg Saint-Jacques, 75674 Paris Cedex 14, France

Junien Claudine, Génétique et Pathologie Fœtale, INSERM U 73, Château de Longchamp, Bois de Boulogne, 75016 Paris, France

Lehn Pierre, Service de Greffes de Moelle, Trèfle 3, Hôpital Saint-Louis, 1, avenue Claude-Vellefaux, 75010 Paris, France

Leserman Lee, Centre d'Immunologie INSERM-CNRS de Marseille-Luminy, Case 906, 13288 Marseille Cedex 9, France

Lévy Jean-Paul, Immunologie et Oncologie des Maladies Rétrovirales, INSERM U.152, Institut Cochin de Génétique Moléculaire, Hôpital Cochin, 27, rue du Faubourg Saint-Jacques, 75014 Paris, France

Lowy Douglas, Laboratory of Cellular Oncology, Blg 37, Room 1B-26, National Institutes of Health, Bethesda, Maryland 20892, États-Unis

Luzzatto Lucio, National Cancer Institute, Royal Postgraduate Medical School, Hammersmith Hospital, Du Cane Road, London, W12 Onn, Royaume-Uni

Mallet Jacques, Laboratoire de Neurobiologie Cellulaire et Moléculaire, CNRS, avenue de la Terrasse, 91198 Gif-sur-Yvette Cedex, France

Mandel Jean-Louis, INSERM U 184, UER Sciences Médicales, 11, rue Humann, 67085 Strasbourg Cedex, France

Mulligan Richard C., Whitehead Institute for Biomedical Research, Nine Cambridge Center, Cambridge, MA 02142, États-Unis

Munnich Arnold, INSERM U 12, Hôpital des Enfants-Malades, Tour Technique Lavoisier, 149, rue de Sèvres, 75743 Paris Cedex 15, France

Perricaudet Michel, Laboratoire de Génétique des Virus Oncogènes, CNRS URA, Institut Gustave Roussy, PR 2, 39, rue Camile Desmoulins, 94805 Villejuif Cedex, France

Piechaczyk Marc, Laboratoire de Biologie Moléculaire, UA CNRS 1191, Génétique Moléculaire, USTL, place E. Bataillon, 34095 Montpellier Cedex 05, France

Ragot Thierry, Laboratoire de Génétique des Virus Oncogènes, Institut Gustave Roussy, PR 2, 39, rue Camille Desmoulins, 94805 Villejuif Cedex, France

Schaison Gérard, Service de Réanimation Hématologique, Unité d'Hématologie Pédiatrique C3, Hôpital Saint-Louis, 1, avenue Claude Vellefaux, 75475 Paris Cedex 10, France

Tambourin Pierre, Section de Biologie, Institut Curie, 26, rue d'Ulm, 75231 Paris Cedex 05, France

Valerio Dinko, TNO Institute of Applied Radiobiology and Immunology, Gene Therapy Section, PO Box 5815, 2280 HV Rijswijk, Pays-Bas

Varet Bruno, INSERM U.152 et Service d'Hématologie, Groupe Hospitalier Cochin, 27, rue du Faubourg Saint-Jacques, 75674 Paris Cedex 14, France

Visser Jan W.M., Department of Cell Biology, TNO Institute of Applied Radiobiology and Immunology, PO Box 5815, 2280 HV Rijswijk, Pays-Bas

Wagner Erwin, Research Institute for Molecular Pathology, Dr Bohr-Gasse 7, A-1030 Vienna, Autriche

Yaniv Moshe, Unité des Virus Oncogènes, Institut Pasteur, 28, rue du Docteur Roux, 75724 Paris Cedex 15, France

Contents
Sommaire

- V   Foreword
- VII *Avant-propos*
- IX   Organizing Committee
  Comité d'organisation
- XI   List of authors and chairmen
  Liste des auteurs et présidents de session

INTRODUCTION

3   **O. Cohen-Haguenauer, M. Boiron**

PROSPECTS FOR GENE THERAPY
LES PERSPECTIVES DE LA THÉRAPIE GÉNIQUE

17   **C.T. Caskey**
Genetic disorders
Maladies génétiques

27   **J.P. Lévy**
HIV infection and gene therapy
Infection par le virus HIV et thérapie génique

33   **M. Girard**
Vaccines
Vaccins

GENE TRANSFER : TOOLS AND MECHANISMS
TRANSFERT DE GÈNES : MOYENS ET MÉCANISMES

51   **L. Stratford-Perricaudet, M. Perricaudet**
Gene transfer into animals : the promise of adenovirus
Transfert de gènes à l'animal : les promesses de l'adénovirus

63 **A.I. Geller, H.J. Federoff**
The use of HSV-1 vectors to introduce heterologous genes into neurons : implications for gene therapy
Utilisation de vecteurs HSV-1 pour introduire des gènes hétérologues dans les neurones : implications pour la thérapie génique

75 **L. Leserman**
Liposomes and cell targeting of nucleic acids
Liposomes et ciblage cellulaire d'acides nucléiques

SOMATIC GENE TRANSFER : DATA
1. HEMATOPOIETIC TISSUES
TRANSFERT DE GÈNES SOMATIQUE : RÉSULTATS
1. TISSUS HÉMATOPOÏÉTIQUES

85 **J.W.M. Visser, M.P.W. Einerhand, D. Valerio**
Four reasons for purifying stem cells for gene therapy
Quatre raisons de purifier les cellules souches hématopoïétiques pour la thérapie génique

95 **H.E. Broxmeyer, C. Carow, G. Hangoc, P.C. Hendrie, S. Cooper**
Hematopoietic stem and progenitor cells in human umbilical cord blood
Cellules souches hématopoïétiques et progéniteurs dans le sang de cordon ombilical humain

103 **C. Bordignon, G. Ferrari, S. Rossini, R. Giavazzi, E. Gilboa, F. Mavilio**
A human PBL/immunodeficient mouse model for *in vivo* preclinical studies of human gene therapy
Un modèle de souris immunodéficiente tolérant les lymphocytes humains du sang périphérique pour des études précliniques in vivo en vue d'une thérapie génique chez l'homme

113 **E. Braakman, V.W. van Beusechem, B.A. van Krimpen, A. Fischer, R.L.H. Bolhuis, D. Valerio**
Expression of adenosine deaminase in genetically corrected T lymphocytes from an ADA$^-$ SCID patient
Expression de l'adénosine désaminase par les lymphocytes T modifiés génétiquement d'un patient atteint de DICS-ADA$^-$

121 **P. Fraser, D. Talbot, S. Philipsen, S. Pruzina, M. Antoniou, M. Lindenbaum, O. Hanscombe, N. Dillon, F. Grosveld**
The regulation of human globin gene switching
La régulation de la commutation des gènes du locus β-globine chez l'homme

2. OTHER TISSUES
2. AUTRES TISSUS

137 **R.M. Blaese**
Lymphocytes for gene therapy
Lymphocytes et thérapie génique

147 **S.L. Brody, R.G. Crystal**
Gene therapy of the respiratory tract
Thérapie génique de l'arbre respiratoire

159 **P. Briand, C. Cavard, L.D. Stratford-Perricaudet, M. Levrero, I. Makeh, G. Grimber, J.F. Chasse, M. Perricaudet**
Germinal and somatic gene therapy of a liver enzymatic defect in mouse
Thérapie génique germinale et somatique d'un déficit enzymatique hépatique chez la souris

169 **N. Ferry, O. Duplessis, D. Calise, D. Houssin, J.M. Heard, O. Danos**
A procedure for stable gene transfer into the liver
Un procédé de transfert stable de gènes dans le foie

177 **M. Etienne-Julan, P. Roux, S. Carillo, P. Jeanteur, M. Piechaczyk**
Approaches to cell targeting by murine recombinant retroviruses
Ciblage cellulaire par les rétrovirus recombinants murins

185 **M.M. Gottesman, I. Pastan**
The multidrug resistance (MDR1) gene as a selectable marker in gene therapy
Le gène de résistance pléiotropique aux cytotoxiques (MDR1) comme marqueur de sélection pour la thérapie génique

HOMOLOGOUS RECOMBINATION AND ANIMAL MODELS
RECOMBINAISON HOMOLOGUE ET MODÈLES ANIMAUX

195 **J.L. Guénet**
Animal models of human genetic diseases
Modèles animaux de maladies génétiques humaines

209 **M.R. Capecchi**
Homologous recombination and gene targeting on ES cells
Recombinaison homologue et ciblage génique dans les cellules ES

217 **P.L. Schwartzberg, E.J. Robertson, S.P. Goff**
A substitution mutation in the *c-abl* gene introduced into the murine germ line by targeted gene disruption in embryonic stem cells
Une mutation de substitution dans le gène c-abl introduit dans la lignée germinale de souris par interruption génique ciblée

227 **E.F. Wagner**
Transgenic mouse models for bone and vascular diseases and gene transfer into hematopoietic cells
Souris transgéniques comme modèles de maladies de l'os et de l'endothélium vasculaire et transfert de gène aux cellules hématopoïétiques

VACCINES
VACCINS

237 **D. O'Callaghan, A. Charbit, J.M. Clément, P. Martineau, S. Muir, S. Szmelcman, C. Leclerc, M. Hofnung**
Avirulent bacteria expressing heterologous genes : implications for vaccines
Des bactéries avirulentes exprimant des gènes hétérologues : implications pour le développement de vaccins

249 **T. Ragot, M. Eloit, M. Perricaudet**
Recombinant E1A-defective adenoviruses expressing pseudorabies and Epstein-Barr virus glycoproteins induce immunological responses as live vaccines in rabbits and mice
Des adénovirus recombinants défectifs pour E1A et exprimant des glycoprotéines du virus de la pseudorage et du virus d'Epstein-Barr provoquent une réponse immunitaire et constituent des vaccins vivants chez le lapin et la souris

SELECTED POSTERS
COMMUNICATIONS SÉLECTIONNÉES

263 **J.A. Wolff, G. Acsadi, S. Jiao, A. Jani, D. Duke, P. Williams, W. Chong**
Direct gene transfer and expression into rodent striated muscle *in vivo*
Transfert de gènes in vivo par injection directe dans les cellules du muscle strié de rongeur

267 **C. Bonifer, N. Yannoutsis, F. Grosveld, A.E. Sippel**
Determination of DNA-elements necessary for macrophage specific and position independent expression of the chicken lysozyme gene in transgenic mice
Caractérisation dans des souris transgéniques des séquences d'ADN nécessaires à l'expression à la fois spécifique dans les macrophages et indépendante de la position du gène de lysozyme du poulet

271 **B. Quantin, M. Perricaudet, S. Tajbakhsh, M. Buckingham, J.L. Mandel**
Adenovirus as an expression vector in muscle cells. Application to dystrophin
L'adénovirus comme vecteur d'expression dans les cellules musculaires. Applications à la dystrophine

273 **T.J. Velu, R.A. Feldman, E.M. Valverius, P.E. Tambourin, D.R. Lowy**
Highly efficient retroviral vectors derived from Harvey and Friend murine viruses
Vecteurs rétroviraux hautement efficaces, dérivés des virus Harvey et Friend de la souris

275 **F.L. Cosset, J.L. Thomas, M. Afanassieff, C. Legras, R.M. Molina, C. Faure, Y. Chebloune, A. Drynda, C. Ronfort, S. Valsésia, V.M. Nigon, G. Verdier**
Gene transfer into birds using ALV-based retrovirus vectors
Transfert de gènes chez l'oiseau au moyen de vecteurs rétroviraux dérivés du VLA (virus de la leucose aviaire)

279 **J.L. Villeval, D. Metcalf, G.R. Johnson**
Fatal polycythemia induced in mice by dysregulated erythropoietin (Epo) production by hemopoietic cells
Polyglobulie fatale provoquée par une production dérégulée d'érythropoïétine par les cellules hématopoïétiques

283 **D. Cournoyer, M. Scarpa, K. Mitani, K. A. Moore, J.W. Belmont, C.T. Caskey**
Gene transfer of adenosine deaminase into primitive human hematopoietic progenitor cells
Transfert du gène de l'adénosine désaminase dans les précurseurs hématopoïétiques primaires chez l'homme

285 **A. Brandenburger, S.J. Russell, M.K.L. Collins, J. Rommelaere**
Transfer and selective expression of interleukin genes in neoplasic cells by means of recombinant parvoviruses

Transfert et expression sélective de gènes d'interleukines dans les cellules néoplasiques au moyen de parvovirus recombinants

287 **A. Rahemtulla, A. Arabian, W.P. Fung-Leung, M. Schilham, A. Wakeham, T.W. Mak**
Targeted disruption of the murine CD4 gene in the germ-line by homologous recombination
Interruption ciblée par recombinaison homologue du gène CD4 murin dans la lignée germinale

ROUND TABLE : GENE TRANSFER AND HUMAN DISEASES
TABLE RONDE : TRANSFERT DE GÈNES EN PATHOLOGIE HUMAINE
Transcription : O. Cohen-Haguenauer

293 **T. Caskey**
Introduction

295 **Y. Beuzard**
Hemoglobinopathies and human gene transfer in mice
Hémoglobinopathies et transfert de gènes humains chez la souris

298 **A. Fischer**
Severe combined immunodeficiency
Déficit immunitaire combiné sévère

302 **E. Gluckman**
Fetal medicine and cord blood
Médecine fœtale et sang de cordon ombilical

307 **C. Junien**
Tumor suppressor genes
Gènes suppresseurs de tumeurs

310 **G. Schaison**
Gene tranfer and leukemias
Transfert de gènes et leucémies

312 **A. Munnich**
Inborn errors of metabolism
Erreurs innées du métabolisme

317 **D. Houssin**
Gene transfer and liver cells
Transfert de gènes et cellules hépatiques

319 **R. Crystal**
Cystic fibrosis
Mucoviscidose

322 **J.L. Mandel**
Fragile X syndrome
Syndrome de l'X fragile

324 **T. Caskey**
Duchenne muscular dystrophy
Myopathie de Duchenne de Boulogne

329 **J. Mallet**
CNS and neurons
Système nerveux central et neurones

333 **P. Lehn**
Scientific and ethical points to consider for the design of clinical trials of human gene therapy
Problèmes scientifiques et éthiques

340 **L. Luzzatto**
Concluding remarks
Conclusions

347 **M. Boiron**
Closing address
Clôture du Congrès

349 Author index
Index des auteurs

351 List and address of participants
Liste et adresse des participants

Introduction

Introduction

Odile Cohen-Haguenauer [1] and Michel Boiron [2]

[1] Service de médecine nucléaire, [2] Centre Hayem, hôpital Saint-Louis, 1, avenue Claude Vellefaux, 75010 Paris, France

Introduction

These past years, the joint efforts of clinicians and researchers allowed the characterization of the molecular anomalies of genes responsible for human diseases; whether constitutive genetic anomalies, solid or hematopoietic tumors, or infectious diseases due to retroviruses such as AIDS.

This progress is due in part to the major contribution of reverse genetics and to the constant development and evolution of molecular biology techniques : through these two pathways, the pathophysiology of inborn diseases such as cystic fibrosis or Duchenne's muscular dystrophy are now understood.

Identification and cloning of the incriminated genes open the way to prenatal diagnoses or to the detection of persons at risk. However, the ability to perform a diagnosis cannot be satisfying in the absence of therapeutic means. The primary goal of this research is that of therapy.

Several lines of therapeutic research can be considered once the molecular and pathogenetic mechanisms of the disease have been understood ; schematically, they can be classified in two groups : -pharmacologic, where one can tailor specific drugs, based on the functional characteristics of the product of the defective gene ; -or genetic, based on the insertion of transgenes which are introduced in the very cells where the anomaly is being expressed in order to substitute themselves to the endogenous gene. This gene therapy consists in the compensation of a functionally abnormal gene by the introduction of a normal gene which will take over the synthesis of the defective protein.

Several prerequisites are common to all candidate disease for gene therapy :
- the pathogenesis of the disease must be understood at the molecular level and involve a single gene; - the corresponding DNA sequences must be available ; - effective methods of gene delivery must be established ; - the regulatory sequences allowing an appropriate expression of the transfered gene must be known ; - finally, taking into account the difficulties in the execution and the potential cost of this therapy, it seems reasonable to limit its application to severe diseases without adequate therapeutic alternative.

Techniques of gene transfer: the vectors

Different approaches can be considered to deliver a given DNA sequence, called transgene, to the nucleus of a cell where this genetic material has to be stably integrated and potentially be transmitted to the following generations issued from that cell. One can thereby alter a group of cells in order to produce a protein which can be directed towards the deficient organ, such a genetically controlled micro-factory. One can also collect cells, alter them in vitro and re-establish them in the same subject without risk of graft rejection. One can ideally deliver the transgene to the target organ, either directly or by using the specificity of a vectorisation system regarding a particular organ or cell type.

Following the disease one is considering and the cell type implicated, the delivery systems of the transgene or vectors, will not have the same requirements. The scope of available techniques is presented and discussed in a separate session.

If to this day, the retroviruses seemed the most eligible mean for efficient gene transfer, but only in cells undergoing at least one mitotic cycle to obtain integration of the viral genome and its stable expression, new and extremely promising vectors are presented.

Herpes virus derived vectors

These vectors are defective herpes viruses, derived from thermo-sensitive mutants incapable of replicating at temperatures above 31°C and possessing a natural tropism for the cells of the nervous system.

Alfred Geller (Boston, USA) was able to use his herpes vectors, previously tested on nervous cells cell lines in culture, to inject stereotaxically in vivo, in the brain of adult rats ; an expression of the trangene was observed for over 6 weeks, in the neurones surrounding the injection point as in those located at a distance, at the end point of the axonal projections. These tools have possible applications both in the expression of neurotrophic factors in the vicinity of axonal sections or neuronal degeneration, and in Parkinson's disease where an expression of tyrosine hydroxylase (the enzyme limiting the level of dopamine biosynthesis), in the striatum, should be able to effectively relieve the symptoms and offer a promising alternative to fetal cell engraftment.

Adenoviruses

Recombinant adenoviruses offer a first choice alternative to retroviruses when addressing the transfer of a gene into differentiated cells incapable of proliferating, such as neuro-muscular cells ; or when the target cells are not explantable, such as pulmonary epithelial cells. Michel Perricaudet (Villejuif, France) has developed his system of adapting the adenovirus's genome as a cloning and expression vector. Importantly, the recombinant adenoviruses, due to their very high infectious titers and their ubiquity, can be administered *in vivo* ; either intravenously as shown by Pascale Briand (Paris, France) in the ornithine transcarbamylase (OTC) deficiency, with a correction of the liver deficiency in the newborn mouse homozygous for the *spf-ash* mutation ; either by the endotracheal pathway, with air-sprays, aiming the bronchial epithelium in diseases such as the alpha-1 antitrypsin deficiency, where an successful expression could recently be evidenced, or cystic fibrosis in which the success of this stategy would represent the first therapeutic hope in man, as was shown by Ronald Crystal (NIH Bethesda, USA) ; finally by direct intra-muscular injection, in the hope of delivering the gene coding for dystrophin to the musular cells in Duchenne muscular dystrophy, as suggested by the work of Béatrice Quantin and Jean Louis Mandel (Strasbourg, France) with an adenovirus containing a reporter gene which had a significant level of expression in myotubes. Some points, essentially linked to the potential secondary effects of the intravenous or endotracheal administration of recombinant adenoviruses remain to be cleared ; it concerns in particular an eventual immune reaction in a patient receiving repeated doses of virus, but also the possibility of generating an infectious virus in the case of recombination or copackaging with an opportunistic wild type virus.

Liposomes

Liposomes, lipid vesicles carrying the necessary DNA sequences, would theoretically offer an elegant alternative to viral vectors. Indeed, these particles can include in their lipid bilayer proteins which determinants can be expressed on the surface and be specifically identified. Targeting of a particular cell type can be obtained. However, in the present stage of research, as shown by Lee Leserman (Marseille, France), when a liposome penetrates in a cell it follows the metabolic pathway of degradation by the intracellular lysosomes if it has not been captured by macrophages prior to its integration in the targeted cell.

Retroviruses

Retroviruses do have numerous potential utilities for gene transfer. First, by their natural life cycle they integrate efficiently into the host genome and in principle they should be able to express the genes of interest over a long term. They are relatively simple since they contain only three required genes to make the particle itself : *gag*, *pol* and *env*. Their host range which conditions the cell type that they can infect is determined by the *env* protein product. Retroviral vectors that have been used to date for transmission into primates such as humans, are murine retroviruses which are contained in an amphotropic envelope. The retroviral regulatory element is the long terminal repeat (*LTR*) which corresponds to sequences that are found both at the 5' and at the 3' end. Retroviruses can be altered in their ability to express genes through deletions in the *LTRs* (self-inactivating retroviral vectors) ; it also is possible to introduce cis-regulatory sequences in other regions of the viral DNA in order to specifically control and even modulate the expression of the gene which is included.

When one is thinking of using retroviruses as vectors for genes of interest, the only viral sequence which is required in the region framed by the two *LTRs* is the packaging sequence which is able to package the viral RNA into the virions, as opposed to viral proteins which can be provided in *trans* in an auxiliary cell-line. Means are available for trying to eliminate the possibility of transfering helper viruses but still make use of the high efficiency of a virus induced transmission, through the expression of *gag, pol* and *env* : 1°- either from an heterologous promotor such as an SV40 promotor so that the 5' LTR is missing and thereby the possibility for homologous recombination is further reduced when the recombinant virus is put in ;

2°- or even to split the *gag pol* and *env* genes so that *gag* and *pol* are made off of an heterologous promotor from one DNA and the *env* protein is made off of a second independent DNA ; therefore multiple recombinational events would be required in order to regenerate an infectious helper virus. This represents a potentially efficient way of trying to limit the possibilities for generating such a recombinant. This is a single infection-cycle process. The target cell is not producing any virus.

More than one gene can be introduced into retroviruses, and there is a plasticity to the size of the genome that can be packaged. The virus normally makes its protein products through two distinct messenger RNAs ; the *gag-pol* products are made off of a full length messenger RNA and the *env* product is made off of a spliced message. In principle, it should be possible to replace either one gene or the other for gene transfer experiments ; in practice, this has turned out to be rather complicated since when *gag-pol* are replaced with one gene and *env* with the second gene, it has been very unpredictable as to whether one or both of these genes will be expressed. The acceptor and donor splice sites thus seem to be used in a relatively unpredictable manner. Therefore, when there is need for the simultaneous transfer of two genes with the same retroviral vector, in general one of the genes is driven by the retroviral LTR, and the second by an auxiliary promotor. One gene can be used as a selectable marker while the phenotypic activity of the second gene is assessed.

Despite the great interest triggered by the successes of new systems of gene transfer, the progress accomplished with the retroviral vectors deserves all our attention. Indeed, the efficacy of retrovirus mediated transfer has greatly increased ; in particular thanks to the higher infectious titers, jointly with the development of auxiliary lineages presenting garanties of non-generation of replication-competent viruses ; and finally to the use of viral LTRs and constructs which achieve both infection and expression in undifferentiated cells. Retroviruses do not tend to be very target specific ; but there are in principle ways in which this could be managed, either by making changes in the *env* protein or perhaps by altering the cis-regulatory elements that are used for expressing the viral genome.

Classically, these vectors address a cell population obtained in a patient, manipulated in vitro, then reinfused in an autologous fashion. In this context, one ideally should deal with a tissue comprising a population of stem cells from which this tissue derives, or cells capable of proliferating in the absence of stem cell compartment ; in this case, reiteration of viral infections at regular intervals probably become required.

Hematopoietic tissue ; first attempts in human gene therapy.

One of the choice targets for retroviruses remains the hematopoietic tissue, along two lines, presently in full expansion: 1°) the transfer of genes to the totipotent hematopoietic stem cells, which have an almost unlimited self-renewal capacity ; and 2°) the transfer to explanted lymphocytes, expanded in vitro in the presence of interleukin 2 and reinfused to the patients. It is in this framework that the first attempts of gene therapy in man are described.

Indeed, the accessibility of the marrow stem cells to the transgene was not as easy as it had been hoped for, taken into account the high infectious potential of the retroviruses which is followed by an automatic integration in the host cell genome. There are problems at several levels: - the access to the actual pluripotent stem cell, - the insufficient percentage of cells transduced among the marrow population (insufficient infectious viral titer), - regulation of the level of expression of the transgenes as well quantitative as spatiotemporal.

However several hurdles have already been successfully passed as witnessed by several convincing and encouraging reports presented at this meeting.

Stem cell purification and gene transfer

Thus, the purification of pluripotent hematopoietic stem cells, still speculative a few years ago, becomes a reality in the mouse, as reported by Jan Visser (Rijswijk, the Netherlands). In man, the impossibility to utilize experimental hematologic reconstitutions after recipient irradiation as performed in mice, led to the development of experimental systems, such as the establishement of a human originated hemopoiesis in immunodeficient mice, xenograft tolerant ; According to Bruno Péault (Systemics, Palo Alto, USA), the purification of human pluripotent cells becomes highly probable. The SCID-Hu mice murine model also enables to test various pathologies of the hematopoietic tissue such as leukemias or its infection by the AIDS virus ; in this context, numerous pharmacologic tests are set up in order to evaluate the newly developed antiviral candidates.

From another standpoint, Hal Broxmeyer (Indianapolis, USA) presented his attempts at the purification of pluripotent stem cells from cord blood collected at birth.

Allogenic bone marrow transplants performed in collaboration with Eliane Gluckman (Paris, France) were vastly successful, in particular for Fanconi's anemia. These first results could lead to the utilization of this usually discarded material, as a potential basis for allogenic bone marrow transplantation; the induction of immune tolerance towards these cells seems easier to achieve than in the case of later obtained graft material. It seems therefore within reason to try to purify stem cells from this type of material ; these could then be utilized for gene transfer ; preliminary data tend to indicate that the cord blood cells are more permeable to retroviral transfer.

Long-term hematopoietic reconstitution in the animal

Several groups have achieved successful gene transfer into hematopoietic stem cells in mice {Thomas Caskey (Houston, USA) ; Richard Mulligan (MIT, Boston, USA) ; Dinko Valerio (Rijswijk, the Netherlands)} ; the transfered gene was usually that of adenosine deaminase (ADA). The long-term restoral (over 6 months) of irradiated mice engrafted with manipulated marrows was shown; either after pre-treatment of the donor mice by 5-fluorouracile (which eliminates the cells in cycle and thereby decreases the number of target cells for the retroviral infection), or after stem cell purification, only a hundred cells or so being transfered into. These experiments are reported by Denis Cournoyer (Houston, USA and Montreal, Quebec) and Dinko Valerio. In primate and in man, experiments of transfer to stem cells in long-term in vitro cultures are described by Denis Cournoyer, Dinko Valerio and Claudio Bordignon (Milan, Italy). The pre-stimulation of the bone marrow cells by growth factors, particularly by IL3 and IL6 or LIF (leukemic inhibiting factor), 48 hours prior to the addition of the retroviruses seems to greatly favor their integration.

The more acurate knowledge of the regulation of the locus encoding the ß-globin chains and the construction of functional mini-genes adequately regulated are reported by Frank Grosveld (London, UK). This should enable to obtain comparable results in hemoglobinopathies.

Claudio Bordignon further describes an experimental system based on the utilization of BNX mice to show the success of the ADA gene transfer in human lymphocyte populations, with a prolonged life span. Dinko Valerio also reports of highly efficient human ADA ⁻ T lymphocytes targeting after two consecutive selection steps using xylofuranosyl-adenine (Xyl-A) and 2'-deoxycoformycin (dCF).

First attempts at gene therapy in man

These results lead to the setting up of the first experiments of gene therapy in man which are reported by Michael Blaese.

These experiments are performed on lymphocytes, inasmuch as the transfer to hematopoietic stem cells did not seem realistic, considering the present state of research ; furthermore, the transfer into cells with a limited life span, lasting however up to 700 days following manipulation and reinfusion, as was shown by the team of professors Blaese and French-Anderson in the primate, could seem justified in a disease in the absence of therapeutic alternative. In this context, the process of drawing, transducing and reinfusing the manipulated cells must be repeated at regular intervals.

The first authorization to use retrovirus transduced cells was delivered in the United States in the framework of immunotherapy of malignant melanomas ; the team was that of professors Blaese, French-Anderson and Rosenberg. The target cells were tumor infiltrating lymphocytes (TIL), expanded in vitro in the presence of IL2. This experiment was a genetic tagging of these cells in order to verify that they were still capable of being recruited to the site of the tumor after in vitro manipulation. This first experiment was essentially designed to clarify the mechanism of action of these TIL in the anti-tumoral immune reaction, to verify that the retroviral infection did not alter their functional properties or induce any deleterious effect. Actual gene therapy protocols remain to be done, using this cell substrate, in which the transfered gene would encode an anti-tumoral substance such as the tumor necrosis factor (TNF).

The second authorization was delivered in the ADA deficiency, a hereditary disease presenting as a severe combined immunodeficiency, rapidly lethal in the absence of allogenic bone marrow transplant. A treatment of substitution with PEG coupled to the enzyme allows a partial correction, it is however very costly, of uneven efficacy and cannot be discontinued. Two children have benefited to this day from infusions of peripheral blood lymphocytes, manipulated and expanded ex vivo. The results are still too preliminary to conclude as to the efficacy of this protocol ; whether the ability of these cells to express sufficient amounts of enzyme to observe a phenotypic correction, or their survival as functional elements. The children are thus maintained under substitution by PEG-ADA. The regular evaluations seem promising, as well the percentages of circulating lymphocytes expressing the transgene as its level of expression.

However, the final goal of gene therapy in the hereditary diseases of the hematopoietic system is to transduce pluripotent stem cells in view of a single and definitive treatment. The experimental successes in the mouse and the results obtained in the primate lead us to hope for similar success in man.

Prospects of gene therapy in Cancer and in AIDS

Roger Monier (Villejuif, France), recalled the most recent data on the respective roles of oncogenes and of tumor suppressor genes in carcinogenesis ; together with the potential protection against tumor growth through immunization following cytokine gene transfer into mouse tumor cell-lines. Michael Gottesman (NIH, Bethesda, USA) reports on the recent data on MDR genes (or multidrug resistance genes) of pleiotropic resistance to cytotoxic drugs. The marrow of mice transgenic for the human MDR1 gene become resistant to drugs such as adriamycin, colchicine or vinca-alcaloids. The negative consequences of chemotherapy for the marrow could be prevented ; new protocols could be applied, with the possibility of autologous transplantation without aplasia. In addition, the MDR1 gene could be used as a selectable marker in gene therapy.

Jean-Paul Lévy (Paris, France) recounts the possible strategies developed *in vitro* for the gene therapy of AIDS ; with the concept of "intracellular immunization" in which the introduction of mutant "transdominant" genes in the infected cells could allow to inhibit either regulatory proteins, structural proteins or viral receptors. Similarly, the constitutive expression of genes encoding antisense RNAs or anti-viral RNA ribozymes decreases viral production and confers a protection against de novo infection. The forced expression of the TAR sequence is followed by an inhibition of the virus in previously infected cells through a "decoy" of the regulatory proteins. Data concerning the conditional-suicide of infected cells also seem encouraging.

Vaccines

The use of gene transfer technologies to generate new types of vaccines, in particular directed against AIDS, including live vaccines, disabbled bacterias carrying exogenous sequences which encode targeted epitopes is reviewed by Marc Girard and Maurice Hofnung.

Retroviruses and gene therapy in the liver

If, as we have just seen, the archetype of the target for retrovirus-mediated gene transfer is the hematopoietic tissue, Olivier Danos, Jean-Michel Heard (Pasteur Institute, Paris, France) and Didier Houssin (Hôpital Cochin, Paris, France) present a particularly seductive model of hepatocyte transfer *in vivo*, in the rat. Hepatocytes are classically considered as post-mitotic and thus do not divide, save in very special circumstances such as enlarged partial hepatectomy. This surgical act is followed by an intense mitotic stimulus which renders the cells permeable to a retroviral infection and subsequent integration. These researchers took advantage of this observation to transfer a reporter gene into rat hepatocytes. The transgene integration is evidenced in cells of the hepatic parenchyma, typed as hepatocytes. This procedure allows to overcome the difficult problem of the re-establishement of manipulated cells which belong to an organ where architecture and function are related and offers a potential alternative to liver transplantation currently performed in the case of some inborn errors of metabolism.

Animal models and Homologous Recombination

Experimental developments on animal models enable the evaluation of new therapeutic pathways and testing of the different systems of transgene vectorisation and expression ; the information is no longer collected on individual cells in culture but in a complete organism. The eventual deleterious consequences such as the virus-spread or the occurrence of an immune reaction directed against the transgene or its product can be evaluated.

If many animal models were obtained randomly, by chemical mutagenesis as recalled by Doctor Jean-Louis Guenet (Pasteur Institute, Paris, France), new methodologies allowing precise, directed mutations have appeared. The classical technique of transgenesis enabled the creation of some models. However, the surgically precise gene targeting by homologous recombination allows today the achievement of models on order, in particular in recessive transmitted diseases. The effect of precise mutations or deletions can be checked in the homozygous animal by crossing heterozygous mice in which the manipulated progenitor embryonic cells (ES cells, derived from blastocysts), contributed to the germinal lineage. The targeted interruption of a gene brings on the other hand precious informations as to its function.

Mario Capecchi (HHMI, Salt Lake City, USA), who participated to the establishment of this technique, reports on recent work concerning the targeted disruption of *int*-1, *int*-2 and *Hox*-1.5. The absence of expression of the latter, induces a phenotype ressembling a severe human immunodeficiency, DiGeorge syndrome.

Stephen Goff (Columbia Univ., New-York,USA), reports the consequences of the replacement of abl by a mutant allele ; with other than anatomic anomalies of the skull and spleen, total depletion of the marrow B-cell precursors ; thereby underlining the role of the abelson gene product in the differentiation and maturation of B-cells.

Erwin Wagner (IMP, Vienna, Austria) shows his results concerning : 1°) The key role of the proto-oncogene *c-fos* product in bone development ; overexpression of these sequences leading to the formation of bone tumors and chondrosarcomas ; 2°) The factors contributing to angiogenesis, whose presence in malignant tumors seems to rule over the spreading of the tumor and the occurrence of metastases ; 3°) The attempts at the differentiation of ES cells into hematopoietic progenitors ; 4°) The reversal of the hematopoietic disorders in W/W mutant mice, by retroviral transfer of *c-kit* in ES cells followed by the production of chimeras ; the proliferation of mast cells in response to the MGF (Mast cell Growth Factor or SCF for Stem cell Growth Factor, or *c-kit* ligand) is restored.

Gene transfer and Human Diseases

This meeting was conceived as a multidisciplinary forum from which a common reflection and productive collaborations could arise. Indeed, if the basic scientists approach technical aspects and problems pertaining to regulations, the clinicians draw their outlook from their practice of a given disease and it's therapeutic needs.

If the tools used in gene transfer are numerous, each of them presenting advantages and disadvantages, the appropriate stategies must be defined according to the diseases one wishes to consider. Retroviral vectors seem compatible with the transfer into explantable cells, reimplanted after manipulation and able to divide in order to integrate the transgene, as is true for hematopoietic cells. Most organs have a defined architecture rendering impossible the stuctured re-establishement of cells after *ex vivo* manipulation.

As many genetic diseases interest this type of organ, and especially the most frequent ones, i.e. cystic fibrosis and Duchenne muscular dystrophy, vectorisation, mode and route of administration of the therapeutic DNA sequences are the subject of debate in each of the diseases.

A round table was held in order to examine the relevance of the gene transfer therapeutic approach in human pathology, the content of which is reprinted here. It includes : hemoglobinopathies, severe combined immunodeficiencies, fetal medicine, tumor suppressor genes and cancer, leukemias, inborn errors of metabolism, liver, cystic fibrosis, fragile X syndrome, Duchenne muscular dystrophy, CNS and neurons and ethics.

The participation of scientists, physicians and surgeons involved in these multiple lines of research concerning various domains of practice, allowed : - on one hand, to evaluate of the common problems and aims ; - on the other, to define specific questions pertaining to some diseases in which there are problems related as well to the accessibility of the deficient organs or tissues as to the regulation of the expression of the newly introduced gene ; - lastly to underline continuing difficulties, in particular the innocuity of these manipulations or the ethical problems thus brought forth.

Prospects for gene therapy

Les perspectives de la thérapie génique

Genetic disorders

C. Thomas Caskey

Institute for Molecular Genetics and Howard Hughes Medical Institute, Baylor College of Medicine, Houston, TX 77030, USA

ABSTRACT

The human genome contains 50,000–100,000 genes and mutations in many of these result in a disease phenotype or carrier status. In theory a wide range of inherited disorders could be corrected by the addition of a functional gene into the appropriate cell type, together with proper expression. I will discuss some of the requirements for a genetic disease to be considered a candidate for gene transfer therapy, some of the disorders for which advances have been made in this area, and some of the potential difficulties. Much progress has been made but we can expect more.

INTRODUCTION

For a genetic disease to be considered a candidate for gene transfer, its pathophysiology should be well understood at the molecular level and functional DNA sequences must be available for gene transfer. It is also necessary to have an efficient means of delivery of the gene and regulatory sequences for the appropriate expression of the transferred gene. In general, candidate diseases are single-gene disorders of recessive or X-linked inheritance in which the function of the defective gene can be supplemented or replaced by a functional copy. At the present time, due to the experimental nature of the gene therapy approach, candidate diseases are generally lethal with no adequate treatment available.

CANDIDATE TISSUES AND GENETIC DISORDERS

Bone marrow

Bone marrow transplantation is a well established form of therapy for a number of inherited and acquired disorders and is therefore an obvious tissue for consideration of gene therapy. The entire lympho/hematopoietic system appears to be derived from a limited number of hematopoietic stem cells which can be obtained by bone marrow aspiration, manipulated as required and then reimplanted into a matched recipient or the original donor. These stem cells therefore represent very attractive vehicles to carry out gene therapy. In theory, all disorders that affect cell lineages derived from the hematopoietic system could be corrected by this approach.

The disease that has received the most attention regarding the possibility of gene transfer is a form of severe combined immune deficiency (SCID) caused by deficiency of the enzyme adenosine deaminase (ADA). This disease meets all the proposed criteria for the use of gene therapy: The disease is uniformly lethal if untreated, thus justifying an experimental approach. Matched bone marrow transplantations can produce a cure but the procedure is occasionally ineffective because of graft failure or rejection. Replacement of the enzyme itself via blood transfusion or conjugated to polyethylene glycol can yield some improvement, suggesting that precise control of replacement gene expression may not be necessary. Both cDNA and genomic sequences are available from the

ADA gene and transfer of ADA activity has been successfully achieved in cultured cells.

Our group is working on gene transfer into pluripotent stem cells (in theory requiring only one or a few infusions) resulting in expression in all hematopoietic cell lineages. Defective retroviruses have been successfully used to transduce long term *in vivo* expression of human ADA in mice (Moore **et al.**, 1990). The transferred gene was expressed for the six-month experimental period in the absence of detectable helper virus. Human enzyme was expressed at levels comparable to endogenous murine ADA (15-50% of endogenous) after full reconstitution. Since 25% of the normal ADA level in blood has been shown to be an effective therapy, the levels achieved in mice should be sufficient for treatment.

High efficiency gene transfer of human ADA into primitive human hematopoietic progenitors has also been demonstrated. Immediately after gene transfer, the infection efficiency of clonogenic progenitors was 90% in normal bone marrow. In order to identify more primitive hematopoietic progenitors, infected bone marrow was maintained in myeloid long term culture (LTC). After nine weeks in LTC, the ADA provirus was present, on average, in 34% of clonogenic cells. Pre-existing clonogenic cells are not maintained in LTC for longer than 5 weeks suggesting successful gene transfer into primitive hematopoietic progenitors related to the hematopoietic stem cells. Enriched stem cell populations are now being used in these studies which are targeted towards clinical trials of gene transfer into human hematopoietic stem cells, the goal ultimately being a therapy for ADA deficiency and other inherited hematopoietic disorders.

Liver

The correction of several inborn errors of metabolism would require that the transgene be expressed in the presence of cofactors or other enzymes of multi-step metabolic pathways that, in certain cases, are only found in the liver. To date, three human disease-related genes (α_1-antitrypsin, phenylalanine hydroxylase and low-density lipoprotein receptor) have been expressed in primary hepatocytes following retroviral-mediated gene transfer. Efficient methods of DNA-mediated gene transfer into adult rat hepatocytes have also been described. The major challenge now is to develop techniques that would allow the reimplantation of genetically modified hepatocytes. The long-term survival of rat hepatocytes implanted into the spleen or the peritoneum has been reported, offering hope that this might eventually be accomplished. However, this approach would probably require a partial hepatectomy to obtain cells in sufficient number and therefore appears undesirably invasive. Another unclear aspect is whether all hepatocytes (in the child or in the adult) retain sufficient proliferative potential to produce long lasting progeny, and therefore to be an appropriate target for a stable gene transfer, or whether this quality is restricted to a limited number of 'hepatic stem cells'. Studies of the early stages of rat hepatocarcinogenesis suggest that a type of epithelial cell lining the bile ducts, designated the 'oval' cells, may constitute a pool of stem cells giving rise to both the ductal epithelial cells and the immature hepatocytes. If so, gene transfer strategies to hepatocytes might need to be optimized for that subtype of cells to offer a long-term benefit.

Another approach to the correction of metabolic diorders that normally require hepatic cofactors or multi-step pathways is the identification of other tissues that can reproduce the entire metabolic pathway and might be more amenable to genetic manipulations. This approach is illustrated by the correction of ornithine transcarbamylase deficiency in sparse fur (*spf*) mice by expression of a transgene in the small bowel epithelium (Jones **et al.**, 1990). Although an optimal method of gene delivery to the small bowel epithelium has not yet been established, this type of observation offers other options to the difficult task of genetically manipulating the liver.

Ornithine transcarbamylase deficiency is a severe X-linked disorder of urea metabolism. Affected males usually present in the newborn period with hyperammonemic coma and frequently die from the disease. Survivors of the initial neonatal insult commonly are mentally retarded and have to be maintained with life-long dietary and pharmacologic management. We are currently developing both retrovirus and adeno-associated virus vector systems for transfer of the human cDNA into target cells. Several retroviral vectors capable of transducing and expressing the human OTC cDNA have been created. As the backbone for the constructs we have utilized both the N2 virus and a new generation of self-inactivating viruses (gen- vectors; Soriano **et al.**, 1991, J. Virol. in press). The most promising of the vectors, ΔN2OTC, has been used to infect primary *spf* hepatocytes *in vitro* and the provirus can be found in up to 35% of the infected cells. Only partial correction of the enzyme defect in the transduced cells was achieved. For this reason different vectors in which strong hepatic promoters are driving OTC expression are currently being tested. Adeno-associated virus vectors have several potential advantages for gene therapy experiments. They are non-pathogenic in animals and man, they appear to integrate site-specifically in the human genome (chromosome 19), very high titers have been reported, they possess tropism for a wide range of species and tissues (including intestine) and there is no interference from viral promoters after integration. This vector has been employed to transduce G418 resistance into Hepa 16 cells, a murine hepatoma line, in our laboratory. Several constructs containing the human OTC cDNA are currently being tested in both hepatoma cells and primary hepatocytes.

Muscle

The prime candidate for a gene therapy approach among the diseases affecting the muscular system appears to be Duchenne muscular dystrophy (DMD). DMD, an X-linked recessive disorder, is the most common inherited muscular disease. Mutations of the dystrophin gene are responsible for both DMD and a less severe form of the disease, Becker muscular dystrophy. The dystrophin gene has recently been isolated, leading to the development of very sensitive and reliable methods of carrier detection and prenatal diagnosis. However, since approximately one third of all cases are due to new mutations (and therefore are not amenable to prenatal diagnosis), and also a portion of the known or potential carriers elect to not use this information in their decision to continue or terminate a pregnancy, there remains a pressing need to improve the treatment of these patients. Although other approaches such as allogeneic muscle cell transplantation are being considered, gene therapy might be the ultimate solution. A valuable tool in the development of this strategy and in the functional studies of the dystrophin molecule is the existence of an animal model for DMD, the *mdx* mouse.

Investigators in our laboratory have recently isolated a full length clone containing the coding sequence of the mouse dystrophin gene (Lee *et al.*, 1991). Its expression in mammalian cells produces a protein indistinguishable from that of muscle dystrophin by western analysis, and the cell membrane location is consistent with that of the native protein. It is therefore now possible to use the *mdx* animal model to test gene therapy strategies for DMD. Work is already in progress to express the dystrophin sequence in transgenic *mdx* animals and to confirm its ability to correct the dystrophin deficiency. Preliminary studies indicate that one line of these *mdx* transgenic mice shows expression of the recombinant dystrophin in skeletal and cardiac muscle. Evaluation of the transgene expression on reversing the histological, biochemical and muscle pseudohypertrophy defects of the *mdx* mouse is currently in progress.

An efficient system of gene delivery to the muscular system has not yet been defined. One additional difficulty in the case of DMD is the large size of the dystrophin cDNA (approximately 14 kb), which is above the size limitation of most viral vectors. One possibility would be to introduce the gene by physical methods into cultured myoblasts derived from *mdx* mice, and then to reinject these cells into the affected muscles. The fate of these cells following transplantation and the extent to which this might improve the function of the muscles in which these cells are injected, however, needs to be investigated in animals. A conceptually related approach would be to directly inject expression vectors into the muscles. One group has recently reported successful gene transfer following direct *in vivo* injection of RNA and DNA expression vectors into mouse muscle cells (Wolff *et al.*, 1990). After injection of a DNA expression vector, the reporter gene was expressed in muscle for a least two months. After a single injection into individual quadriceps muscles, approximately 1.5% of the cells that comprise the entire muscle (10-30% of the cells within the injection area) expressed the reporter gene. While this kind of approach may eventually allow us to improve the muscular strength and quality of life of DMD patients, it would seem difficult to use it to improve the cardiac and respiratory functions.

Since these functions generally determine the life-expectancy of DMD patients, a method that could deliver the gene *in vivo* to all muscles would be highly desirable. It might be possible to develop a system of *in vivo* delivery that would be targeted to muscle-specific receptors. Alternatively, a less specifically targeted vector could include regulatory elements that would restrict its expression to muscle cells.

Central nervous system

One of the criteria mentioned above for considering gene therapy for a genetic disorder is that the pathophysiology be well understood and this is often achieved by means of an animal model. A devastating neurological human disease, Lesch-Nyhan syndrome, results from deficiency of the purine metabolism enzyme hypoxanthine-guanine phosphoribosyltransferase (HPRT). Transgenic mice deficient in HPRT have been generated in an attempt to further understand Lesch-Nyhan syndrome but do not display any symptoms (Hooper *et al.*, 1987; Kuehn *et al.*, 1987). Mice have an enzyme in the same purine metabolism pathway, urate oxidase, which is lacking in the human, and it has therefore been proposed that the presence of urate oxidase in mice might provide protection against the toxic effects of HPRT-deficiency. A gene-targeting approach was used to 'knock-out' by homologous recombination the urate oxidase gene in transgenic mice and these mice are currently being evaluated. Breeding of urate oxidase-deficient mice with HPRT-deficient mice will produce animals deficient in both enzymes and the possibility of an animal model for human HPRT-deficiency. HPRT-deficiency in the human serves as an example of a disorder where it is inappropriate to consider gene therapy until we better understand the nature of the disease.

CONCLUSIONS

There has been considerable progress in the field of gene transfer with the ultimate goal of developing procedures for gene replacement therapy of human inherited disease. Viral delivery vectors are more efficient and safer, long-term expression of transgenes in bone marrow has been achieved, and clinical trials for human therapy have been approved. There is still much to be done, however, before we can consider gene therapy a routine treatment for genetic disease.

ACKNOWLEDGEMENTS

C.T.C. is a Howard Hughes Medical Institute Investigator. The assistance of Drs. Belinda Rossiter, Markus Grompe, Cheng-Chi Lee, Kohnosuke Mitani and Xiang-Wei Wu in preparing this manuscript is appreciated.

REFERENCES

Hooper, M., Hardy, K., Handyside, A., Hunter, S., and Monk, M. (1987): HPRT-deficient (Lesch-Nyhan) mouse embryos derived from germline colonization by cultured cells. Nature 326: 292-295.

Jones, S.N., Grompe, M., Munir, M.I., Veres, G., Craigen, W.J., and Caskey, C.T. (1990): Ectopic correction of ornithine transcarbamylase deficiency in sparse fur mice. J. Biol. Chem. 265: 14684-14690.

Kuehn, M.R., Bradley, A., Robertson, E.J., and Evans, M.J. (1987): A potential animal model for Lesch-Nyhan syndrome through introduction of HPRT mutations into mice. Nature 326: 295-298.

Lee, C.C., Pearlman, J.A., Chamberlain, J.S., and Caskey, C.T. (1991): Expression of recombinant dystrophin and its localization to the cell membrane. Nature 349: 334-336.

Moore, K.A., Fletcher, F.A., Villalon, D.K., Utter, A.E., and Belmont, J.W. (1990): Human adenosine deaminase expression in mice. Blood 75: 2085-2092.

Wolff, J.A., Malone, R.W., Williams, P., Chong, W., Acsadi, G., Jani, A., and Felgner, P.L. (1990): Direct gene transfer into mouse muscle in vivo. Science 247: 1465-1468.

RESUME : Le génome humain contient entre 50 et 100 000 gènes et des mutations touchant nombre de ceux-ci conduisent à un phénotype pathologique ou à un statut de porteur sain susceptible de transmettre le trait. Un large éventail de maladies héréditaires pourrait théoriquement être corrigé par l'addition d'un gène fonctionnel dans les cellules appropriées suivi d'une expression adéquate. Je discuterai ici certains des pré-requis permettant de considérer une maladie génétique comme un candidat potentiel pour la thérapie par transfert génétique, certaines des pathologies pour lesquelles des avances ont pu être faites dans ce domaine, et certaines difficultés potentielles. Des progrès substantiels ont déjà pu être réalisés mais de nombreux restent à attendre.

HIV infection and gene therapy

Jean-Paul Lévy

Immunologie et Oncologie des Maladies Rétrovirales. INSERM U 152, Institut Cochin de Génétique Moléculaire. Hôpital Cochin, 27, rue du Faubourg Saint-Jacques, 75014 Paris, France

The idea to protect an individual against a viral infection by genetically induced resistance of his own cells looks crasy if we think in terms of acute viral infections. On the contrary, as recently suggested by D. Baltimore (1988), this could be valuable in the case of the HIV Infection for several reasons : 1) This infection induces a chronic disease which result in full blown AIDS, after a mean of 10 years or more. During this very long latency the immune T cell repertoire is progressively destroyed but one could imagine that a gene therapy could save at least a part of this repertoire. This would not solve all the problems which are encountered in the course of an HIV infection, notably the involvement of the central nervous system and the developpement of lymphomas, but a gene therapy might possibly avoid the complete immunodeficiency which finally kills most of HIV infected patients. 2) The virus infects preferentially T lymphocytes and monocytes which are among the most suitable targets for gene therapy. 3) : Antiviral drugs remain poorly efficient. Even, if in the following years improvements can be expected with the appearance of new families of drugs, it is clear that the development of an effecient antiviral therapy of AIDS will probably be a very long story. It is therefore logical to consider other approaches, at least to determine whether they are "in vitro gimmick" or realistic models for new forms of therapy (Baltimore, 1988).

I. PRESENT LIMITATIONS IN AIDS THERAPY

Three classes of antiviral drugs could play a role in the treatment of HIV infections : a) Antiviral substances which would avoid cell infection ; b) Drugs inhibiting the production of infectious viruses by infected cells ; c) Toxins specifically killing HIV-infected cells.

Using drugs of the first class : we are able to partly inhibit the viral infection by reverse-transcriptase inhibitors. All the drugs currently employed are nucleosides analogues but other reverse-transcriptase inhibitors, the Tibos, are at the beginning of their clinical trials. The efficiency of nucleosides is clear but limited and we know that they will not definitely control the disease. The same will be probably true for Tibos if they prove a real in vivo efficiency. On the other hand, one can try to inhibit the virus cell penetration by blocking either cell recognition through the viral receptor, or the fusion of viral enveloppe and cell membrane. In theory this can be realized by substances like soluble CD4 molecules, sulfated polysaccharides or anti-env antibodies. All these products are at the beginning of their trials in human beings. Some of them finally might turn to be useful but their present efficiency appears rather limited and strong improvements would be necessary for real clinical applications. At the present time, we don't know whether or not they will be usefull in the futur. All other targets of antiviral drugs which would avoid cell infection, as for example the viral DNA integration step remain for the moment hypothetical.

Similarly, our present capability to avoid the formation of infectious viruses by infected cells remains very limited. The use of antisens oligonucleotides, including ribozymes, is only experimental and many problems will have to be solved before one can really imagine their application in human beings. Futhermore, developement of drugs capable to inhibit regulatory proteins like TAT or Rev remains an assumption. Substances, which would block viral RNA dimerisation and/or encapsidation by interacting with the nucleocapside (p15), or drugs inhibiting capsid formation, by interaction with the gag-p24 protein, could perhaps be designed in the futur but they don't exist. Interferons on the contrary do exist but their use in HIV infection has been disappointing. Finally, our only hope for the near future lies in the development of protease inhibitors. Some of them will enter in phase I clinical trials in 1991 and a consistent improvement of AIDS therapy may possibly appear with this new family of drugs but their real in vivo efficiency remains presently unpredictable.

Toxins specifically killing HIV-infected cells represent the third class of possible antiviral drugs to be designed in the futur. Here again, however they remain only experimental.

Due to the tremendous involvement of hundred of laboratories in the world, it is likely that new anti-HIV drugs will become a reality in the coming 5 to 10 years. Nevertheless, the problems to be solved are huge enough to make advisable the search for new ways. Gene therapy must be considered as a parallel track, with formidable obstacles. It is clear however that it must be explored because the results we shall obtain with more conventional approaches remain unforseable.

II. GENE THERAPY AND INFECTION BY HIV

The concept of "intracellular immunization" (Baltimore, 1988) has been proposed as an application to viral diseases of the functional inactivation of genes by dominant negative mutations (Herskowitz, 1987). It could be applied in already infected persons in the aim to render a part of their lymphocytes and macrophages resistant to HIV infection. This would therefore be a true immunization process allowing a part of the T cell repertoire to escape HIV induced killing. As far as an autologous graft of in vitro transformed hematopoietic precursors cells will be necessary, including a preliminary treatment by cytotoxic drugs or irradiation, to give space for these precursors, this treatment will not be acceptable for uninfected people or even perhaps for recently infected patients. However, the development of new procedures of gene transfer could modify the problem. Retroviruses or adenoviruses might be valuable vectors. Adenoviruses, for example, are known to infect T lymphocytes, and they do not induce severe diseases in human beings. One may imagine, if conventional antiviral drugs approaches would remain unsuccessful, that such vectors might finaly represent a useful tools not only for intracellular immunization in advanced patients (to limit the consequences of the viral infection) but perhaps also for a possible curative treatment of recently infected people. Their use as a kind of vaccination would remain on the contrary very questionnable as far as these viral vectors integrate the cellular DNA.

III. NEGATIVE DOMINANT MUTANTS AND HIV INFECTION

As proposed by Herskowitz (1987) and D. Baltimore (1988) at least two kinds of viral proteins might be inhibited by the introduction of transdominant mutant genes in infected cells : regulatory monomeric or oligomeric proteins and structural multimeric proteins.

After the initial contribution of Friedman et al (1988) showing that the expression of a truncated viral transactivator of Herpes simplex virus type 1 (HSV-1) selectively impedes the lytic infection of transformed cells by HSV-1, two groups have reported preliminary data suggesting a possible application to the HIV-1 model. Malim et al (1989) have shown that a mutant of the Rev gene, the product of which is determinant in viral mRNA nuclear export, can transdominantly inhibit the

Rev function in a transitory expression system. Cotransfection by the mutant gene induces a dramatic inhibitory effect on HIV-1 genes expression. The results of these experiments can be interpreted as a probable competitive inhibition by the mutant protein which would have kept its ability to associate with viral RNA but not its functional site, as already suggested in the HSV-1 VP16 model (Friedman et al 1988). This system however has not been tested in HIV-1 infected cells, so that we ignore whether or not the level of mutant Rev expression would be sufficient to protect against HIV-1. Similarly, Green et al (1989), in an experimental system of microinjected Hela cells with transitory expression of a CAT gene under the control of an HIV-1 LTR, have shown that mutant TAT peptides can competitively inhibit the viral LTR transactivation induced by their normal counterpart. Here, again we still ignore whether or not mutant genes expressing the same mutant peptides in infected cells would be efficient, but these experiments, together with the results of Malim et al (1989) suggest that the concept of negative dominant regulatory gene could be successfully applied to HIV infected cells, as it has been for HSV-1 infected cells in vitro.

To inhibit the production of infectious virions by HIV infected cells, another possibility, with a probable higher efficiency, would be the use of dominant negative mutants of a multimeric structural protein. As emphasized by Trono et al. (1989) a moderate level of expression would be sufficient with such mutants to obtain a strong inhibitory effect. This idea has been applied by these authors to block HIV-1 replication in a transcient assay, by transfection of the gag or p17+p24 mutants genes. Furthermore, cells constitutively expressing such mutants of the gag p24 capsidial protein showed an impaired ability to support HIV-1 replication. It is possible that the viral replication could be inhibited at different steps including viral assembly, viral release, virion stability or even viral entry and/or uncoating in a second generation of infected cells. The concept of intracellular immunization is strongly supported by such experiments which have now to be confirmed in an in vivo model.

It should be also mentionned that the use of a cellular gene encoding a modified viral receptor could be also interesting, in the aim to thwart the HIV replication in infected cells, as suggested by Buonocore and Rose (1990). These authors have used a CD4 mutant gene coding for a soluble CD4 molecule expressing the KDEL retention signal for the endoplasmic reticulum. In cells expressing this mutant the Env protein gp160 was trapped by CD4 mutant molecules in the reticulum and did not appear at the cell surface. Moreover, the fusion with other $CD4^+$ cells, which represent a part of the HIV induced cytopatic effect was inhibited. The viral production however was not tested in these experiments. Note that the major advantage of such a system lies on the sequence conservation of the viral gp 120 domain interacting with CD4 molecules, so that one may suppose that any isolate of HIV-1 or HIV-2 could be inhibited by the same mutant.

IV. GENE THERAPY BY EXPRESSION OF ANTISENS OLIGONUCLEOTIDES OR RIBOZYMES

As already discussed above, oligonucleotides, notably antisens or ribozymes, might become antiviral drugs in the futur but only if we shall be able to solve the major problems encountered in their use, including : a) oligonucleotide stability ; b) cell targetting, penetration and acces to the convenient cellular compartment ; c) obtention of sufficient concentrations of oligonucleotides in infected cells to fully inhibit the viral RNAs. The last point seems to be specially critical. At the present time we still ignore whether or not we shall be able to get over these obstacles and therefore whether or not such molecules could effectively become antiviral drugs in a conventional meaning. It could possibly be more efficient to induce a stable expression of genes coding for antisens viral RNA in normal bone marrow precursor cells which would be later engrafted in their autologous donor. Here again the results woul be an intracellular immunization but at the RNA level. Very few data are available in the HIV-1 modele, nevertheless Sarver et al (1990) have reported that the transfection of Hela-$CD4^+$ cells with a gene coding for an hammerhead antigag-ribozyme could induce a substantial reduction of HIV-1 gag RNA expression in these cells after viral infection. The levels of p24-Gag protein were reduced by 50 to 100 times. Moreover, the level of proviral DNA was also reduced by 100 times, suggesting that the ribozyme was able not only to reduce the viral production by infected cells but also to provide a protection against de novo viral infection by cleavage of incoming viral RNAs. These results suggest that a gene therapy using either bone marrow graft of in vitro transformed precursor cells or viral vectors, could possibly be realized not only with dominant negative mutants but also with antisens or ribozymes encoding genes.

V. GENE THERAPY BY OVEREXPRESSION OF DECOY VIRAL RNA

The RNA TAR sequence being the normal target of the TAT-induced transactivation phenomenon, an over-expression of the normal TAR sequence could constitute a decoy for TAT and/or TAT associated cellular regulatory proteins involved in the viral LTR transactivation. The procedure, which consists in transfecting not an antisens but a sens TAR gene, has recently been realized in CEM cells by Sullenger et al. (1990). Using a retroviral vector in which a t-RNA^{met}-TAR hybrid sequences was inserted in both LTR, these authors have obtained a very high level of cellular expression resulting in a 98-99 % inhibition of p24 expression in HIV-1 infected cells. Moreover, HIV-1, HIV-1, HIV-2 or SIV TAT proteins interacting with HIV-1 TAR this inhibitory system offers the advantage of not being limited by the virus variability.

VI. GENE THERAPY BY HIV-1 DEPENDANT TOXINS

Selective killing of HIV-infected cells is difficult. The production of drugs which would be toxic for these cells but not for uninfected cells remains questionable. On the other hand, immunotoxins or toxins associated with soluble CD4 molecules, can be used but the specificity of targetting remains uncertain as well as the in vivo efficiency. Moreover, the cell surface markers allowing recognition of these cells, specially ENV molecules, are produced relatively late in the virus cycle so that only cells already engaged in virus production could be killed. Surface markers of an earlier stage of HIV infection would be necessary but they lack. Therefore, another approach for toxin therapy seems to be required and here againt, this approach coul be a gene therapy. One of the most efficient way to treat HIV infections could be to introduce in cells a suicide order which would function only in HIV infected cells. The principle of such experiments consists in introducing in CD4 lympocytes or macrophages, a lethal gene coding, for example for the ricin α chain or another toxin, under the control of a viral LTR. In theory such a gene would remain silent except if a TAT gene is expressed in the same cell, allowing toxin synthesis and cell suicide. A double control would however be required to lock any TAT latent expression of the lethal gene. This could be obtained, for example by introducing a retention sequence and a Rev-target RRE sequence in the toxin mRNA to prevent its export to the cytoplasm in the absence of the viral Rev protein. This approach could strongly limit the virus spreading, especially in recently infected persons if infected cells might be selectively destroyed at the early phase of viral infection. The use of viral vectors to transfer lethal TAT and/or Rev-dependent genes without having to perform an autologous bone marrow graft could strongly improve this approach. Recently, Venkatesch et al (1990) have reported that a conditionally cytotoxic HSV-1 thymidine kinase gene (HSV-1 tk) under the transcriptionnal control of an HIV-1 LTR can be introduced in HeLa also cells by an adenovirus vector. Target HeLa cells expressing a TAT gene, produced the HVS-1-tk gene which appeared to be lethal in the presence of the guanoside-analog gancyclovir. More than 98 % of HeLa-Tat cells were killed. Several points however remain to be solved : a) the results were less clear with another human cell of lymphoïd origin, Jurkatt ; b) some toxicity clearly existed for normal cells and c) we ignore whether or not HIV-1 infected cells would be killed and if yes, if they could be destroyed before virus production. Nevertheless, this results suggests that an adenovirus which is known to replicate in T lymphocytes might drive an efficient toxin in recently infected cells allowing their destruction as soon as they will produce HIV-1 early RNAs. D. Klatzman will present in this meeting data supporting the hypothesis that conditionaly expressed toxins might be in the futur a valuable tool for a gene therapy of AIDS.

CONCLUSION

The Gene therapy of AIDS is obviously in its infancy but at least four kinds of approaches can be imagined. Preliminary experimental data, reported in 1989-1990, suggest that they might be efficient at least in vitro but only some of them have been applied to the control of HIV-replication. Further demonstrations will be necessary using either dominant negative mutant genes, or virus-dependant toxins or genes expressing antisens, ribozymes or sens viral sequences. Moreover, in vivo models must be explored either in murine systems or in lentivirus infected macaques or cats. A gene therapy of AIDS is not a creasy idea : its futur developpment will primarily depend on the succes or failure of antiviral drugs in the following ten years. Perhaps must me remember however, that if we finally succeed, such a therapy will be accessible for developping countries only. In Africa, in which millions of humans beings will die, it will certainly remain mythical for long periods of time.

REFERENCES

Baltimore, D. (1988): Intracellular imunization. Nature 335: 395-396.
Buenocore, L. and Rose, J.K. (1990): Prevention of HIV-1 glycoprotein transport by soluble CD4 retained in the encoplasmic reticulum. Nature 345: 627-628.
Friedman, A.D., Triezenberg, S.J., McKnight, S.L. (1988): Expression of a truncated viral transcriptor selectively impedes lytic infection by its cognate virus. Nature 335: 452-455.
Green, M., Ishino M., Loewarstein, P.M. (1989): Mutational analysis of HIV-1 TAT minimal domain peptides : identification of transdominant mutants that suppress HIV-LTR-driven gene expression. Cell 58 : 215-223.
Herskowitz, I. (1987): Functionnal inactivation of genes dominant by negative mutations. Nature 329: 219-222.
Malim, M.H., Bölinlein, S., Hauber, J., Cullen, B.R. (1989): Functional dissection of the HIV-1 Rev trans-activator. Derivation of a trans-dominant repressor of Rev function. Cell 58: 205-214.
Sarver, N., Cantin, E.M., Chang, P.S., Zaia, J.A., Ladne, P.A., Stephens, D.A., Rossi, J.J. (1990): Ribozymes as potential anti-HIV-1 therapeutic agents. Science 247: 1222-1225.
Sullenger, B.A., Gallardo, H.F., Ungers, G.E., Gibbon, E. (1990): Overexpression of TAR sequences renders cells resistant to human immunodeficiency virus replication. Cell 63: 601-608
Trono, D., Feinberg, M.B., Baltimore, D. (1989). HIV-1 Gag mutants can dominantly interfere with the replication of the wild-type virus. Cell 59: 113-120.
Venkatesh, L.H., Avens, M.Q, Subramanian, T., Chinnadurai, G. (1990): Selective inhibition of toxicity to human cells expressing human immunodeficiency virus type 1 TAT by a conditionally cytotoxic adenovirus vector. Proc. Nat. Acad. Sc. USA. 87: 8746-8750.

RESUME : L'idée de protéger un individu au moyen d'une résistance génétiquement induite de ses propres cellules pourrait constituer une approche intéressante dans le cas de l'infection par le virus HIV pour plusieurs raisons : 1) Une partie du répertoire T pourrait être ménagé protégeant ainsi du déficit immunitaire profond responsable de la mort de la plupart des patients ; 2) Le virus affecte préférentiellement les lymphocytes T et les monocytes qui font partie des cellules cibles les plus accessibles au transfert de gène ; 3) Les drogues anti-virales demeurent globalement peu efficaces. Si la thérapie génique du SIDA en est à ses premiers balbutiements, quatre types d'approches différentes peuvent être imaginées, qu'il s'agisse : soit des gènes mutants négatifs dominants, soit des toxines conditionnelles dépendant de la présence du virus dans les cellules, soit des gènes exprimant des anti-sens, des ribozymes ou enfin de ceux commandant l'hyperexpression de séquences virales. Des expériences préliminaires suggèrent qu'une efficacité potentielle pourrait être obtenue, tout au moins in-vitro, cependant, seules quelques unes ont été appliquées au contrôle de la réplication du virus HIV. Des preuves supplémentaires de l'efficacité de cette approche devront être apportées. Des modèles animaux in-vivo devront de plus être étudiés (soit systèmes murins, soit macaques ou chats infectés par des lentivirus). Le développement futur d'une thérapie génique du SIDA dépendra avant tout des succès ou des échecs des drogues antivirales dans les dix ans qui viennent. La question se posera alors de savoir dans quelle mesure ce type de traitement sera économiquement accessible aux malades.

Vaccines

Marc Girard

Département de Virologie, Institut Pasteur, 28, rue du Docteur Roux, 75724 Paris Cedex 15, France

SUMMARY

The applications of gene transfer to the field of vaccines are reviewed. A heap of new recombinant live vaccines and subunit vaccines is under development, although much effort is still to be made before their immunogenicity is fully optimized. In addition, the new field of intracellular immunization fosters a great many hopes for the future.

INTRODUCTION

Most vaccines are based on the principle that the injection of an attenuated or inactivated pathogenic microorganism, or of appropriate antigens from that microorganism will elicit in the host a specific protective immunity comparable to that observed after natural infection.

Many of the current viral vaccines are composed of live viruses which are attenuated for their host. These vaccines induce long lasting immunity after a single injection (except the oral poliomyelitis vaccine which requires 3-5 administrations to provide 100 % coverage) and are relatively cheap. BCG, a bacterial vaccine, shares the same properties (Table 1).

Table 1 - Live, attenuated human vaccines

Organism	Agents	
	Current vaccines	Under trial
Viruses	Vaccinia (smallpox) Measles Yellow fever Mumps Polio (OPV) Adenovirus Rubella Varicella-Zoster	Cytomegalovirus Hepatitis A Dengue Japanese encephalitis Herpes simplex (HSV-2) Rotavirus Influenza
Bacterias	BCG S. typhi (Ty21a)	V. cholerae S. typhi (aroA)

As demonstrated by Louis Pasteur with Bacillus anthracis, Pasteurellas and rabies virus, bacterias and viruses that have lost their pathogenicity upon ageing or treatment with heat or chemical agents make also efficient vaccines.

Table 2 - Inactivated human vaccines

Organism	Agents	
	Current vaccines	Under trial
Viruses	Polio (IPV) Influenza Rabies Japanese encephalitis Tick-borne encephalitis	Hepatitis A
Bacterias	V. cholerae B. pertussis S. typhi S. paratyphi	V. cholerae + B sub-unit

Several inactivated virus vaccines are available to-day (Table 2) and most are quite effective, but they are more expensive than live virus vaccines because larger doses of viral antigen and a higher number of injections are required. The situation is less bright for inactivated bacterial vaccines. To the exception of B. pertussis (which suffers other disadvantages) the use of inactivated bacterial preparations has been disappointing.

The search has been, therefore, for simpler vaccines, made only of one (or a few) subunit antigen(s). Gaston Ramon discovered in 1923 that heat and formalin treatments converted bacterial toxins into highly immunogenic and inoffensive toxoids that could be used as effective vaccines (Table 3). Another type of bacterial subunit vaccine is that made of the polysaccharides from the capsule of certain bacterias. Vaccines composed of these polysaccharides are however ineffective in young children below 2 years of age, because of lack of maturation of the immune system. Coupling of the polysaccharide to a protein moiety has allowed vaccinologists to overcome this problem.

Table 3 - Sub-unit vaccines

Organism	Agents	
	Current vaccines	Under trial
Viruses	Hepatitis B Influenza	
Bacterias	H. influenzae S. pneumoniae N. meningitidis S. typhi (Vi Ag) Tetanus Diphteria	B. pertussis

In the case of viral vaccines, the only successful subunit vaccine is that made from the surface antigen of hepatitis B virus (HBsAg). Attempts at developing other subunit viral vaccines have not met with similar success, because of the low immunogenicity of isolated viral antigens (envelope glycoproteins or capsid proteins). Several formulations are under development in an attempt to solve this problem.

Two domains of application of gene transfer to the field of vaccines can be distinguished ; one is that of the live recombinant vaccines, which are made of live, attenuated viral or bacterial vectors capable of expressing one or more genes from other micro-organisms while retaining infectivity (for a review, see WHO, 1990). The other is that of sub-unit recombinant vaccines which are made of purified antigens produced by DNA recombinant technology in heterologous expression systems such as bacterias, yeasts, or mammalian cells. The coming of age of genetic engineering and the potential it offers for the cloning and expression of viral or bacterial genes has led to a heap of candidate vaccines that have been developed in recent years as a direct product of gene transfer. In addition, a new potential field for the prevention of diseases has recently opened, that of intracellular immunization (Baltimore, 1988). The purpose of this approach is to render target cells refractory to virus replication. Although no immune response is involved in the process, it is, at the cellular level, a form of preventive immunization. Development in these different domains will be reviewed, with emphasis on AIDS.

LIVE RECOMBINANT VACCINES

The development of safe, effective, live recombinant vaccines involves the use of an attenuated bacterial or viral strain which serves as a vector and which is made capable of expressing the protective antigens of the pathogen against which protection is sought. A list of the most commonly used vectors is given in table 4.

Table 4 - Potential vectors for live recombinant vaccines

Viruses	Bacterias
Vaccinia virus	BCG
Fowlpox virus	S. typhimurium
Canarypox virus	S. typhi
Adenoviruses	E. coli
Herpes virus	
Varicella-zoster virus	
Picornaviruses	
Flaviviruses	

Vaccinia virus as a vector

To date, the most successful approach has been using vaccinia virus (VV) as the recombinant vector (Panicali and Paoletti, 1982 ; Smith et al, 1983). This virus has a large DNA genome into which foreign genes can be inserted without compromising its capacity to replicate. It induces both humoral and cellular immunity, it is cheap to manufacture, heat and dehydratation resistant, and easy to administer. At least 17 different viral as well as bacterial and parasitic antigens have been expressed in VV recombinants, among which the envelope glycoproteins from rabies virus, Hepatitis B virus (HBV), Herpes simplex virus (HSV), Epstein-Barr virus, influenza virus, respiratory syncitial virus, parainfluenzae type 3 virus, dengue virus, human immunodeficiency virus (HIV), simian immunodeficiency virus (SIV) or different antigens from Plasmodium falciparum. VV double or multiple recombinants have also been constructed, for example with influenza and herpes simplex virus genes.

The most successful achievement so far, in terms of practical applications of recombinant VV to the field of vaccines, is that of the recombinant rabies-VV constructed by Kiény et al (1984) which expresses the rabies G glycoprotein (Lathe et al, 1985). A single injection of the recombinant rabies-VV was sufficient to induce high titers of neutralizing antibodies in animals and to provide protection against an infectious virus challenge by the intracerebral route (Wiktor et al, 1984). More remarkable, a single dose of recombinant rabies-VV by the oral route was sufficient to elicit a protective immunity against rabies (Bricou et al, 1986). This has prompted the use of the recombinant virus in baits for the vaccination of animals such as foxes, skunks or raccoons, that propagate rabies and spread the virus in the wild. Several experiments in the field are under way to demonstrate the efficacy of the procedure (for a review, see Lecocq, this volume).

A VV-rinderpest construct expressing the hemagglutinin (HA) and fusion (F) surface proteins of rinderpest virus (RPV) has similarly been shown very effective in providing protective immunity against RPV in cattle. Its use in Africa to vaccinate wild ungulate animals against RPV is under consideration A VV-measles recombinant expressing the HA and F proteins of measles virus has recently been constructed ; it should be tested presently in humans.

Recombinant VV technology has also been applied to the expression of HIV envelope glycoprotein gp160. HIV-VV recombinants show however little humoral immune potency (Girard et al, 1989) and, probably for that reason, were not able to provide protection of chimpanzees against challenge with HIV (Hu et al, 1987 ; Girard et al, 1989). The weak humoral immunogenicity of recombinant HIV-VV for apes has been confirmed in human volunteers. Recombinant VV were however able to induce or to prime a strong cellular immune response both in chimpanzees (Zarling et al, 1987 ; Van Eedenburg et al, 1989) and in humans (Corey, personal communication ; Zagury et al, 1988). These results suggest that recombinant VV expressing the HIV envelope glycoproteins could be useful for priming the response of the immune system to booster injections of HIV envelope antigen or synthetic peptides.

Recombinant VV expressing the gag pol gene of HIV were able to induce the formation and budding of HIV-like particles out of infected cells, even in the absence of the viral envelope glycoprotein (Flexner et al, 1988 ; Gowda et al, 1989 ; Shioda and Shibuta, 1990). Cells doubly-infected with recombinant VV expressing the gag-pol and env genes excreted into the culture supernatants genome-less HIV particles, complete with envelope spikes (Karacostas et al, 1989 ; Haffar et al, 1990). These particles contained RNA reacting with a gag specific probe, but not with an env specific probe, and were devoid of infectivity. There is reason to believe the RNA inside the particle could be the gag-pol mRNA. Recombinant VV carrying the gag-pol and env genes represent an interesting new type of vaccine. They could be used either in vivo as a live virus vaccine or in vitro as a safe source of material for the development of inactivated HIV vaccines from infected cell culture supernatants. It will be of interest to test their efficacy in a protection test on chimpanzees.

VV has also been used as a vector for the manufacture of live recombinant vaccines against experimental tumors. Thus, a recombinant VV expressing the polyomavirus middle T antigen was able to provide mice with 100 % protection against a polyoma induced tumor (Lathe et al, 1989). Interestingly, antibodies seemed to play no role in protection. Whether vaccination could be similarly successful against other tumorogenic viruses, such as human papillomaviruses or human T lymphotropic virus remains to be determined.

The use of recombinant vaccinia viruses in humans has however been met with little enthusiasm, because of the fear of local vaccination reactions and of possible complications such as fatal progressive vaccinia, eczema vaccinatum, and post-vaccinial encephalopathy, which are known to have occurred in the past with frequencies of about 3×10^{-6}, 60×10^{-6} and 120×10^{-6} or lower per primary vaccination, respectively. Complications were very rare in revaccinations, however. Also, the inactivation of the TK gene of the VV vector has been shown to decrease its neurovirulence by close to 4 logs, thus rendering recombinants potentially much less hazardous than the VV virus strains that were used to vaccinate against smallpox a quarter of a century ago.

Other virus vectors

The live vector technology has been applied to other virus vectors as well (table 4). Fowl poxvirus and canary poxvirus are of special interest. These viruses have the remarkable property that they do not multiply in mammalian cells and are, therefore, devoid of the undesirable side effects of VV. They can nevertheless express foreign antigens in an efficient manner, which makes them prime candidates for use as live recombinant vectors. Several live recombinant canary poxvirus vaccines are under development to-day.

Adenoviruses type 4 and 7 make up another type of vector of interest. They are currently in use in the US Army as an oral vaccine against acute respiratory illnesses . Recombinant adenovirus vaccines containing a cloned foreign gene have been developed (McDermott et al, 1989). For example, the HBsAg gene has been inserted into the E3 region of adenovirus type 4 and 7 (Molnar-Kimber et al, 1989). The vaccine was shown to provide partial protection to chimpanzees against an infectious HBV challenge. Recombinant adenovirus vaccine expressing the HIV env and rev genes have also been developed. Co-expression of rev was found to be required for full expression of env. Recombinant adenovirus expressing the F glycoprotein of respiratory syncitial virus provided protection to cotton rats against a virus challenge. However, adenoviruses have a small DNA genome, which limits their gene-carrying capacity. They exhibit potential pathogenicity for the respiratory tract, which makes them difficult to use in children and infants. And their restricted host range makes the assessment of their efficacy in animal model systems difficult.

Attenuated polioviruses are attractive vectors, because the three-dimensional structure of their capsid and its antigenicity as well as the organization of their genome are well known, and because there is ample experience of the virus as a live virus vaccine in humans. The strategy for using poliovirus as a vector for foreign antigens relies on the use of infectious cDNA. Chimeric poliovirus type 1 particles were engineered which expressed type 2 or type 3 antigenic sites (Burke et al, 1988 ; Martin et al, 1988 ; Murray et al, 1988). Sequences from Coxsackie virus, human papillomavirus (HPV), HIV (Evans et al, 1989) and Chlamydia trachomatis have also been inserted into poliovirus type 1 capsids.

A problem with this approach is that only limited foreign amino acid sequences can be inserted (the largest insert so far is 22 amino acids long) which could induce a monospecific antibody response, and, in turn, favor the emergence of escape mutants. Also, there is reason to believe that the basal level of immunity to poliovirus in a human population vaccinated against poliomyelitis would much hamper the use of poliovirus chimeras. Other picornaviruses are therefore developed as potential replacement vectors. For unknown reasons, not all poliovirus chimeras have been able to elicit an immune response to the inserted sequence. More work has to be done to understand this phenomenom.

Finally, the possibility of using herpes viruses as vectors has been studied. An attenuated HSV-1 strain has been engineered to express hetero-logous antigens. Two HSV-1 virus strains, R7017 and R7020, express HSV-2 D, G, and I glycoproteins and part of the E glycoprotein, and can efficiently be used as live virus vaccine to induce protection against HSV-2 diseases (Meignier et al, 1988).

Bacterias as vectors

Another type of live recombinant vaccines makes use of live, attenuated bacterias as a vehicle in which foreign antigens can be expressed. This approach is based on the observation that mutations that suppress the virulence of pathogenic bacterias often leave enough of their invasivity to let them induce a protective immune response when administered alive to their host (for reviews, see Hofnung, 1988 ; WHO, 1990 ; and Oral Immunization using recombinant bacteria, 1990).

At present, Escherichia coli and Salmonella typhimurium are the bacterial strains the most frequently used. Salmonella typhi attenuated mutants such as the Ty21a strain have also been tested. Current efforts to construct aroA-aroC or cya-crp deletion mutants of S. typhi should provide improved carrier strains for oral vaccines of humans. A number of foreign antigens have been expressed in these bacterias, such as the B sub-unit of the E. coli heat-stable toxin, E. coli heat-labile toxin, Plasmodium berghei circumsporozoite protein (Sadoff et al, 1988), the Shigella flexneri 2a O polysaccharide side chain, etc...

Expression of a foreign protein is however often toxic to bacterias. A solution to this problem is to first identify the antigenic determinant(s) or epitope(s) of the foreign antigen which are critical for protection and to have them expressed by genetic insertion within a recipient bacterial protein such as a surface protein. For example, neutralization antigenic site 1 of poliovirus, a stretch of 10 amino acids from capsid polypeptide VP1, was expressed either in the periplasm or at the surface of E. coli as a hybrid MalE or LamB protein, respectively. Injection to rabbits of live recombinant E. coli expressing such hybrid polio-bacterial proteins was shown to result in induction of anti-poliovirus neutralizing antibodies (Charbit et al, 1988 ; see also Hofnung, this volume). Only a few sites in the carrier bacterial protein allow insertion of the foreign epitope without affecting the activity of the protein and therefore the viability of the recombinant hosts. Thus, a seach for permissive sites has to be made for every protein before hybrid constructs can be successfully prepared.

Another promising bacterial species to be used as a vehicle and for which many hopes have been voiced (Bloom, 1986) is Bacillus Calmette-Guérin (BCG), the avirulent derivative of Mycobacterium bovis that has been in use as a live attenuated vaccine against tuberculosis for close to 70 years. The vaccine is remarkably cheap, it can be given at birth, induces very few serious side effects, and elicits a strong cell-mediated immunity that can last for up to 50 years. In addition, the vaccine has superb adjuvant activity. The development of a host-vector system using BCG had to await the ability to transform or transduce Mycobacterias, which was achieved recently (see for example Snapper et al, 1988). Since then, several foreign antigens have been expressed successfully and a foreign antigen secretion system has been developed (Matsuo et al, 1990). It remains however to be determined if recombinant BCG will be effective in eliciting substantial immunity and protection, particularly against diseases where B-cell responses are important.

RECOMBINANT SUB-UNIT VACCINES

The genes of a pathogen coding for antigens involved in the induction of a protective immune response can be transferred to plasmids, and their products expressed in and purified from bacteria, yeasts or mammalian cells.

Similarly, portions of these genes which encode critical antigenic determinants can be expressed in the same systems, either as such or in the form of hybrid fusion proteins. The VPI capsid protein of foot-and-mouth disease virus, the B sub-unit of the cholera toxin, HSV-1 envelope glycoprotein D, antigens from Plasmodium falciparum, HBsAg, the envelope glycoprotein gp110 of HIV have been cloned and expressed in such a fashion, just to name a few. Expression systems can be either constitutive, i.e. made of recombinant cells which express the foreign antigen continuously, or inducible, in which case expression is transient only. Inducible systems offer evident advantages when expression of the foreign protein is toxic to the cell. Another possibility in such a case is to have the protein excreted into the cell culture medium.

As an alternative to transient expression systems, foreign antigens can also be expressed using viruses as vectors. Thus, recombinant vaccinia viruses that were engineered to express the gp160 envelope glycoprotein of HIV have been used in cell cultures in fermentors to generate mass quantities of the antigen (Kieny et al, 1988 ; Barrett et al, 1989). Deletion of the hydrophobic transmembrane portion of viral surface antigens allow the recombinant molecules to be excreted by the infected cells into their culture medium, from which they can then be purified readily. Another system makes use of recombinant baculoviruses that are grown on insect cells in culture (Luckow and Summers, 1988). This system is remarkable for its high yields, but mass cultivation of insect cells still remains an unsolved problem. Also, glycosylation of proteins by insect cells is different from that by mammalian cells (Wells and Compans, 1990).

The first sub-unit vaccine for human use to be developed from a purified recombinant antigen was the HBV vaccine made of HBsAg expressed from either yeast or CHO cells (for a review, see Tiollais et al, 1985). The advantage of HBsAg is that it naturally forms particles which are relatively immunogenic and only need to be adsorbed onto aluminium hydroxyde to make up a potent vaccine (André et al, 1989). Most other purified antigens do not possess the immune potency of the antigenic structures from which they are derived and thus have to be potentiated by strong adjuvants. Incomplete Freund's adjuvant (IFA) is one of the most powerful adjuvants, but its use in humans is not accepted, in spite of lack of retrospective long-term side effects (Zanetti et al, 1987). Other adjuvants such as MDP-base oil emulsions, immuno stimulating complexes (Hoglund et al, 1989), and liposomes are under active development (Stewart-Tull, 1989).

It has been our experience that high titers of HIV neutralizing antibodies could be induced in chimpanzees by the injection of recombinant HIV gp160 followed by a synthetic oligopeptide with the sequence of the principal neutralization epitope of gp160, provided both preparations were mixed with the MDP-base adjuvant SAF-1. The neutralizing antibody response obtained was correlated with protection against experimental HIV infection (Berman et al, 1990 ; Girard et al, 1991).

Considerable progress has been made in the development of a new generation of vaccines. The science for optimizing their immunogenicity still remains however to be developed (Zanetti et al, 1987).

INTRACELLULAR IMMUNIZATION

The mutation of regulatory genes may yield proteins that exhibit a <u>dominant negative phenotype</u> : when the gene carrying such a mutation is expressed, its product interferes in a dominant fashion with the function of the parental gene product (Herskowitz, 1987). The phenomenom has been observed with eukaryotic transcriptional <u>trans</u>-activators (Hope & Struhl, 1986) and extended to viral <u>trans</u>-activators (Wachsman et al, 1987 ; Friedman et al, 1988 ; Triezenberg et al, 1988). Thus the expression of a <u>trans</u>-dominant mutant of the VP16 <u>trans</u>-activator of HSV-1 led to resistance to HSV-1 infection on a normally susceptible murine cell population (Friedman et al, 1988). This antiviral approach, which has been called <u>intracellular immunization</u> by Baltimore (1988), is of great potential interest for the control of virus infections.

At least two possible mechanisms of actions have been suggested to explain dominant negative phenotypes (Heskowitz, 1987). When the protein is multimeric, the mutant defective molecules might be able to form mixed, non functional multimers with the wild-type molecules and hence inhibit the function of the latter in a <u>trans</u>-dominant manner. In the case of <u>trans</u>-activating factors, mutations that affect the "activation domain" of the protein, but not its "binding domain" (for a review, see Ptashne, 1988), result in mutant proteins which are believed to compete with the wild-type protein for binding to the appropriate cellular or viral target, yet are incapable of activating transcription once binding has occurred. Examples of possible intracellular immunization as applied to HIV are described below (see also Levy, this volume).

HIV-1 encodes two <u>trans</u>-acting nuclear regulatory proteins, Tat and Rev (for a review, see Cullen, 1991), the functional expression of which is required for virus replication (Fisher et al, 1986 ; Dayton et al, 1986 ; Feinberg et al, 1986 ; Sodroski et al, 1986). The Tat protein acts at the transcriptional level, perhaps as an anti-terminator (Kao et al, 1987). Its target is a 44 nucleotide RNA stem loop structure at the 5' end of viral RNA, the Tat responsive element (TAR) (Muesing et al, 1987 ; Kao et al, 1987). The <u>rev</u> gene product, in contrast, functions post-transcriptionnally by activating the nuclear export of the incompletely spliced mRNAs which encode Gag and Env. In the absence of Rev protein, or if the <u>rev</u> gene product is inactive, the only mRNAs that are exported to the cytoplasm are the fully spliced mRNAs that encode the viral regulatory proteins, among which Tat and Rev itself (Malim et al, 1989). The Rev protein functions in a highly sequence-specific manner by interaction with its RNA target sequence, the Rev responsive element (RRE), a 234 nucleotide RNA stem loop structure present within the HIV-1 <u>env</u> gene (Malim et al, 1989a).

Both the <u>tat</u> gene and the <u>rev</u> gene are potential targets for the generation of dominant negative mutants. In the case of the <u>tat</u> gene, such a possibility was analyzed by Green et al (1989) using a microinjection assay to introduce a bacterial chloramphenicol acetyl transferase (CAT) gene under the control of the HIV-1 LTR into the nuclei of HeLa cells that were subsequently treated with "minimal domain" Tat peptides. Peptides Tat 1-86, Tat 37-62 or Tat 37-72 all triggered the formation of CAT mRNA, as measured by <u>in situ</u> hybridization. Substitution of alanine for 41Lys, 46Ser or 47Tyr in these peptides yielded peptides that behave as <u>trans</u>-dominant antagonists of the wild-type Tat peptides in the same assay. These Tat mutant peptides, and specially the 41Lys substitution peptides, could be taken up by cells and block the function of Tat, suggesting that a <u>tat</u> gene containing these trans-dominant mutations and transferred to hematopoietic stem cells through a suitable vector could be effective in intracellular immunization against HIV-1 (Green et al, 1989).

In the case of the rev gene, the possibility of generating trans-dominant mutations was explored by Malim et al (1989b). Deletion of the C-terminal part of the Rev protein or substitution of amino acids 78Leu and 79Glu (mutant M10), resulted in defective Rev proteins that were able to inhibit wild-type Rev function in trans. Similarly, rescue of a rev provirus from COS cells by transfection with the wild-type rev gene expression vector was blocked in a competitive manner by co-expression of the trans-dominant mutants. Trans-dominant rev mutants could thus be choice candidates for the intracellular immunization of lymphoid cells from AIDS infected individuals.

A similar observation has been made with HTLV-1, the rex gene product of which mimicks that of the HIV-1 rev gene product and can actually substitute for it, although the two proteins do not possess apparent amino acid sequence homology (Rimsky et al, 1988). It was found that cotransfected rex trans-dominant mutants inhibited the rescue of a rev⁻ HIV-1 provirus by wild-type Rex protein supplied in trans (Rimsky et al, 1989). More recently, a trans-dominant negative HTLV-1 rex mutant was shown to block both the HTLV-1 rex and the HIV-1 rev gene functions, suggesting this mutant could have the potential to exert antiviral activity against both HTLV-1 and HIV-1 in double-infected individuals (Böhnlein et al, 1991).

A third distinct potential target for the generation of dominant negative mutants is the gag gene, which encodes the core proteins of HIV. The product of the HIV gag gene, Pr55^{gag}, is cleaved by the virally encoded protease to generate mature viral proteins p17(p18), p24(p25), and p15. The latter seems to be associated with the viral RNA ; p17 is believed to line the interior of the viral envelope ; and p24 constitutes the shell of the tubular core of HIV (Geldelblom et al, 1987 ; Mervis et al, 1988 ; Veronese et al, 1988). Negative dominant HIV Gag mutants were generated by deletion or insertion of a few amino acids at the p17/p24 cleavage site or in p24, respectively (Trono et al, 1989). Cotransfection of the DNA of these mutants with that of wild-type HIV was shown to reduce dramatically the yield of wild-type virus in a transient expression assay using COS cells. When stable HeLa cell lines expressing the CD4 molecule at their surface and selected for constitutive expression of such HIV Gag mutants were infected with wild-type HIV, the yield of infectious virus was reduced more than 3000 fold. It was suggested that the cells had been made refractory to HIV multiplication through formation of chimeric Gag multimers containing a mixture of wild-type and mutant Gag molecules which either made them unable to carry out the steps of viral assembly and/or release, or resulted in the formation of non infectious viral particles.

The actual efficacy of the intracellular immunization approach in vivo remains to be tested. However, the approach is facilitated in the case of HIV by the fact that HIV infection is largely an infection of cells (T4 lymphocytes and monocytes/macrophages) that are derived from haematopoietic stem cells. Thus, provided the appropriate dominant negative mutant gene is placed under the control of transcriptional elements that function when the stem cell matures to T cells or monocytes/macrophages, intracellular immunization could become a real AIDS therapy for seropositive individuals (Baltimore, 1988).

For diseases other than AIDS, intracellular immunization will probably be of lesser use in view of its cost, of the practical difficulties of the method, and of the fact that it is an individualistic approach to disease control. However, in the case of animals, one could imagine to combine intracellular immunization and transgenesis, which would result in the production of animals refractory to disease, in the same way as one can obtain to-day plants that display resistance to viruses. This is quite obviously for the future, but the future may soon be here.

ACKNOWLEDGEMENTS

It is a pleasure to acknowledge the efficient editorial help of C. Rousselet and C. Avrameas.

REFERENCES

Andre, F.E., Goilan, C., and Piot, P. (1989): Development and clinical studies with a recombinant DNA hepatitis B vaccine. In Vaccines for sexually transmitted diseases, eds A. Meheus and R.E. Spier, pp. 128-133. London: Butterworths.

Barrett, N., Mitterer, A., Mundt, W., Eibl, J., Eibl, M., Gallo, R.C., Moss, B., and Dorner, F. (1989): Large-scale production and purification of a vaccinia recombinant-derived HIV-1 gp160 and analysis of its immunogenicity. AIDS Res. Hum. Retrovirus 5: 159-171.

Berman, P.W., Groopman, J.E., Gregory, T., Clapham, P.R., Weiss, R.A., Ferriani, R., Riddle, L., Shimasaki, C., Lucas, C., Lasky, L.A., and Eichberg, J.W. (1990): Human immunodeficiency virus type 1 challenge of chimpanzees immunized with recombinant envelope glycoprotein gp120. Proc. Natl. Acad. Sci. USA. 85: 5200-5204.

Baltimore, D. (1988): Intracellular immunization. Nature (London) 335: 395-396.

Bloom, B.R. (1986): Learning for leprosy: a perspective on immunology and the Third World. J. Immunol. 137: 2831-2834.

Böhnlein, S., Pirker, F.P., Hofer, L., Zimmermann, K., Bachmayer, H., Böhnlein, E., and Hauber, J. (1991): Transdominant repressors for human T-cell leukemia type 1 Rex and human immunodeficiency virus type 1 Rev function. J. Virol. 65: 81-88.

Bricou, J., Kieny, M.P., Lathe, R., Lecocq, J.P., Pastoret, P.P., Soulebot, J.P., and Desmettre, P. (1986): Oral vaccination of the fox against rabies using a live recombinant vaccinia virus. Nature (London) 322: 373-375.

Burke, K.L., Dunn, G., Ferguson, M., Minor, P.D., and Almond, J.W. (1988) Antigenic chimaeras of poliovirus as potential new vaccines. Nature (London) 334: 81-82.

Chanock, R.M., Murphy, B.R., Collins, P.L., Coelingh, K.V.W., Olmsted, R.A., Snyder, M.H., Spriggs, M.K., Prince, G.A., Moss, B. , Flores, J., Gorziglia, M., and Kapikian, A.Z. (1988): Live viral vaccines for respiratory and enteric tract diseases. Vaccine 6: 129-133.

Charbit A., Van der Werf, S., Mimic, V., Boulain , J.C., Girard, M., and Hofnung, M. (1988): Expression of a poliovirus neutralization epitope at the surface of recombinant bacteria: first immunization results. Ann.Inst.Pasteur/Microbiol. 139: 45-58.

Cullen, B.R. (1991): Human immunodeficiency virus as a prototypic complex retrovirus.J.Virol. 65: 1053-1056.

Dayton, A.I., Sodroski, J.G., Rosen, C.A., Goh, W.C., and Haseltine, W.A. (1986): The trans-activated gene of the human T cell lymphotropic virus type III is required for replication. Cell 44: 941-947.

Evans, D.J., McKeating, J., Meredith, J.M.., Burke, K.L, Katrak, K., John, A., Ferguson, M.,

Minor, P.D., Weiss, R.A., and Almond, J.W. (1989): An engineered poliovirus chimaera elicits broadly reactive HIV-1 neutralizing antibodies. Nature (London) 339: 385-388.

Feinberg, M.B., Jarrett, R.F., Aldovini, A., Gallo, R.C., and Wong-Staal, F. (1986): HTLV-III expression and production involve complex regulation at the levels of splicing and translation of viral RNA. Cell 46: 807-817.

Fischer, A.G., Feinberg, M.B., Josephs, S.F., Harper, M.E., Marselle, L.M., Reyes,G., Bonda, M.A., Aldovini, A., Debouk, C., Gallo, R.C., and Wong-Staal, F. (1986): The trans-activator gene of HTLV-III is essential for virus replication. Nature (London) 320: 3367-371.

Flexner, C.,Broyles, S.S., Earl, P., Chakrabarti, S., and Moss, B. (1988): Characterization of human immunodeficiency virus gag/pol gene products expressed by recombinant vaccinia viruses. Virology 166: 339-349.

Friedman, A.D., Triezenberg, S.J., and McKnight, S.L. (1988): Expression of a truncated viral trans-activator selectively impedes lytic infection by its cognate virus. Nature (London) 335: 452-454.

Gelderblom, H.R., Hausman, E.H.S., Ozel, M., Pauli, G., and Koch, M.A. (1987): Fine structure of human immunodeficiency virus (HIV) and immunolocalization of structural proteins. Virology 156: 171-176.

Girard, M., Kieny, M.P., Pinter, A., Barré-Sinoussi, F., Nara, P., Kolbe, H., Kusumi, K., Chaput, M., Reinhart, T., Muchmore, E., Ronco, J., Kaczorek, M.,Gomard, E., Gluckman,J .C., and Fultz, P.N. (1991): Immunization of chimpanzees confers protection against challenge with human immunodeficiency virus. Proc.Natl.Acad.Sci.USA 88: 542-546.

Girard, M., Kieny, M.P., Gluckman, J.C., Barre-Sinoussi, F., Montagnier,L., and Fultz, P.N. (1989): Candidate vaccines for HIV. In Vaccines against sexually transmitted diseases, eds A. Meheus and R.S. Spier, pp. 227-237. London: Butterworths .

Gowda, S., Stein, B.S., Steimer, K.S. , and Engelman, E.G. (1989): Expression and processing of human immunodeficiency virus type 1 gag and pol genes by cells infected with a recombinant vaccinia virus. J.Virol. 63: 1451-1454.

Green, M., Ishino, M., and Lowestein, P.M. (1989): Mutational analysis of HIV-1 Tat minimal domain peptides : identification of trans-dominant mutants that suppress HIV-LTR-driven gene expression. Cell 58: 215-223.

Haffar, O., Garrigues, J., Travis, B., Moran, P., Zarling, J., and Hu, S.L. (1990): Human immunodeficiency virus-like, non replicating gag-env particles assemble in a recombinant vaccinia virus expression system.J.Virol. 64: 2653-2659.

Herskowitz, I. (1987): Functional inactivation of genes by dominant negative mutations. Nature (London) 329: 219-222.

Hofnung, M. (1988): Génie génétique et tendances dans la recherche de nouveaux vaccins.C.R.Soc.Biol. 182: 141-157.

Hoglund, S., Dalsgaard, K, Lovgren, K., Sundquist, B., Osterhaus, A., and Morein, B. (1989): ISCOMs and immunostimulation with viral antigens. In Subcellular Biochemistry ed J.R. Harris, vol.15, pp. 39-68. London: Plenum Press .

Hope, I.A. , and Struhl, K. (1986): Functional dissection of an eukaryotic transcriptional activator protein, GCN4 of yeast. Cell 46: 885-894.

Hu, S.L., Fultz, P.N., McClure, H.M., Eichberg, J.W., Thomas, E.K., Zarling, J., Singhal, M.C., Kosowski, S.G., Swenson, R.B., Anderson, D.C., and Todaro, G. (1987): Effect of immunization with a vaccinia-HIV env recombinant on HIV infection of chimpanzees. Nature (London) 328: 721-723.

Kao, S.Y., Calman, A.F., Luciw, P.A., and Peterlin, B.M. (1987): Anti-termination of transcription within the long terminal repeat of HIV-1 by tat gene product. Nature (London) 330: 489-493.

Karacostas, V., Nagashima, K., Gonda, M., and Moss, B. (1989): Human immunodeficiency virus-like particles produced by a vaccinia virus expression vector. Proc.Natl.Acad.Sci. USA 86: 8964-8967.

Kieny, M.P., Lathe, R., Drillien, R., Spehner, D., Skory, S., Schmitt, D., Wiktor, T., Koprowski, H., and Lecocq, J.P. (1984): Expression of rabies virus glycoprotein from a recombinant vaccinia virus. Nature (London) 312: 163-166.

Kieny, M.P., Lathe, R., Riviere, Y., Dott, K., Schmitt, D., Girard, M., Montagnier, L., and Lecocq, J.P. (1988): Improved immunogenicity of the HIV env protein by cleavage site removal. Prot.Eng. 2: 219-226.

Lathe, K, Kieny, M.P., Lecocq, J.P., Drillien, R., Wiktor, T., and Koprowski, H. (1985): Immunization against rabies using a vaccina-rabies recombinant virus expressing the surface glycoprotein. In Modern approaches to vaccines, eds R.A. Lerner, R.M. Chanock and F. Brown, pp.157-162. Cold Spring Harbor, N.Y.: Cold Spring Harbor Laboratory Press.

Luckow, V.A., and Summers, M.D. (1988): Trends in the development of baculovirus expression vectors. Bio Technology 6: 47-55.

McDermott, M.R., Graham, F.L., Hank, T., and Johnson, D.C. (1989): Protection of mice against lethal challenge with Herpes simplex virus by vaccination with an adenovirus vector expressing HSV glycoprotein B. Virology 169:244-247.

Malim, M.H., Hauber, J., Le, S.Y., Maizel, J.V., and Cullen, B.R. (1989 a): The HIV-1 rev trans-activator acts through a structured target sequence to activate nuclear export of unspliced viral mRNA. Nature (London) 328: 254-257.

Malim, M.H., Böhnlein, S., Hauber, J. , and Cullen, B.R. (1989 b): Functional dissection of the HIV-1 rev trans-activator. Derivation of a trans-dominant repressor of rev function. Cell 58: 205-214.

Martin, A., Wychowski, C., Couderc, T., Crainic, R., Hogle, J.M. , and Girard, M. (1988): Engineering a poliovirus type 2 antigenic site on a type 1 capsid results in a chimaeric virus which is neurovirulent for mice. EMBO J. 7: 2839-2847.

Matsuo, K, Yamaguchi, R., Yamazaki, A., Tasaka, H., Terasaka, K., Totsuka, M., Kobayashi, K., Yukitake, H., and Yamada, T. (1990): Establishment of a foreign antigen secretion system in mycobacteria. Infect.Immun. 58: 4049-5054.

Meignier, B., Longnecker, R., and Roizman, B. (1988): R7017 and R 7020 Herpes simplex virus recombinant prototype vaccine strains: animal studies. In Vaccines 88 , eds R.M.Chanock, R.A.Lerner, F.Brown and H.J. Ginsberg. pp.199-196. Cold Spring Harbor. N.Y. :Cold Spring Harbor Laboratory Press.

Mervis, R.J., Ahmad, N., Lillehoj, E.P., Raum, M.G., Salazar, F.H.R., Chan, H.W., and Venkatesan, S. (1988): The gag gene products of human immunodeficiency virus type 1: alignment within the gag open reading frame, identification of post-translational modifications, and evidence for alternative Gag precursors. J.Virol. 62: 3993-4002.

Molnar-Kimber, K.L., Lubeck, M.D., Jarocki-Witek, V., Morin, J.E., Chengalvata, M., Dheer, S.K., Mason, B.B., Barton, J., Bhat, B., Stauffer, B., Mizutani, S., Conley, A.J., Davis, A.R., Halgwood, N.L., Najarian, R., and Moore, G.K. (1989) : Characterization and utilization of the E3 region of Ad4 and Ad7 for development of Ad4 and Ad7 recombinant vaccines for Hepatitis-B virus. In Vaccines 89 , eds. R.M. Chanock, R.A. Lerner, F. Brown, and H.J. Ginsberg, pp.193-196. Cold Spring Harbor, N.Y.: Cold Spring Harbor Laboratory Press.

Muesing, M.A., Smith, D.H., and Capon, D.J. (1987): Regulation of mRNA accumulation by a human immunodeficiency virus trans-activator protein. Cell 48: 691-701.

Murray, M.G., Kuhn, R.J., Arita, M., Kawamura, N., Nomoto, A., and Wimmer, E. (1988): Poliovirus type 1/type 3 antigenic hybrid virus constructed in vitro elicits type 1 and type 3 neutralizing antibodies in rabbits and monkeys. Proc.Natl.Acad.Sci.USA 85: 3203-3207.

Oral immunization using recombinant bacteria, an international symposium (1990) eds F. Schödel and M. Hofnung . Res.Microbiol., 141: 743-1025.

Panicali, D., Davis, S.W., and Paoletti, E. (1983): Construction of live vaccines by using genetically engineered poxviruses. Biological activity of recombinant vaccinia virus expressing influenza virus hemagglutin. Proc.Natl.Acad.Sc.USA 80: 5364-5368.

Ptashne, M. (1988): How eukaryotic transcriptional activators work. Nature (London) 335: 683-689.

Rimsky, L.,Hauber, J., Dukovich, M., Malim, M.H., Langlois, A., Cullen, B.R., and Greene, W.C. (1988): Functional replacement of the HIV-1 Rev protein by the HTLV-1 Rex protein. Nature (London) 335: 738-740.

Rimsky, L., Duc Dudon, M., Dixon, E.P., and Greene, W.C. (1989): Trans-dominant inactivation of HTLV-I and HIV-1 gene expression by mutation of the HTLV-1 transactivator. Nature (London) 341: 453-456.

Sadoff, J.C., Ripley-Ballou, W., Baron, L.S., Majarian, W.R., Brey, R.N., Hockmeyer, W.T., Young, J.F., Cryz, S.J., Ou, J., Lowell, G.H., and Chulay, J.D. (1988): Oral Salmonella typhimurium vaccine expressing circumsporozoïte protein protects against malaria. Science 240: 336-338.

Shidda, T., and Shibuta, H. (1990): Production of human immunodeficiency virus (HIV)-like particles from cells infected with recombinant vaccinia viruses carrying the gag gene of HIV. Virology 175: 139-148.

Smith, G.L., Mackett, M., and Moss, B. (1983): Infectious vaccinia virus recombinants that express hepatitis B virus surface antigen. Nature (London) 302: 490-495.

Snapper, S.B, Lugosi, L., Jekkel, A., Melton, R.E., Kieser, T., Bloom, B.R. , and Jacobs, W.R. (1988): Lysogeny and transformation in mycobacteria: stable expression of foreign genes.Proc.Natl.Acac.Sci.USA 85: 6987-6991.

Sodroski, J., Goh, W.C., Rosen, C., Dayton, A., Terwilliger, E., and Haseltine, W. (1986): A second post-transcriptional trans-activator gene required for HTLV-III replication. Nature (London) 321: 412-417.

Steward-Tull, D.E.S. (1989): Selection and suitability of adjuvants. In Vaccines for sexually transmitted diseases, eds A.Meheus and R.E.Spier, pp.17-32. London: Butterworths.

Tiollais, P., Pourcel, C. , and Dejean, A. (1986): The hepatitis B virus. Nature (London) 317: 489-495.

Triezenberg, S.J., Kingsbury, R.C., and McKnight, S.L. (1988): Functional dissection of VP16, the trans-activator of herpes simplex virus immediate early gene expression. Genes Dev. 2: 718-729.

Trono, D., Feinberg, M.B., and Baltimore, D. (1989): HIV-1 gag mutants can dominantly interfere with the replication of the wild-type virus. Cell 59: 113-120.

Van Eendenburg, J.P., Yagello, M., Girard, M., Kieny, M.P., Lecocq, J.P., Muchmore, E., Fultz, P.N., Riviere, Y., Montagnier, L., and Gluckman, J.C. (1989): Cell-mediated immune proliferative responses to HIV-1 of chimpanzees vaccinated with different vaccinia recombinant viruses. AIDS Res.Hum.Retrovirus 5: 41-50.

Veronese, F.D.M., Copeland, T.D., Orozlan, S., Gallo, R.C., and Sarngadharan, M.G. (1988): Biochemical and immunological analysis of human immunodeficiency virus gag gene products p17 and p24. J.Virol. 62: 795-801.

Wachsman, W., Cann, A.J., WIlliams, J.L., Slamon, D.I., Souza, L., Shah, N.P., and Chen, I.S.Y. (1987): HTLV X gene mutants exhibit novel transcriptional regulatory phenotypes.Science 235: 674-677.

Wells, D.E., and Compans, R.W. (1990): Expression and characterization of a functional human immunodeficiency virus envelope glycoprotein in insect cells. Virology 176: 575-586.

Wiktor, T., McFarnan, R., Reagan, K., Dietzschold, B., Curtis, P., Wunner, W., Kieny, M.P., Lathe, R., Lecocq, J.P., Mackett, M., Moss, B., and Koprowski, H. (1984): Protection from rabies by a vaccinia virus recombinant containing the rabies virus

Protection from rabies by a vaccinia virus recombinant containing the rabies virus glycoprotein gene. Proc.Natl.Acad.Sci.USA 81: 7194-7198.

WHO, Programme for Vaccine Development (1990): Potential use of live viral and bacterial vectors for vaccines. Vaccine 8: 425-437.

Zagury, D., Bernard, J., Cheynier, R., Desportes, I., Leonard, R., Fouchard, M., Reveil, B., Ittele, F.D., Lurthuma, Z., Mbayo, K., Wane, J., Salaun, J.J., Goussard, B., Decharzal, L., Burny, A., Nara, P., and Gallo, R.C. (1988): A group-specific anamnestic immune reaction against HIV-1 induced by a candidate vaccine against AIDS. Nature (London) 322: 728-731.

Zanetti, M., Sercarz, E., and Salk, J. (1987): The immunology of new generation vaccines. Immunol Today 8: 18-25.

Zarling, I.M., Eichberg, J.W., Moran, P.A., McClure, J., Shidhar, F., and Hu, S.L. (1987): Proliferative and cytotoxic T-cells to AIDS virus glycoproteins in chimpanzees immunized with a recombinant vaccinia virus expressing AIDS virus envelope glycoprotein. J.Immunol. 139: 988-990.

RESUME

Le transfert de gènes trouve des applications multiples dans le domaine des vaccins et notamment celui des vaccins vivants recombinants utilisant des virus ou des bactéries atténués comme vecteurs, et celui des vaccins sous-unités à base d'antigènes recombinants purifiés. Il faut ajouter à cela le domaine de l'immunisation intracellulaire où les cellules de l'hôte seraient rendues immunes à l'infection par transfert d'une partie appropriée du génome du virus ou de la bactérie contre lesquels on cherche à se protéger. Ces techniques sont appelées à se développer encore et permettent d'espérer des moyens de prévention accrus contre les maladies infectieuses dans le futur.

Gene transfer : tools and mechanisms

Transfert de gènes : moyens et mécanismes

Gene transfer into animals :
the promise of adenovirus

Leslie Stratford-Perricaudet and Michel Perricaudet*

Laboratoire de Génétique des Virus Oncogènes, CNRS, URA 1301, Institut Gustave-Roussy PRII, rue Camille Desmoulins, 94800 Villejuif, France
* Author for correspondence

> Adenovirus has been evaluated as a new gene delivery system applicable to gene therapy. The potential of this virus to accommodate a large piece of DNA and to express a gene in the absence of both viral and cellular replication make this virus an attractive gene transfer system. Specifically, it could provide an effective alternative when the target cells are not amenable to retroviruses. Furthermore, the normal trophism of adenoviruses for the respiratory epithelium suggests a strategy to treat an important genetic disease like cystic fibrosis.

If the ultimate target of gene delivery is an actual living organism, virus-based gene transfer vehicles merit unprecedented attention. This becomes all the more true as genes involved in hereditary disease are continuously being identified and cloned. The dream of one day offering more than diagnosis becomes perpetuated by recent advances in viral transduction of DNA. This strategy capitalizes on the intrinsic ability of viruses to enter cells, bringing their own genetic material with them. Although a retroviral vector has been engineered from a murine leukemia retrovirus and underlies tissue recolonization (the standard means currently in use for transferring genes into living animals), for various reasons, interest is increasing in expression vectors derived from other viruses. Indeed, it is quite evident that retroviruses will have a limited range of action since one of their serious drawbacks is their dependence on host cell division. Many putative targets for gene transfer however, precisely are post-mitotic cells. Due to the success of recombinant adenoviruses in cell culture as high-level expression vectors of a wide variety of biologically active eukaryotic gene products, we have set out to evaluate the feasibility of adenovirus to directly provide an animal with a foreign gene. The current trend focuses on the extraction of cells from the body with their reimplantation following manipulation. Nevertheless, at present, those tissues capable of withstanding such treatment are not numerous. From this viewpoint, the direct administration of a viral vector to an organism could provide the simplest route. We present here an overview of our different attempts to adapt adenovirus as a gene transfer vehicle for various tissues *in vivo*.

BIOLOGY OF ADENOVIRUS

Adenovirus (Ad) genomes are linear, double-stranded DNA molecules about 36 kilobase pairs long. Each extremity of the viral genome has a short sequence, the inverted terminal repeat (ITR), which is necessary for viral replication. Adenoviruses commonly cause latent infection of lymphoid tissue, and are mainly associated with respiratory disease which can reach epidemic proportions in closed populations. Thus, a human vaccine consisting of live Ad types 4 and 7 (Ad 4 and 7) in enteric-coated capsules has been developped.

The genetic organization of the Ad 2 genome is schematized in Fig. 1, where the mRNAs are discriminated according to an early or late phase transcription. It is noteworthy that splicing plays a key role in the temporal expression of functionally similar proteins. Thus, the E1 region (E1A & E1B) encodes proteins responsible for the regulation of transcription of the viral genome and a few cellular genes (Nevins, 1987). A role for the protection of DNA sequences has also been attributed to some of the products of this region (Pilder et al., 1984; White et al., 1984; Lai & Mak, 1982). The expression of the E2 region (E2A & E2B) leads to the synthesis of viral replicative functions (a DNA-binding protein, a DNA polymerase, and a terminal protein which primes replication) (Kelly, 1984; Stillman, 1985). The products encoded by the E3 region prevent cytolysis by cytotoxic T cells and tumor necrosis factor (Wold & Gooding, 1989; Ginsberg et al., 1989). The functions associated with the E4 proteins are more diversified since they are involved in DNA replication, late gene expression, and host cell shutoff (Falgout & Ketner, 1987; Halbert et al., 1985; Weinberg & Ketner, 1986; Yoder & Berger, 1986; Sandler & Ketner, 1991). The products of the late genes, including the majority of virion capsid proteins, are expressed only after significant processing of a single primary transcript issued from the major late promoter (MLP) (Berget et al., 1977; Chow et al., 1977). The MLP (located at 16.8 map units (mu)) is particularly efficient during the late phase of infection, and all the mRNAs issued from this promoter possess a 5' tripartite leader sequence which makes them preferential messages for translation.

ADAPTATION OF ADENOVIRUS AS A CLONING VECTOR

The well-characterized molecular genetics of adenovirus, as well as its handy manipulation, render this virus an advantageous vector for gene transfer both in cell culture and in animals. Other criteria responsible for a growing interest in Ad follow :
(1) The knowledge of its genetic organization allows substitution of a large piece of viral DNA by foreign sequences.
(2) Recombinant adenoviruses are structurally stable and no rearranged virus can be observed after extensive amplification.
(3) This virus appears to be linked only to mild diseases since there is no known association of human malignancies with adenoviral infection. Moreover, no side effects have been reported following vaccination of U.S. recruits with wild-type adenovirus (Couch et al., 1963; Top et al., 1971), demonstrating its safety and efficacy for human use.

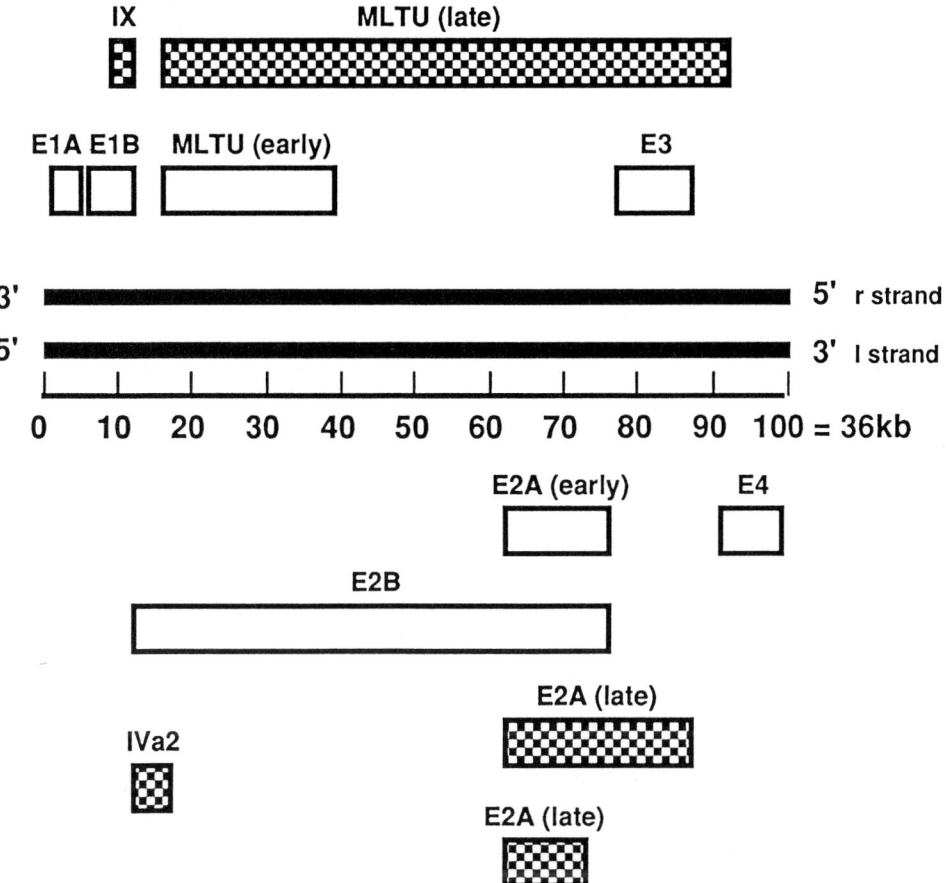

Fig.1. The adenovirus genome and its transcription units. The early transcription units (E1A, E1B, E2A, E2B, E3, E4, and MLTU early) are represented by white boxes, whereas the late ones (IX, IVa2, E2A, and MLTU late) are shown as checkered boxes. The promoter of the major late transcription unit (MLTU) is active both early and late after infection; however, only a subset of the MLTU genes is expressed during the early phase. The genes of the E2A transcription unit are also transcribed during the late phase, but from different promoters. The viral genome covers 36 kb and is divided into 100 map units.

STRATEGY FOR THE GENERATION OF RECOMBINANT ADENOVIRUSES

The cloning of foreign DNA sequences into adenovirus takes advantage of the dispensability of the E3 region for viral propagation in cell culture, (Kelly & Lewis, 1973; Jones & Shenk, 1978), and relies on 293 cells which express the viral products of the E1 region. The 293 cell line, obtained following transformation of primary human embryonic kidney cells by the E1 region of Ad 5, provides constitutively the E1 products (Graham et al., 1977). Consequently, an adenovirus deleted for both regions E1 and E3, will be able to carry up to 7 kb of foreign DNA, and can be grown to high titers in 293 cells.

In order to efficiently express the cloned foreign gene, we have made use of the major late promoter in association with the tripartite leader sequence to drive the transcription of the coding sequence. To this end, a cassette plasmid called pMLP-AdK7 was designed for the cloning of foreign genes downstream from the transcription-translation regulatory signals (MLP & tripartite leader) (Fig.2). Such a plasmid allows the construction of recombinant adenoviruses by homologous recombination between an enzyme-restricted adenovirus genome and the Ad sequences (9.4 - 17 mu) which flank the 3' end of the cloned gene (Fig. 3).

SYNTHESIS, PROCESSING, AND TRANSPORT OF PROTEINS

The dramatic impairment of replication of E1A-defective recombinant adenoviruses would undoubtedly carry over to gene expression; or would it ? This had yet to be proved. In an attempt to answer this important question, infection of various cell types was carried out with a recombinant adenovirus harboring a reporter gene. Thus, the hepatitis B virus (HBV) surface antigen (HBsAg) gene placed under the control of the MLP was cloned in the E1 region of adenovirus. Equivalent constructs retaining a functional E1A gene were used as controls in the experiment. The infection of a wide spectrum of cell lines showed an efficient synthesis of the reporter gene product, whatever the tissue or species origin of the cell line infected, and irrespective of the presence of the E1A products (Table 1). These results show that a high level of synthesis can be obtained even in the absence of efficient viral replication and transcription of early viral genes (Levrero et al., 1991).

Several recombinant adenoviruses harboring genes coding for protein necessitating various post-translational modifications for their activity were used to demonstrate if such alterations could effectively be obtained from polypeptides issued from adenoviral vectors. Infection of cells with the recombinant virus carrying the gene encoding the HBsAg led to an accumulation in the cell culture medium of spherical, 22nm particles of HBsAg with a buoyant density of 1.2. In contrast, after infection of cells with a recombinant adenovirus engineered to express the Epstein- Barr virus (EBV) membrane antigen gp340/gp220, the glycoproteins were found correctly inserted within the plasma membrane of the host cell. Additionally, both classes of proteins (HBsAg and gp340/gp220) were correctly glycosylated and appeared physically identical to the authentic products synthesized by HBV and EBV.

The process of proteolytic cleavage of peptides entails the precise folding of the substrate which thereby becomes active. The

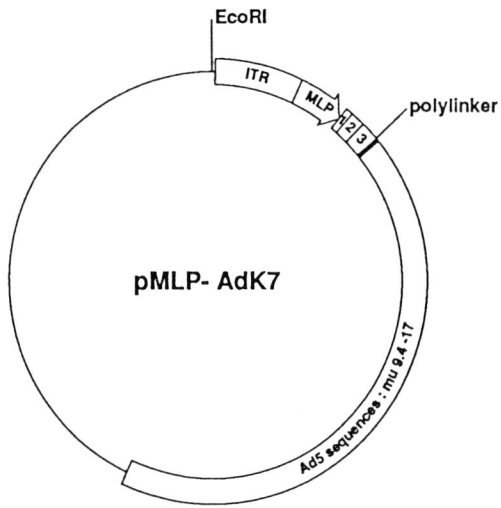

Fig.2. The pMLP-AdK7. This plasmid is a pML2 derivative containing several sequences from adenovirus permitting the construction of recombinant viral genomes carrying a foreign gene controlled by the MLP. Flanked by an EcoRI site and a polylinker are the following:
455bp of the very left-end of Ad5 which provide the ITR and the packaging sequences with the E1A enhancers; the MLP from the Ad2 genome followed by the tripartite leader sequence cloned from a cDNA. Downstream from the polylinker are inserted Ad5 sequences (mu 9.4-17) through which the plasmid can recombine with the Ad5 genome to generate the recombinant virus. The foreign gene inserted within the polylinker will contain the complete coding region through the polyadenylation site.

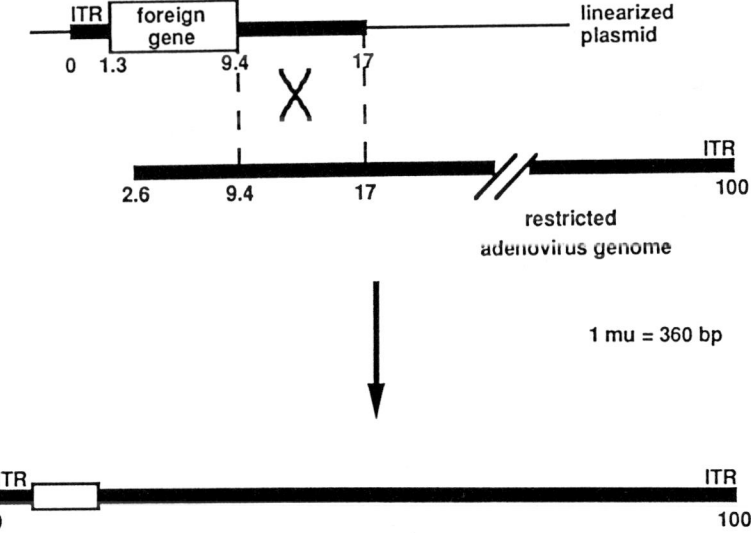

Fig.3. Generation of a recombinant adenovirus by in vivo recombination. Recombinant adenoviruses are constructed by replacing the internal E1 region of adenovirus by foreign sequences through a recombination process between the linearized plasmid and the restricted adenovirus genome.

biogenesis of ornithine transcarbamylase (OTC), a nuclear- coded mitochondrial protein, begins with the transport of a precursor protein into the mitochondrial matrix, followed by the cleavage of its leader peptide. The mature OTC subunits can then be assembled into enzymatically active homotrimers. Because the use of a recombinant adenovirus carrying the gene coding for OTC leads to the production of an active enzyme, it may be deduced that the OTC thus synthesized is a true replica of the cell-generated product. These types of observations demonstrate that post-translational modifications of proteins generated by recombinant adenoviruses occur faithfully.

GENE TRANSFER INTO ANIMALS

The efficiency with which recombinant adenoviruses in cell culture express the foreign gene they carry, even in the absence of the immediate early gene products E1A and E1B, prompted us to evaluate the efficacy of such a tool in animals.

Can the success of the in vitro gene transfer process be duplicated in animals? Can non-dividing cells be infected and express the gene? Is the yield of the foreign gene product important enough to induce an immune response, or better yet, to relieve an enzymatic deficiency, at least temporarily ? In an effort to assess the degree of effectiveness of replication-deficient adenoviruses, answers to these types of questions were sought.

A recombinant adenovirus which directs the synthesis of HBsAg in cell culture was first used to evaluate gene expression in animals. For this, rabbits were intravenously inoculated with highly purified preparations of recombinant adenovirus, and the expression of HBsAg was indirectly monitored by following the appearance of specific antibodies in the blood. Although no HBsAg particles could be detected in the sera following the inoculation, the ease with which antibodies could be assayed evidenced a substantial synthesis of HBsAg after the infection (Ballay et al., 1985). The elicitation of specific antibodies in inoculated rabbits provided the first line of evidence that a gene may be expressed in an animal on account of a recombinant adenovirus.

Although the production of specific antibodies clearly demonstrates that gene transfer can be obtained via the use of recombinant adenoviruses, it is important to show that gene transfer may be extended to DNA sequences encoding other than immunogenic proteins. Can Adenovirus be used to deliver directly to an organism an enzyme-encoding gene ? In search of the answer, different recombinant viruses were constructed and used to infect postnatal animals. With the purpose of delivering a specific gene to a particular tissue, we tried to preferentially infect either muscle, lung, or liver. Such specific targets would also serve to reveal any host restrictions associated with Adenovirus.

The intramuscular injection into mice of a β-galactosidase-encoding recombinant adenovirus, with the subsequent incubation of the tissue with X-gal chromagen, indicated an efficient infection of these cells and a substantial expression of the transduced β-galactosidase gene several days post-infection. The detection of stained myotubes clearly demonstrated the ability of a recombinant adenovirus to infect skeletal muscle cells. Importantly, it also

Table 1. Levels of expression of HBsAg after infection with the recombinant adenovirus. Cells were infected at a multiplicity of infection of 10 plaque-forming units per cell; supernatants were collected 120h post-infection, and tested for HBsAg reactivity as described (Ballay et al., 1985). Levels are given as ng HBsAg/10^6 cells.

ORIGIN	CELL LINE	AdS(E1A⁻)	AdS(E1A⁺)
HUMAN	293	6000	3900
	HeLa	1540	1150
	HepG2	1850	1430
	Raji	450	2150
	EBV lymphoblastoid	1050	1780
SIMIAN	VERO	11,600	5430
MOUSE	NIH3T3	850	780
	L	430	170
RABBIT	RK13	950	860
	537	480	250

indicates that adenovirus can transduce a gene directly into post-mitotic cells.

The recombinant adenovirus harboring the OTC gene was used to target expression in the liver of OTC-deficient mice (Stratford-Perricaudet et al., 1990). In this model, gene transfer is documented by measuring the enzymatic activity of one of the catalysts of the urea cycle. Some of the OTC-deficient mice inoculated with the virus exhibited an increased hepatic OTC activity as a result of the expression of the OTC gene carried by the virus. Another, albeit indirect, demonstration of the increased presence of OTC specifically in the liver was a substantial drop in orotic acid present in the urine of these mice. Indeed, one of the consequences of the OTC deficiency is the accumulation of carbamoyl phosphate which then saturates the pyrimidine biosynthetic pathway, thereby, yielding orotic acid. The existence of the OTC-deficient mouse offered an opportunity to begin to assess the feasibility of liver-directed genetic therapies. Partial correction of the metabolic consequences of the defect demonstrates successful adenoviral-mediated gene transfer into hepatic tissue in vivo.

Because adenovirus is trophic for the respiratory system we sought to exploit this natural route of infection to deliver a gene to the lung. A recombinant adenovirus expressing the gene for human α_1-antitrypsin (α_1-AT) was constructed (Gilardi et al., 1990) and used as a model to evaluate gene transfer to this organ specifically. After intratracheal instillation of the recombinant virus it was demonstrated that gene delivery was possible to the cotton rat respiratory epithelium in vivo (Rosenfeld et al., 1991).

DISCUSSION AND PERSPECTIVES

The adaptation of adenovirus as an expression vector for heterologous genes has provided an additional means to faithfully overproduce gene products in vitro. Because adenovirus is capable of infecting a wide variety of cell types in culture, it may prove realistic to use such a vector to target any organ in vivo. Thus far, we have found that adenovirus can deliver a gene in vivo to various tissues. It may be possible to circumscribe the infection simply by locally administering the recombinant viruses; however, further studies are necessary to determine the extent of dissemination of infection when chosen organs are aimed. In addition, thorough control of expression of transferred genes could be achieved through the use of tissue-specific regulatory elements.

Adenovirus vectors might constitute an interesting gene delivery vector for the airway cells of the lung. It has already been shown that adenoviral-mediated gene transfer to respiratory epithelium is possible. The delivery of therapeutic genes such as α_1-AT or cystic fibrosis might even be obtained by inhalation of recombinant adenoviruses in an aerosol. Use of a spray would prove advantageous due to the turnover of these cells and the subsequent need for repetitive delivery. Moreover, most of these airway epithelial cells proliferate only slowly, or not at all, making the use of retrovirus vectors (that require proliferation of the target cells for expression of the transduced gene) inappropriate.

The targeted expression in non-dividing cells is, on the whole, an objective which cannot be reached using retrovirus vectors. The transduction and expression of genes in neurons and striated muscles require development of new types of vectors. In this context, reported expression of β-galactosidase following injection of the recombinant adenovirus in muscle of mice is particularly noteworthy, and suggests that the transfer of genes responsible for neuromuscular diseases might be achieved this way.

Somatic gene therapy of specific deficiencies, like OTC deficiency, might be performed by intestine-targeted gene transfer (Jones et al., 1990). The use of adenovirus as a live vaccine delivered to man as an encapsulated form, has shown its capability to efficiently infect the intestinal epithelium without any side effects. This makes adenovirus a suitable vector for such gene transfer procedures.

If it proves appropriate to consider Adenovirus as a gene transfer vector for man, development of new adenovirus-based vectors, limiting the contribution of viral genes, will have to be undertaken. With this purpose in mind, construction of viruses harboring the foreign gene(s) bordered only by the ITRs, is now in progress in our laboratory. Further safety aspects will also need to be entertained before human trials can be envisaged.

REFERENCES

Ballay, A., Levrero, M., Buendia, M.A., Tiollais, P., & Perricaudet, M. (1985): In vitro and in vivo synthesis of the hepatitis B virus surface antigen and of the receptor for polymerized human serum albumin from recombinant human adenovirus. EMBO J. 4 : 3861-3865.

Berget, S.M., Moore C., & Sharp P. (1977): Spliced RNA segments at 5' terminus of adenovirus 2 late mRNA. Proc. Natl. Acad. Sci. USA 74 : 3171-3175.

Chow, L.T., Roberts, J.M., Lewis, J.B., & Broker T.R. (1977): A map of cytoplasmic RNA transcripts from lytic adenovirus type 2 determined by electron microscopy of RNA DNA hybrids. Cell 11: 819-836.

Couch, R.B., Chanock, R.M., Cate, T.R. Lang, D.J., Knight, V., & Huebner, R.J. (1963) : Immunization with types 4 and 7 adenovirus by selective infection of the intestinal tract. Am. Rev. Resp. Dis. 88 : 394-403.

Falgout, B. & Ketner, G. (1987) : Adenovirus early region 4 is required for efficient virus particle assembly. J. Virol. 61: 3759-3768.

Gilardi, P., Courtney, M., Pavirani, A., & Perricaudet, M. (1990) : Expression of human α 1-antitrypsin using a recombinant adenovirus vector. Febs Letters 267 : 60-62.

Ginsberg, H.S., Lundholm-Beauchamp, U., Horswood, R.L., Pernis B., Wold, W.S.M., Chanock, R.M., & Prince, G.A. (1989) : Role of early region 3 (E3) in pathogenesis of adenovirus disease. Proc. Natl. Acad. Sci. USA 86 : 3823-3827.

Graham, F.L., Smiley, J., Russell, W.C., & Nairn, R. (1977) : Characteristics of a human cell line transformed by DNA from human adenovirus 5. J. Gen. Virol. 36 : 59-72.

Halbert, D.N., Cutt, J.R., & Shenk, T. (1985) : Adenovirus early region 4 encodes functions required for efficient DNA replication, late gene expression and host cell shutoff. Virol. 56 : 250-257.

Jones, N. & Shenk, T. (1978) : Isolation of deletion and substitution mutants of adenovirus type 5. Cell 13 : 181-188.

Jones, S.N., Grompe, M., Munir, M.I., Veres, G., Craigen W.J., & Caskey, C.T. (1990). Ectopic correction of ornithine transcarbamylase deficiency in sparse fur mice. J. Biol. Chcm. 265 : 14684-14690.

Kelly, T.J. & Lewis, A.M.. (1973) : Use of non-defective adenovirus-simian virus 40 hybrids for mapping the SV40 genome. J. Virol. 12 : 643-652.

Kelly, Jr. T.J., (1984) : Adenovirus DNA replication. In The Adenovirus, ed. H.S. Ginsberg, pp. 271-308. New York : Plenum Press.

Lai Fatt, R.B. & Mak, S. (1982) : Mapping of an adenovirus function involved in the inhibition of DNA degradation. J. Virol. 42 : 969-977.

Levrero, M., Barban, V., Manteca, S., Ballay, A., Balsamo, C., Avantaggiati M.L., Natoli, G., Skellekens, H., Tiollais,P., & Perricaudet, M. (1991) : Defective and nondefective adenovirus vectors for expressing foreign genes in vitro and in vivo. Gene (in press).

Nevins, J.R. (1987) : Regulation of early adenovirus gene expression. Microbiol. Rev. 51 : 419-430.

Pilder, S., Logan, J., & Shenk, T. (1984) : Deletion of the gene encoding the adenovirus 5 early region 1B 21,000-molecular-weight polypeptide leads to degradation of viral and host cell DNA. J. Virol. 52 : 664-671.

Rosenfeld, M.A., Siegfried, W., Yoshimura, K., Stier, L.E., Paavo, P.K., Stratford-Perricaudet, L.D., Perricaudet, M., Jallat, S., Pavirani, A., Lecocq, J.-P., & Crystal, R.G. (1991) : In vivo transfer of a functional human α_1-antitrypsin cDNA directly to the respiratory epithelium with a recombinant adenovirus vector. Science (in press).

Sandler, A.B. & Ketner, G. (1991). The metabolism of host RNAs in cells infected by an adenovirus E4 mutant. Virology 181: 319-326.

Stillman, B.W. (1985) : Biochemical and genetic analysis of adenovirus DNA replication in vitro. In <u>Genetic Engineering: Principles and Methods</u>, ed. J.K. Setlow & A. Hollaender, pp. 1-27. New York : Plenum Press.

Stratford-Perricaudet, L.D., Levrero, M., Chasse, J.F., Perricaudet, M., & Briand, P. (1990) : Evaluation of the transfer and expression in mice of an enzyme-encoding gene using a human adenovirus vector. Human Gene Therapy 1 : 241-256.

Top, F.H., Jr., Buescher, E.L., Bancroft, W.H., & Russell, P.K. (1971) : Immunization with live types 7 and 4 adenovirus vaccines. II. Antibody response and protective effect against acute respiratory disease due to adenovirus type 7. J. Infect. Dis. 124 : 155-160.

Weinberg, D.H. & Ketner, G. (1986) : Adenoviral early region 4 is required for efficient viral DNA replication and for late gene expression. J. Virol. 57 : 833-838.

White, E., Grodzicker, T., & Stillman, B.W. (1984) : Mutations in the gene encoding the adenovirus early region 1B 19,000-molecular-weight tumor antigen cause the degradation of chromosomal DNA. J. Virol. 52 : 410-419.

Wold, W.S.M. & Gooding, L.R. (1989) : Adenovirus region E3 proteins that prevent cytolysis by cytotoxic T cells and tumor necrosis factor. Mol. Biol. Med. 6 : 433-452.

Yoder, S.S. & Berget, S.M. (1986) : Role of adenovirus type 2 early region 4 in the early-to-late switch during productive infection. J. Virol. 60 : 779-781.

RESUME : L'adénovirus a été évalué comme un nouveau moyen de délivrer des gènes avec un développement possible vers la thérapie génique. La capacité de ce virus à contenir un large fragment d'ADN et à exprimer un gène en l'absence à la fois de réplication virale et de divisions cellulaires font de celui-ci un système de transfert génétique séduisant. Il pourrait, en particulier, constituer une alternative efficace lorsque les cellules cibles du transfert ne sont pas accessibles aux rétrovirus. De plus, le tropisme naturel des adénovirus pour l'épithélium respiratoire conduit à élaborer une stratégie de traitement pour la mucoviscidose (ou fibrose kystique du pancréas), maladie génétique d'importance.

The use of HSV-1 vectors to introduce heterologous genes into neurons : implications for gene therapy

A.I. Geller [1]* and H.J. Federoff [2]

[1] *Division of Cell Growth and Regulation, D8110A Dana Farber Cancer Institute, 44 Binney Street, Boston, MA 02115, USA;* [2] *Department of Medicine, Albert Einstein College of Medicine, Bronx, NY 10461, USA*

*Author for correspondence

We have recently developed a defective Herpes Simplex Virus One (HSV-1) vector system that provides a method to deliver heterologous genes into cells of the nervous system, including post-mitotic neurons (Geller and Breakefield, 1988; Geller and Freese 1990; Freese et. al., 1990). As described in this paper, HSV-1 vectors can be used to introduce genes into neurons in culture and in the adult mammalian brain. The potential applications of this gene transfer methodology are numerous; ranging from the study of gene product function within neurons to the modification of neuronal physiology, *in situ*, in the normal and pathologic central nervous system (CNS). The molecular biology of defective HSV-1 vectors, their utilization for the manipulation of gene expression in neurons, and their potential applications for human gene therapy are the focus of this paper.

The life cycle of wild type HSV-1.

To fully appreciate the characterisitics of HSV-1 vectors, a discussion of the HSV-1 life cycle is beneficial. The genome of HSV-1 is a linear molecule of 150 kb of double stranded DNA which encodes about 75 genes. An HSV-1 virus particle is a layered structure which consists of (from the inside out) DNA, an icosohedral protein capsid, a protein layer named the tegument, and a lipid bilayer obtained from the nuclear membrane of an infected cell, viral encoded glycoproteins are embedded in this membrane (Spear and Roizman, 1981). These glycoproteins mediate a fusion event between the lipid bilayer of the virus and the plasma membrane of the newly infected cell, delivering the remainder of the virus particle into the cytoplasm. While the details of this fusion event have not been elucidated, its generality may account for the wide host range of HSV-1. Once inside the cell, the HSV-1 DNA finds its way to the nucleus where its genes are transcribed in a regulated cascade (Spear and Roizman, 1981). The five immediate early (IE) genes, encoding the major viral regulatory proteins, are expressed initially. The IE proteins turn-on the expression of the early genes which encode the DNA replication machinery. The late genes are expressed after DNA replication; these gene encode most of the components of the virus particle and the enzymes which assemble the particle.

When wt HSV-1 infects neurons, a presumed molecular switch is activated early in the life cycle which permits HSV-1 to enter a latent state (Stevens, 1975). Once in the latent state, the lytic cycle is repressed such that the virus persists indefinitely in the neuron in a benign state. The precise molecular mechanism of the lytic--latency switch is not well understood (Stevens et. al., 1987; Deatly et. al., 1987). Injection of wt HSV-1 into the brain causes a lytic infection, resulting in the production of progeny virus, thereby spreading the infection throughout the brain and subsequently killing the animal.

In contrast, intracerebral injection of certain temperature sensitive (ts) mutants results in a latent infection (Watson et. al., 1980). The mutant protein is functional at 31 $^\circ$C, but not at body temperature, 37 to 39 $^\circ$C. Thus, the lytic cycle can operate in tissue culture at 31 $^\circ$C but not *in vivo* at 37 $^\circ$C. By choosing an appropriate ts mutant which blocks the lytic cycle at the IE stage, it is possible to infect cells with HSV-1 at 37 $^\circ$C and not produce cell damage. Furthermore, since these ts mutants do not grow *in vivo*, the infection is limited to cells around the injection site and neurons which project to the injection site; the infection does not spread throughout the brain (Watson et. al., 1980).

Deletion mutants (DeLuca et. al., 1985; Patterson and Everett, 1990), which contain a deletion in an essential gene of HSV-1 such as the IE3 gene, are similarly unable to produce a lytic infection except in a complementing cell line. The IE3 gene is the major regulatory gene of HSV-1; deletion mutants in the IE3 gene express the four other IE genes and perhaps one or two early genes but they do not replicate their DNA or produce progeny virus (DeLuca et. al., 1985). The deletion mutant is grown in a cell line which contains the deleted gene integrated into the cell's genome (DeLuca et. al., 1985; Patterson and Everett, 1990). In a subsequent section we describe the use of ts and deletion mutants as components of the packaging system used to produce defective HSV-1 virus. Because deletion mutants essentially do not revert, they may be useful for packaging defective virus that will be used for human gene therapy studies.

HSV-1 AS A VECTOR FOR GENE TRANSFER.

Gene delivery directly into post-mitotic cells, by transfection with naked DNA or infection with retroviral vectors, has not yet been obtained. However, a vector system based on HSV-1 is well suited for gene transfer into neurons (Freese et. al., 1990). HSV-1 has a number of advantages (Spear and Roizman 1981): 1) HSV-1 can infect post-mitotic neurons in adult animals or in culture; 2) HSV-1 can infect many different cell types such as fibroblasts, macrophages, glia, and neurons in many different organisms, including humans, non-human primates, rodents, and birds; 3) HSV-1 can be maintained indefinitely in neurons in a latent state (Stevens, 1975); 4) While in the latent state, expression of viral genes is limited to a latency associated transcript(s) and perhaps some IE genes (Stevens et. al., 1987; Deatly et. al., 1987) and thus, DNA replication and the production of viral progeny does not occur; 5) viral genes are transcribed by the cellular RNA polymerase II (Spear and Roizman, 1981), suggesting that cellular promoters in HSV-1 vectors could be appropriately regulated, and; 6) The 150 kb genome of HSV-1 suggests that HSV-1 vectors could be constructed to accommodate large genes.

THE PROTOTYPE DEFECTIVE HSV-1 VECTOR.

A defective HSV-1 vector (Geller and Breakefield, 1988; Geller and Freese, 1990; Fig. 1) contains a transcription unit composed of a promoter, a gene and processing elements. Second, it contains two HSV-1 sequences that support propagation of the vector in a virus stock. Third, it possesses bacterial plasmid sequences that support growth in *E. coli*. Our prototype vector, pHSVlac, places the *E. coli Lac Z* gene under the control of the HSV-1 IE

4/5 promoter, a constitutive promoter that functions in many cell types. The *Lac Z* gene encodes a bacterial ß-galactosidase absent from mammalian cells, and by using convenient assays its expression can be readily detected in infected cells.

The experimental procedure for using HSV-1 vectors (Geller et. al., 1990) is shown in Fig. 2. The vector is constructed in *E. coli* employing standard molecular biological techniques. Vector DNA is then packaged into HSV-1 particles (Geller, 1988): vector DNA is transfected by calcium phosphate coprecipitation into M64A cells (carrying an integrated copy of the HSV-1 IE3 gene; Patterson and Everett, 1990) and the cells are subsequently

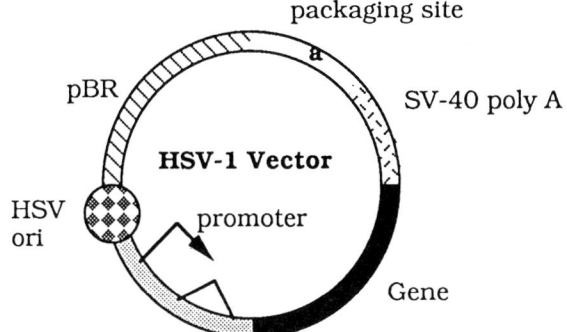

Fig. 1. The structure of a prototype defective HSV-1 vector (Freese et. al., 1990). The vector contains three kinds of genetic elements. **1.** Two sequences required for growth of the vector in a HSV-1 virus stock: A HSV-1 origin of DNA replication ori_s (circle filled with diamonds) supports replication of vector DNA. The HSV-1 **a** sequence (clear segment) contains the packaging site, responsible for subsequently packaging vector DNA into HSV-1 particles. **2.** A transcription unit in the vector is composed of the HSV-1 IE 4/5 promoter (arrow), the intervening sequence following that promoter (triangle), a gene (black segment), and the SV-40 early region polyadenylation site (dotted segment). **3.** pBR322 sequences (diagonal line segment) support growth in *E. coli*.

superinfected with the HSV-1 strain 17 D30EBA, carrying a deletion in IE3 gene (Patterson and Everett, 1990). The cells are then incubated and the resulting virus stock is used for expression experiments. Transformed cell lines or normal cells in primary culture are infected with virus containing the vector and incubated; after an appropriate period of time, expression is analyzed. To infect a group of neurons *in vivo*, virus is delivered directly into the brain of adult animals by stereotactic injection.

pHSVlac STABLY EXPRESSES ß-GALACTOSIDASE IN NEURAL CELL LINES, CULTURED NEURONS, AND IN THE ADULT RAT BRAIN.

In a series of studies with pHSVlac virus, we have demonstrated the potential of using defective HSV-1 vectors for delivery of genes into dividing neural cell lines, post-mitotic neurons in primary culture, and neurons in the adult rat brain. With our protocol, cells in culture are infected with pHSVlac virus, and one day later expression of the *Lac Z* gene product is detected using an *in situ* enzymatic assay employing the chromogenic substrate 5-bromo-4-chloro-3-indolyl-ß-D-galactoside (X-Gal). We have observed expression of ß-galactosidase in a number of dividing neural cell lines, including N1E-115 mouse adrenergic neuroblastomas, NS-20Y mouse cholinergic neuroblastomas, PC12 rat pheochromocytomas, AtT-20 mouse pituicytes, GH4 rat pituicytes, SK-N-BE (2) human neuroblastomas and Hs 683 human glioma (Geller, 1991). Furthermore, the expression of ß-galactosidase was observed one day after infection with pHSVlac in two differentiated neural cell lines: PC12 cells treated with NGF, and N1E-115 cells treated with dibutyryl cAMP (Geller, 1991).

The expression of ß-galactosidase from pHSVlac was also observed in primary cultured neurons from many regions of the nervous system. When peripheral neurons from superior cervical ganglia and dorsal root ganglia were infected with pHSVlac virus, those expressing ß-galactosidase were identified by X-GAL staining, as shown in Fig. 3 (Geller and Breakefield, 1988). Infection of cultured neurons from different CNS regions also resulted in ß-galacotosidase expression. In these cultures, ß-galacotosidase expression was detected by a double immunofluorescent assay: ß-galactosidase immunoreactivity was detected using a rabbit anti-*E. coli* ß-galactosidase antibody; neurofilament immunoreactivity was detected using a mouse anti-neurofilament antibody. Using this assay, expression of ß-galactosidase, one day after pHSVlac infection, was shown

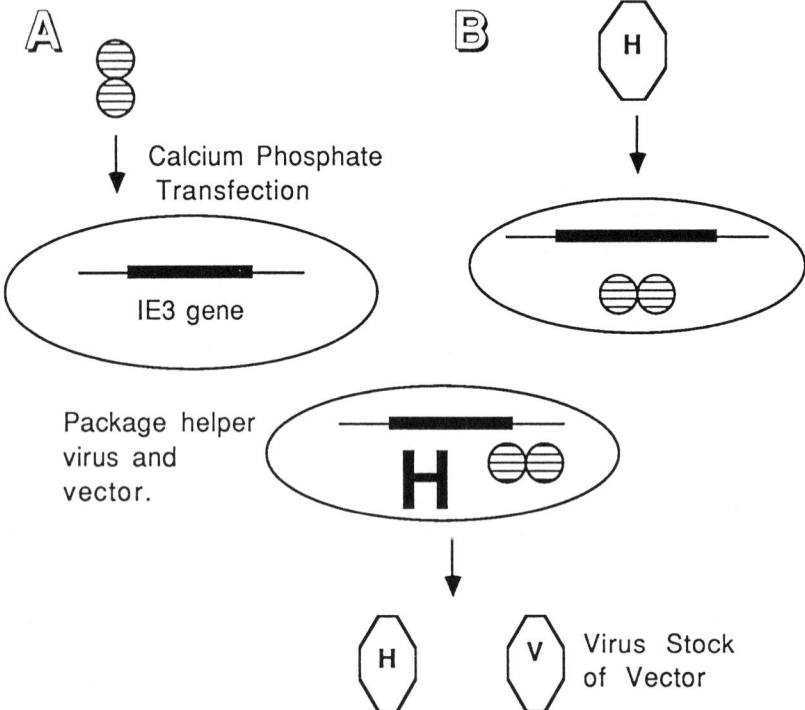

Fig. 2. Diagram of the experimental procedure with defective HSV-1 vectors (Geller et. al., 1990). **A.** To package vector DNA into HSV-1 particles (Geller, 1988) M64A cells (Patterson and Everett, 1990) are transfected with vector DNA using the calcium phosphate procedure (Graham and Van der Eb, 1973). **B.** The cells are superinfected with helper virus, a deletion mutant of HSV-1, D30EBA (Patterson and Everett, 1990); the cells are then incubated. **C.** The resulting virus stock contains identical HSV-1 particles, containing either the vector DNA or the DNA of the helper virus. Virus containing the vector can then be used to infect cells and stably express a gene (Freese et. al., 1990). Cells can be infected in culture, including immortalized cell lines or primary cultures of normal cells such as neurons. Alternatively, virus can be delivered into an animal; for example, neurons in the adult rat brain are infected following stereotactic injection of virus into the desired site.

in cultured neurons from spinal cord, cerebellum, thalamus, striatum, hippocampus, occipital cortex, temporal cortex, and frontal cortex (Geller and Freese, 1990).

To demonstrate that pHSVlac DNA persisted in neurons and stably expressed ß-galactosidase, we infected cultured neurons from sensory ganglia, striatum, total neocortex, and hippocampus with pHSVlac virus, and maintained the infected cultures for at least two weeks. pHSVlac DNA persisted in these cells for at least two weeks and could be recovered following superinfection with HSV-1. Furthermore, pHSVlac was stably maintained within the cells that were originally infected, and was not transmitted horizontally to other cells. Expression of ß-galactosidase was demonstrated up to two

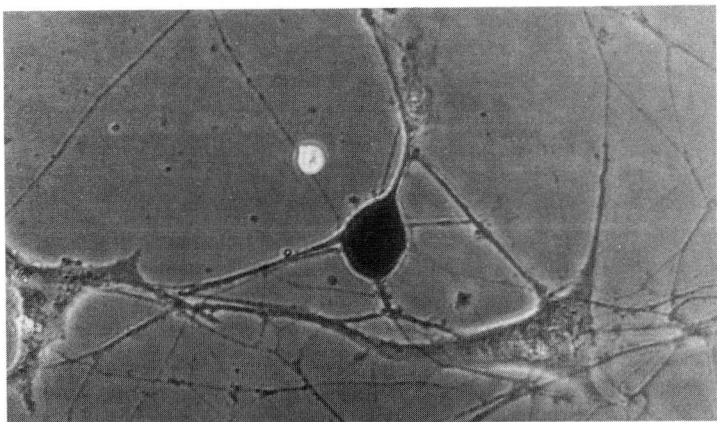

Fig. 3. Expression of ß-galactosidase from pHSVlac in cultured dorsal root ganglia cells. Virus containing pHSVlac was prepared (Geller, 1988) using HSV-1 strain 17 ts K as helper virus (Geller and Breakefield, 1988). The titer was 1×10^6 plaque forming units (pfu) of ts K /ml and 8×10^5 infectious particles of pHSVlac /ml. Cultures prepared from newborn rat dorsal root ganglia were treated with 10^{-5}M cytosine arabinoside for 1 day. On day 10 cultures contained 3 to 8×10^5 cells per 35-mm plate; cultures were then infected with 0.1 ml pHSVlac, incubated for 1 day, and ß-galactosidase enzyme was detected with X-gal (Geller and Breakefield, 1988). The width of the photomicrograph represents 230 microns.

weeks following pHSVlac infection of the cultures (Geller and Breakefield, 1988; Geller and Freese, 1990). Several *in vivo* experiments demonstrated that, following stereotactic injection of pHSVlac virus into the brain of adult rats, ß-galactosidase was expressed in neurons surrounding the injection site (hippocampus, occipital cortex, and superior colliculus), as well as in distant neurons whose axons project to the injection site (Sabel et. al., 1989). Expression was maintained for at least 6 weeks, suggesting that pHSVlac could escape immune surveillance and be retained in a transcriptionally active state. In contrast to wt HSV-1, pHSVlac did not spread throughout the brain, indicating that the production of pHSVlac virus did not occur.

In summary, pHSVlac can infect and stably express a heterologous gene in many different types of neurons, both *in vitro* and *in vivo*. These results suggest that HSV-1 vectors might be used to perform gene therapy. To illustrate how HSV-1 vectors may be designed for a particular application, we will first discuss the components of the vector system that are amenable to experimental control.

DESIGNING DEFECTIVE HSV-1 VECTORS: PARAMETERS SUBJECT TO EXPERIMENTAL MANIPULATION.

In designing HSV-1 vector experiments, one should consider the three variables subject to manipulation (Freese et. al., 1990). These are first, the number and location of the cells infected; second, the promoter used in the vector; and third, the gene expressed by the vector. The location of the cells infected is determined by several factors including the site of injection; the location of neurons which project to the injection site; the number of virus particles in the inoculum; and the extent of diffusion of the virus in the extracellular space before infection. Thus, one can control which cells are infected by choosing the site of injection and the number of virus particles injected. The promoter used in the vector is the second variable subject to experimental control. pHSVlac contains the HSV-1 IE 4/5 promoter, a constitutive promoter which functions in most cell types. However, replacement of the IE 4/5 promoter with tissue specific promoters will allow one to restrict expression of a gene in the vector to a chosen cell type. For example, the human neurofilament L promoter (Julien et. al.,1987) can restrict expression to neurons (Federoff et. al.,1990). The gene expressed by the vector is the third variable amenable to experimental manipulation. The *Lac Z* gene in pHSVlac may be replaced with virtually any gene. For example, one could use a gene encoding a secreted product such as a growth factor or a peptide hormone. Alternatively, one could use a gene encoding an enzyme or a receptor.

In summary, there are three variables which can be manipulated when using HSV-1 vectors *in vivo*. First, the injection site determines which cells are infected. Second, the promoter determines in which of the infected cells the gene is expressed. Third, the gene that is expressed will modify cellular, and perhaps the organism's physiology, in a predictable fashion.

ADVANTAGES OF HSV-1 VECTORS FOR GENE TRANSFER INTO NEURONS.

Prior to the development of defective HSV-1 vectors, several approaches were used to deliver genes into cells, but none are effective with post-mitotic cells. The low efficiency of DNA-mediated gene transfer and problems surrounding microinjection into somatic cells make these approaches impractical for gene transfer into primary cells or to cells *in vivo*. Retrovirus vectors (Mann et al., 1983)) are more useful for expressing genes in primary cells because gene transfer is efficient. Retroviral vectors possess both selectable genes and convenient restriction sites for insertion of heterologous genes, pose little biological hazard, and have a broad host cell range. However, retroviruses require at least one mitotic cycle for proviral genome integration and stable expression; consequently, retrovirus vectors are ineffective for gene transfer into post-mitotic neurons. The production of transgenic mice, has been used to study gene regulation, to elucidate oncogene function, to ablate a cell type during development, and to correct genetic disorders (Palmiter and Brinster, 1985). This approach has provided much useful information; however, transgenic mice result in delivery of a foreign gene into every cell in the organism. Although the use of a cell-type specific promoter has made it possible to target gene expression to all cells capable of using that promoter, the transgenic technology does not permit the investigator to achieve a regional localization of gene product expression that is desirable for many experiments. Moreover, transgenic methods can not be applied in a "therapeutic" manner to correct a gene defect in an already affected individual animal.

POTENTIAL APPLICATION OF HSV-1 VECTORS FOR GENE THERAPY.

Altering the physiologic response to axotomy: Using HSV-1 vectors to express neurotrophic factors.

Modification of neuronal physiology by the expression of recombinant neurotrophic factor genes from HSV-1 vectors may provide a powerful new approach to understanding the actions of neurotrophic factors in the intact nervous system and explore their potential for ameliorating the sequelae secondary to nerve injury. Because neurotrophic factors are secreted proteins, their action is not limited to the cells that synthesize the factor. Thus, the expression of a neurotrophic factor gene from a HSV-1 vector should result in an effect on a greater number of cells than the number of infected cells. Each member of the family of neurotrophic factors that includes the well studied nerve growth factor (NGF; Thoenen et al.,1987), brain derived neurotrophic factor (BDNF; Lindsay et al.,1985; Hofer and Barde, 1988) and neurotrophin 3 (NT-3; Hohn et al.,1990; Rosenthal et al., 1990), promote the survival of particular types of developing neurons (reviews: Snider and Johnson, 1989; Barde, 1989). In the adult CNS, a trophic role for NGF has been demonstrated for the group of ascending basal forebrain cholinergic neurons that synapse on NGF-producing hippocampal neurons. When these cholinergic neurons are disconnected from their NGF-producing target cells by axotomy, they degenerate and their content of choline acetyltransferase (ChAT) decreases (Gage et. al., 1986; Kromer, 1987). Restoration of the number of ChAT positive neurons by the administration of exogenous NGF (Gage et. al., 1986; Kromer, 1987) or the transplantation of fibroblasts genetically engineered to secrete NGF (Rosenberg et. al., 1988) indicate that augmented NGF supply to axotomized neurons has potential pharmacologic benefit. Therefore, the ability to increase the neurotrophic factor supply to damaged neurons by the expression of a neurotrophic factor gene from a HSV-1 vector may be a means to ameliorate the sequelae of neuronal injury.

For example, consider a HSV-1 vector in which a NGF cDNA is placed under the control of the IE 4/5 promoter. Injection of this virus into the basal forebrain region of rats that had undergone fimbria-fornix transection is expected to result in a local increase in NGF production. The restoration of ChAT content in basal forebrain cholinergic neurons would be evidence of a "therapeutic" effect. In a similar manner, one can consider the design and use of HSV-1 vectors to express other neurotrophic factors such as NT-3 and BDNF. Through the use of these vectors it should be possible to determine whether neuron function and/or survival following CNS injury can be improved.

Using HSV-1 vectors to alter the production of dopamine in neurons: Relevance to Parkinson's Disease.

Parkinson's disease is a neurodegenerative disorder that results from the death of dopaminergic neurons in the substantia nigra and the consequent depletion of dopamine within the corpus striatum, a post-synaptic target of substantia nigral neurons (Yahr and Bergmann, 1987). The therapeutic approaches used for Parkinson's disease have focused on the repletion of dopamine levels in the striatum. Clinical and basic research efforts have used precursor loading (L-DOPA; Cotzias et. al., 1967; Yahr et. al., 1969; Rossor et. al., 1980; Martin, 1971), dopamine agonists (such as bromocryptine), tissue transplants (fetal or autologous adrenal chromaffin; Freed et. al., 1987; Lindvall et. al., 1987), and implantable dopamine delivery systems (either polymeric or pump systems), with varying degrees of success (Yahr and Bergmann, 1987). Ideally, the reconstitution of dopamine biosynthesis might be achieved by gene therapy. Given that tyrosine hydroxylase is the rate limiting enzyme in dopamine biosynthesis, expression of the tyrosine hydroxylase gene (O'Malley et al., 1987) within neurons in, or projecting to, the striatum might increase striatal dopamine levels. Moreover, gene therapy for Parkinson's disease would not require the use of human fetal tissue.

To explore the possibility of treating Parkinson's disease with recombinant HSV-1 vectors, the human tyrosine hydroxylase gene was inserted into a HSV-1 vector, termed pHSVth. pHSVth causes the production and regulated release of dopa and dopamine from cultured striatal neurons. Infection of neurons in or projecting to the striatum with such a vector might cause an increased localized conversion of tyrosine to L-DOPA, with a consequent increase in dopamine levels in the striatum. Two well established animal models for Parkinson's disease could be used to test this approach; both models are produced by administration of a neurotoxin. Injection of 6-OH-dopamine directly into the substantia nigra of rats results in destruction of dopaminergic neurons which project to the striatum, eliciting a sterotypical rotational behavior. Alternatively, administration of MPTP to primates results in a Parkinsonian syndrome, that is characterized biochemically by dopamine depletion in the nigrostriatal system (Yahr and Bergmann, 1987). Both of these animal models provide a behavioral test to assess recovery of dopaminergic function following 'therapy" with pHSVth virus.

An initial attempt at gene therapy of Parkinson's disease has been reported: The tyrosine hydroxylase gene was transfected into fibroblasts, which in turn were transplanted adjacent to the striatum in animal models. Partial biochemical recovery of dopaminergic function was observed (Horellou et. al., 1990; Uchida et. al., 1990; Wolff et. al., 1989).

SUMMARY AND IMPLICATIONS.

The development of the defective HSV-1 methodology for introducing genes into neurons *in vitro* and *in vivo* has a number of important implications. Virtually any gene can be inserted into a defective HSV-1 vector, including those encoding gene products missing or mutated in neurodegenerative diseases. This methodology makes it possible to deliver a gene to a localized brain region, and by employing particular *cis-* acting genetic elements, the expression of the gene can be restricted to a specific cell type, thus adding a critical level of control. Ongoing experiments in basic neurobiology and applied neurology are exploring the power and general utility of this methodology.

Acknowledgements: A.I.G. was supported by Alkermes Inc, and the American Health Assistance Foundation; H.J.F. was supported by N.I.H. grant HD 27226.

References

Barde, Y. (1989) Trophic factors and neuronal survival. Neuron 2: 1525-1534.
Cotzias, G.C., Van Woert, M.H., Schiffer, L.M. (1967) Aromatic amino acids and modification of parkinsonism. N. Engl. J. Med. 276: 374-379.
Deatly, A.M., Spivack, J.G., Lavi, E., and Fraser, N.W. (1987) RNA from an immediate early region of the type 1 herpes simplex virus genome is present in the trigeminal ganglia of latently infected mice. Proc. Natl. Acad. Sci. USA 84: 3204-3208.

DeLuca, N.A., McCarthy, A.M., and Schaeffer, P.A. (1985) Isolation and characterization of deletion mutants of herpes simplex virus type 1 in the gene encoding immediate-early regulatory protein ICP4. J. Virol. 56: 558-570.

Federoff, H.J., Geller, A.I., and Lu, B. (1990) Neuronal specific expression of the human neurofilament L promoter in a HSV-1 vector. Abs. Soc. Neurosci. 16: 154.2.

Freed, W.J., Perlow, M.J., Karoum, F., Seiger, A., Olson, L., Hoffer, B.J., and Wyatt, R.J. (1987) Restoration of dopaminergic function by grafting of fetal rat substantia nigra to the caudate nucleus: long-term behavioral, biochemical, and histochemical studies. Ann. Neurol. 8: 510-519.

Freese, A., Geller, A. I., and Neve, R. (1990) HSV-1 vector mediated neuronal gene delivery: Strategies for molecular neuroscience and neurology. Biochem. Pharm. 40: 2189-2199.

Gage, F. H., K. Wictorin, W. Fischer, L. R. Williams, S. Varon and A. Bjorklund. (1986) Life and death of cholinergic neurons: in the septal and diagonal band region following complete fimbria fornix transection. Neurosci. 19: 241-256.

Geller, A.I. (1988) A new method to propagate defective HSV-1 vectors. Nucleic Acids Res. 16: 5690.

Geller, A.I., and Breakefield, X.O. (1988): A defective HSV-1 vector expresses Escherichia coli ß-galactosidase in cultured peripheral neurons. Science 241: 1667-1669.

Geller, A.I. and Freese, A. (1990) Infection of cultured central nervous system neurons with a defective herpes simplex virus 1 vector results in stable expression of Escherichia coli ß-Galactosidase. Proc. Natl. Acad. Sci. USA 87: 1149-1153.

Geller, A.I., Keyomarski, K., Bryan, J., and Pardee, A.B. (1990) An efficient deletion mutant packaging system for defective HSV-1 vectors; potential applications to neuronal physiology and human gene therapy. Proc. Natl. Acad. Sci. USA. 87: 8950-8954.

Geller, A.I., Freese, A., During, M.J., and O'Malley, K. (1990a) Expression of the human tyrosine hydroxylase gene in cultured fibroblasts and striatal neurons from a HSV-1 vector; possible gene therapy for Parkinson's Disease. J. Cell Biol. 111: 339a.

Geller, A.I. (1991) A system, using neural cell lines, to characterize HSV-1 vectors containing genes which effect neuronal physiology, or neuronal promoters. J. Neurosci. Methods 36: 91-103.

Graham, F.L., and Van der Eb, A.J. (1973) A new technique for the assay of human adenovirus DNA. Virol. 52: 456-467.

Hofer, M.M. and Barde, Y. (1988) Brain-derived neurotrophic factor prevents neuronal death in vivo. Nature 331: 261-262.

Hohn, A., Leibrock, J., Bailey K., and Barde, Y. (1990) Identification and characterization of a novel member of the nerve growth factor/brain-derived neurotrophic factor family. Nature 344: 339-341.

Horellou, P., Brundin, P., Kalen, P., Mallet, J., and Bjorklund, A. (1990) In vivo release of Dopa and dopamine from genetically engineered cells grafted to the denervated rat striatum. Neuron 5: 393-402.

Julien, J.P., Tretjakoff, I. Beaudet, L., and Peterson, A. (1987) Expression and assembly of a human neurofilament protein in transgenic mice provide a novel neuronal marking system. Genes and Dev. 1: 1085-1095.

Kromer, L.F. (1987) Nerve growth factor treatment after brain injury prevents neuronal death. Science 235: 214-217.

Lindsay, R.M., Thoenen, H. and Barde, Y. (1985) Placode and neural crest-derived sensory neurons are responsive at early developmental stages to brain-derived neurotrophic factor. Dev. Biol. 112: 319-328.

Lindvall, O., Backlund, E.O., Farde, L, Sedvall, G., Freedman, R., Hoffer, B., Nobin, N.,

Seiger, A., and Olson, L. (1987) Transplantation in Parkinson's disease: two cases of adrenal medullary grafts to the putamen. Ann. Neurol. 22: 457-468.

Mann, R., Mulligan, R.L., and Baltimore, D. (1983) Construction of retrovirus packaging mutant and its use to produce helper-free defective retrovirus. Cell 33: 153-159.

O'Malley, K.L., Anhalt, M.J., Martin, B.M., Kelsoe, J.R., Winfield, S.L., and Ginns, E.I. (1987) Isolation and characterization of the human tyrosine hydroxylase gene: Identification of 5' alternative splice sites responsible for multiple mRNAs. Biochemistry 26: 6910-6914.

Martin, W.E. (1971) Adverse reactions during treatment of Parkinson's disease with levodopa. J.A.M.A. 216: 1979-1983.

Palmiter, R.D., and Brinster, R. (1985) Transgenic Mice. Cell 41: 343-345.

Paterson, T., and Everett, R.D. (1990) A prominent sereine-rich region in Vmw175, the major transcriptional regulator protein of herpes simplex virus type 1, is not essential for virus growth in tissue culture. J. Gen. Virol. 71: 1775-1783.

Rosenberg, M.B., Friedmann, T., Robertson, R.C., Tuszynski, M., Wolff, J.A., Breakefield, X.O., and Gage, F.H. (1988) Grafting genetically modified cells to the damaged brain: restorative effects of NGF expression. Science 242: 1575-1578.

Rosenthal, A., Goeddel, D.V., Nguyen, T., Lewis, M., Shih, A., Laramee, G.R., Nikolics K., and Winslow, J.W. (1990) Primary structure and biological activity of a novel human neurotrophic factor. Neuron 4: 767-773.

Rossor, M.N., Watkins, J., Brown, M.J., Reid, J.L., and Dollery, C.T. (1980) Plasma levadopa, dopamine and therapeutic response following levadopa therapy of parkinsonian patients. J. Neurol. Sci. 46: 385-392.

Sabel, B., Martin, C., Waldmann, C., Freese, A., and Geller, A. I. (1989) Gene transfer into neurons of the adult rat brain. Abs. Soc. Neurosci. 15: 8.4.

Snider, W. D. and E. M. Johnson. (1989) Neurotrophic molecules. Ann. Neurol. 26: 489-506.

Spear, P.G., and Roizman, B. (1981) Herpes Simplex Viruses. In DNA Tumor Viruses, ed. J. Tooze, pp. 615-746. N.Y.: Cold Spring Harbor Labs.

Stevens, J.G. (1975) Latent herpes simplex virus and the nervous system. Curr. Top. Microbiol. Immunol. 70: 31-50.

Stevens, J.G., Wagner, E.K., Devi-Rao, G.B., Cook, M.L., and Feldman, L.T. (1987) RNA complementary to a herpesvirus alpha gene mRNA is prominent in latently infected neurons. Science 235: 1056-1059.

Thoenen, H., Bandtlow, C. and Heuman, R. (1987) The physiological function of nerve growth factor in the central nervous system: comparison with the periphery. Rev. Physiol. Biochem. Pharmacol. 109: 146-178.

Uchida, K., Ishii, A., Kaneda, N., Toya, S., Nagatsu, T., and Kohsaka, S. (1990) Tetrahydrobiopterin-dependent production of L-dopa in NRK fibroblasts transfected with tyrosine hydroxylase cDNA:future use for intracerebral grafting. Neurosci. Lett. 109: 282-286.

Watson K., Stevens J.G. Cook, M.L., and Subak-Sharpe, J.H. (1980) Latency competence of thirteen HSV-1 temperature-sensitive mutants. J. Gen. Virol. 49: 149-159.

Wolff, J.A., Fisher, L.J., Xu, L., Jinnah, H.A., Langlais, P.J., Iuvone, P.M., O'Malley, K.L., Rosenberg, M.B., Shimohama, S., Friedmann, T., and Gage, F.H. (1989) Grafting fibroblasts genetically modified to produce L-dopa in a rat model of Parkinson's Disease. Proc. Natl. Acad. Sci. USA. 86: 9011-9014.

Yahr, M.D., Duvoisin, R.C., Schear, M.J., Barrett, R.E., and Hoehn, M.M. (1969) Treatment of parkinsonism with levodopa. Arch. Neurol. 21: 343-354.

Yahr, M.D., and Bergmann, K.J. (eds) (1987) Parkinson's Disease. N.Y.: Raven Press.

RESUME : Le développement d'une méthodologie basée sur l'utilisation de vecteurs HSV-1 défectifs afin d'introduire des gènes dans des neurones in-vitro et in-vivo, a de nombreuses implications potentielles. En théorie, n'importe quel gène peut être inséré dans un vecteur HSV-1 défectif, y compris ceux qui codent pour des produits qui soit font défaut soit sont mutés dans le cadre de maladies dégénératives du système nerveux. Cette technologie devrait permettre de délivrer un gène à une partie localisée du cerveau en ajoutant, en particulier, des éléments de régulation génétique agissant en cis. L'expression du gène transduit peut être limitée à un type particulier de cellules conférant ainsi la possibilité de contrôler le niveau d'expression, un élément déterminant à considérer. Les expériences de neurobiologie fondamentale et de neurologie appliquée en cours explorent le potentiel et les champs d'application de cette méthodologie.

Liposomes and cell targeting of nucleic acids

Lee Leserman

Centre d'Immunologie INSERM-CNRS de Marseille-Luminy, Case 906, 13288 Marseille Cedex 9, France

SUMMARY

Nucleic acids encapsulated in liposomes are protected against degradation and may be fixed to different cell types *in vitro* by various ligands. Modification of the lipid composition of the liposomes renders them less stable in endocytic vesicles, with augmented delivery of their contents into cells, at the cost of an increased fragility in biological fluids in general. Limiting factors in the application of liposome-encapsulated nucleic acids *in vivo* are associated with the difficulty in access to target tissue and potential immunogenicity of the liposomes or their contents.

Liposomes are of interest in gene therapy because of their capacity to encapsulate and protect nucleic acids, the possibility of their use *in vivo*, and the absence of the dangers associated with infectivity, which remain at least a theoretical problem for retroviruses. Liposomes used for gene transfer are of two distinct types. Those most recently introduced have positively charged amphiphiles as components of their structure (Felgner et al. 1987). Mixture of these liposomes with DNA, which is negatively charged, will result in association of the DNA with the liposome surface. A residual positive charge permits electrostatic interaction between liposomes and eukaryotic cells, which are themselves negatively charged. This may be followed by penetration of the complex and release of the DNA into the cell. Release may be via several mechanisms, including endocytosis, fusion, and a poorly characterized perturbation of the membranes of the cell surface or of endocytic vesicles (Wang and Huang 1987; Leventis and Silvius 1990). This technique has also been applied to the delivery of RNA into cells (Malone et al. 1989). The relative ease of application of this method is counterbalanced by several inconvenient features:

1) Since the nucleic acids are on the outside of the liposomes, they may be subject to degradation by nucleases present in biological milieu.
2) The amphiphiles responsible for the binding of DNA have detergent-like properties (indeed, some are detergents (Pinnaduwage et al. 1989)), and consequently these liposomes have appreciable toxicity for certain cell types.
3) The charge on the liposome is susceptible to neutralization by charged elements present in serum, rendering this approach impractical in vivo except under carefully defined conditions of direct injection into the target tissue (See Felgner and Rhodes 1991 for a recent review). Another charged amphiphile used for transfection (lipopolyamine) forms liposomes in water, but forms a non-liposomal DNA-lipid complex in medium containing physiologic ion concentrations. Thus, the molecular species of lipopolyamine responsible for transfection is not a liposome (Behr et al. 1989; Loeffler et al. 1990).
4) Finally, no selectivity for a particular cell type has been reported for this technology, though the success of the attachment of transferrin to DNA-polylysine conjugates for purpose of targeting (Wagner et al. 1990) suggests that this may be technically possible.

The second, more conventional form of liposome-mediated delivery dates from the earliest years after the description of liposomes. In this approach the genes (or other form of nucleic acid) of interest are encapsulated in the aqueous spaces of the liposomes during liposome formation. (For a review of the early literature on liposome-mediated transfection see Ostro and Giacomoni (1983); more recent studies are reviewed in Mannino and Gould-Fogerite (1988)). Several liposome formation techniques suitable for this purpose are described in detail in an excellent recent methods book (New 1989). Encapsulation of nucleic acids in liposomes is relatively inefficient. This is compensated by protection of the nucleic acids against degradation by nucleases, which do not have access to the interior of the liposomes.

The emphasis in current transfection strategies is to construct liposomes which mimic the cell binding and fusogenic properties of viruses, since naked liposomes are of little value in transfecting most cell types, at least *in vitro* (Uchida 1988; Lapidot and Loyter 1990). Liposome uptake by specific cells may be augmented *in vitro* and *in vivo* by virtue of various ligands which may be attached to, or associated with, the liposome surface. These include antibodies directed at cell-surface determinants or ligands for which the cells have receptors (Leserman and Machy 1987). Numerous additional parameters are of importance in determining if and to what extent liposome contents are delivered to their sites of action. These include such characteristics of the liposomes as size, lipid composition, nature of the encapsulated molecule, type of ligand used for targeting and its linkage to the liposome. Uptake of liposomes depends on the cell type as well as the target molecule (Machy *et al.* 1982; Machy and Leserman 1983; Matthay *et al.* 1989). Cells which expressed a non-endocytosed cell surface molecule could be stably transfected, albeit with low efficiency, by the combination of liposomes bound to that determinant via antibody and subsequent electroporation. This occurred under conditions in which the concentration of liposome-encapsulated gene was too low to permit transfection in the absence of the targeting antibody. This technique would potentially permit transfection of a sub-population of cells for which a specific antibody was available, but it is obviously limited to *in vitro* studies (Machy *et al.* 1988). Facilitation of delivery of liposome contents into cells may be achieved by the addition of viral proteins which promote fusion or other perturbation of target cell membranes (Tikchonenko *et al.* 1988; Uchida 1988; Gould-Fogerite *et al.* 1989; Lapidot and Loyter 1990). Liposomes combining features of specific binding via antibodies and enhanced fusion, via "fusogenic" lipids have been described, (Wang and Huang 1989). These liposome systems may be less stable than conventional liposomes. This instability is due to the requirement that they are made by dialysis from detergent-containing solutions, and thus contain residual detergent, or contain proteins or lipids that undergo transitions in response to changes in pH or via juxtaposition with membranes. These conditions are likely to be encountered *in vivo* at sites other than the designated target.

Although the parameters which control delivery of liposome contents into cells are complex, appropriately composed antibody-bearing liposomes containing cytotoxic drugs may kill 100% of cells expressing the target molecule, permitting this technique to be used for the selection of rare mutants not expressing the target molecule (Schmitt-Verhulst *et al.* 1987; Leserman *et al.* 1989). Liposomes of identical composition targeted by the same antibodies have been used to extend the information gained in studies on drug delivery to the problem of transport of nucleic acids. Liposomes were made containing poly- and oligo nucleotides, including synthetic, double-stranded polynucleotides such as poly (rI).poly (rC) (Milhaud et al. 1989). These liposomes, by virtue of their capacity to induce interferon production, very efficiently kill L929 cells, which are particularly sensitive to interferon. Liposomes containing antisense oligodeoxynucleotides (15 base pairs) complementary to the initiation codon and four downstream codons of myc mRNA, which encodes a protein necessary for proliferation, can also kill essentially all L929 cells in culture. Liposome-encapsulated control oligonucleotides of the same base composition in scrambled order are non-toxic under the same conditions, as are liposomes containing authentic antisense, but lacking the relevant targeting antibody (Leonetti et al. 1990; Leserman et al. 1991). More recently, antibody-targeted liposomes have been used to successfully transport long (greater than 1 kilobase) RNA sequences complementary to HIV mRNA into HIV-infected lymphoid cells, with subsequent reduction in viral titers (Renneisen et al. 1990). These results indicate that nucleic acids may be delivered into cells by liposomes efficiently and in an active form. The percentage of cells which may be transfected transiently or permanently by liposome encapsulated genes are more the consequence of problems related to integration or expression of the gene than of problems in the delivery system.

Targeting to a particular cell or tissue requires contact; liposomes will not bind specifically to cells they cannot encounter. Liposomes are virus sized, so they are vulnerable to various protective mechanisms which presumably evolved to remove viruses and other infectious agents from the circulation. Though parenterally administered liposomes have been used to successfully deliver transiently expressed genes to the liver, this is the principle site of clearance of liposomes by tissue macrophages (Nicolau et al. 1983; Soriano et al. 1983; Kaneda et al. 1989). Recent developments suggest that liposomes may be fabricated to reduce uptake by the liver, which increases their chances to be targeted to other sites accessible to the circulation (Maruyama et al. 1990). The capacity of these liposomes to leave the circulation or to transport nucleic acids into cells has not been evaluated.

The final barrier remains the problem of an active host response against the liposomes or their contents. Many of the immune mechanisms which protect against infection will equally well protect against transfection. A large literature is devoted to the immune response against virally encoded peptides and the cells expressing them. The individual congenitally lacking the gene product replaced by liposome-mediated or other gene therapy will presumably mount an immune response against that gene product, since he is not tolerant, and may not distinguish it from a viral protein (Weatherall 1991). This difficulty for long term gene replacement may, however, be an opportunity for use of liposome-encapsulated nucleic acids for immunization (Felgner and Rhodes 1991).

ACKNOWLEDGEMENTS

The Centre d'Immunologie de Marseille-Luminy is Unité Mixte de Recherche 004 of the Centre National de la Recherche Scientifique and Unité 136 of the Institut National de la Santé et de la Recherche Médicale.
Some of the experiments from my laboratory discussed in this paper were also supported by grants from the Agence Nationale de Recherches sur le SIDA (ANRS) and the Association pour la Recherche sur la Cancer (ARC).

REFERENCES

Behr, J.-P., Demeneix, B., Loeffler, J.-P., and Perez-Mutul, J. (1989): Efficient gene transfer into mammalian primary endocrine cells with lipopolyamine-coated DNA. *Proc. Natl. Acad. Sci. USA* 86, 6982-6986.
Felgner, P.L., Gadek, T.R., Holm, M., Roman, R., Chan, H.W., et al. (1987): Lipofection: A highly efficient, lipid-mediated DNA-transfection procedure. *Proc. Natl. Acad. Sci. USA* 84, 7413-7417.
Felgner, P.L., and Rhodes, G. (1991): Gene therapeutics. *Nature* 349, 351-352.
Gould-Fogerite, S., Mazurkiewicz, J.E., Raska Jr., K., Voelkerding, K., Lehman, J.M., et al. (1989): Chimerasome-mediated gene transfer *in vitro* and *in vivo*. *Gene* 84, 429-438.
Kaneda, Y., Iwai, K., and Uchida, T. (1989): Introduction and expression of the human insulin gene in adult rat liver. *J. Biol. Chem.* 264, 12126-12129.
Lapidot, M., and Loyter, A. (1990): Fusion-mediated microinjection of liposome-enclosed DNA into cultured cells with the aid of influenza virus glycoprotiens. *Exp. Cell Res.* 189, 241-246.
Leonetti, J.-P., Machy, P., Degols, G. Lebleu, B., and Leserman, L. (1990): Antibody-targeted liposomes containing oligodeoxyribonucleotides complementary to viral RNA selectively inhibit viral replication. *Proc. Natl. Acad. Sci. USA.* 87, 2448-2451.

Leserman, L., Degols, G., Machy, P., Leonetti, J.-P., Mechti, N., et al. (1991): Targetting and intracellular delivery of antisense oligonucleotides interfering with oncogene expression. In *Prospects for antisense nucleic acid therapy of cancer and viral infections*, ed. E. Wickstrom, In press. New York: Alan R. Liss, Inc.

Leserman, L., Langlet, C., Schmitt-Verhulst, A.-M., and Machy, P. (1989): Positive and negative liposome-based immunoselection techniques. In *Vesicular Transport*, ed. A. Tartakoff, pp. 447-471. New York: Academic Press.

Leserman, L., and Machy, P. (1987): Ligand targeting of liposomes. In *Liposomes: from biophysics to therapeutics*, ed. M. Ostro, pp. 157-194. New York: Marcel Dekker, Inc.

Leventis, R., and Silvius, J.R. (1990): Interaction of mammalian cells with lipid dispersions containing novel metabolizable cationic amphiphiles. *Biochim. Biphys. Acta.* 1023, 124-132.

Loeffler, J.P., Barthel, F., Feltz, P., Behr, J.P., Sassone-Corsi, P., et al. (1990): Lipopolyamine-mediated transfection allows gene expression studies in primary neuronal cells. *J. Neurochem.* 54, 1812-1815.

Machy, P., and Leserman, L.D. (1983): Small liposomes are better than large liposomes for specific drug delivery in vitro. *Biochim. Biophys. Acta* 730:, 313-320.

Machy, P., Pierres, M., Barbet, J., and Leserman, L.D. (1982): Drug transfer into lymphoblasts mediated by liposomes bound to distinct sites on H-2 encoded I-A, I-E and K molecules. *J. Immunol.* 129, 2098-2102.

Machy, P., Lewis, F. McMilan, L., and Jonak, Z.L. (1988): Gene transfer from targeted liposomes to specific lymphoid cells by electroporation. *Proc. Natl. Acad. Sci. USA* 85, 8027-8031.

Malone, R.W., Felgner, P.L., and Verma, I.M. (1989): Cationic liposome-mediated RNA transfection. *Proc. Natl. Acad. Sci. USA* 86, 6077-6081.

Mannino, R.J., and Gould-Fogerite, S. (1988): Liposome mediated gene transfer. *BioTechniques* 6, 682-690.

Maruyama, K., Kennel, S.J., and Huang, L. (1990): Lipid composition is important for highly efficient target binding and retention of immunoliposomes. *Proc. Natl. Acad. Sci. USA* 87, 5744-5748.

Matthay, K.K., Abai, A.M., Cobb, S., Hong, K., Papahadjopoulos, D., et al. (1989): Role of ligand in antibody-directed endocytosis of liposomes by human T-leukemia cells. *Cancer Res* 49, 4879-4886.

Milhaud, P.G., Machy, P., Lebleu, B., and Leserman, L. (1989): Antibody-targeted liposomes containing poly (rI).poly (rC) exert a specific antiviral and toxic effect on cells primed with interferons α/β or γ. *Biochim. Biophys. Acta.* 987, 15-20.

New, R.R.C., Ed. (1989): *Liposomes: a practical approach*, The practical approach series. Oxford: Oxford Univ. Press.

Nicolau, C., Le Pape, A., Soriano, P., Fargette, F., and Juhel, M.F. (1983): *In vivo* expression of rat insulin after intravenous administration of liposome-entrapped gene for rat insulin. *Proc. Natl. Acad. Sci. USA* 80, 1068-1072.

Ostro, M., and Giacomoni, D. (1983): Liposomes as a tool in molecular biology: a comparison to other methodologies. In *Liposomes*, ed. M. Ostro, pp. 145-208. New York: Marcel Dekker.

Pinnaduwage, P., Schmitt, L., and Huang, L. (1989): Use of a quaternary ammonium detergent in liposome mediated DNA transfection of mouse L-cells. *Biochim. Biophys. Acta* 985, 33-37.

Renneisen, K., Leserman, L., Matthes, E., Schröder, H.C., and Müller, W.E.G. (1990): Inhibition of expression of Human Immunodeficiency Virus-1 *in vitro* by antibody-targeted liposomes containing antisense RNA to the env region. *J. Biol. Chem.* 265, 16337-16342.

Schmitt-Verhulst, A.-M., Guimezanes, A., Boyer, C., Poenie, M., Tsien, R., et al. (1987): Pleitropic loss in activation pathways in a T cell receptor α chain deletion variant of a cytolytic T cell clone. *Nature* 325, 628-631.

Soriano, P., Dijkstra, J., Legrand, A., Spanjer, H., Landos-Gagliardi, D., et al. (1983): Targeted and non-targeted liposomes for *in vivo* transfer to rat liver cells of a plasmid containing the preproinsulin I gene. *Proc. Natl. Acad. Sci. USA* 80, 7128-7131.

Tikchonenko, T.I., Glushakova, S.E., Kislina, O.S., Grodnitskaya, N.A., Manykin, A.A., et al. (1988): Transfer of condensed viral DNA into eukaryotic cells using proteoliposomes. *Gene* 63, 321-330.

Uchida, T. (1988): Introduction of macromolecules into mammalian cells by cell fusion. *Exp. Cell. Res.* 178, 1-17.

Wagner, E., Zenke, M., Cotten, M., Beug, H., and Birnstiel, M.L. (1990): Transferrin-polycation conjugates as carriers for DNA uptake. *Proc. Natl. Acad. Sci. USA* 87, 3410-3414.

Wang, C.Y., and Huang, L. (1987): Plasmid DNA absorbed to pH-sensitive liposomes efficiently transforms the target cells. *Biochem. Biophys. Res. Commun.* 147, 980-985.

Wang, C.-Y., and Huang, L. (1989): Highly efficient DNA delivery mediated by pH-sensitive immunoliposomes. *Biochemistry* 28, 9508-9514.

Weatherall, D.J. (1991): Gene therapy in perspective. *Nature* 349, 275-276.

RESUME

Les acides nucléiques encapsulés dans les liposomes sont protégés contre les dégradations et peuvent être fixés à différents types cellulaires *in vitro* par des ligands variés. La modification de la composition des liposomes permet leur déstabilisation dans les vésicules d'endocytose, avec une amélioration du relargage de leur contenu dans les cellules, au prix d'une augmentation de leur fragilité dans les fluides biologiques. Les facteurs limitant leur application *in vivo* sont la difficulté d'accéder aux tissus cibles et l'immunogenicité potentielle des liposomes ou leur contenu.

Somatic gene transfer : data
1. Hematopoietic tissues

Transfert de gènes somatique : résultats
1. Tissus hématopoïétiques

Four reasons for purifying stem cells for gene therapy

Jan W.M. Visser*, Mark P.W. Einerhand and Dinko Valerio

Department of Cell Biology, TNO Institute of Applied Radiobiology and Immunology, Lange Kleiweg 151, PO Box 5815, 2280 HV Rijswijk, The Netherlands
* Author for correspondence

Genes are successfully transfered to pluripotent hemopoietic stem cells and long term expression of such genes in the recipients of the stem cells has been documented by several investigators (Belmont et al., 1988; Beusechem et al., 1990; Dick et al., 1985; Keller and Snodgrass, 1990; Lim et al., 1987; Magli et al., 1987; Valerio et al., 1989). These successes are only partly based on the knowledge about stem cells as it was gathered by experimental hematologists for several decades. Their assays and definitions of such cells had to be modified concomitantly with the development of gene therapy protocols using hemopoietic stem cells, because of a number of new observations. The CFU-S (colony forming unit-spleen) test could not be accepted any more as a stem cell assay after it became clear that the assay detects a heterogeneous population of early hemopoietic cells, and that spleen colonies can be formed by other cells than pluripotent stem cells (Magli et al., 1983; Baines and Visser, 1983; Visser et al., 1984; Bertoncello et al., 1985; Mulder et al., 1985). Recent evidence based on the analysis of cells that provide long-term chimerism after transplantation indicates that stem cells can be largely separated from CFU-S (Jones et al., 1990; Ploemacher and Brons, 1989; Sluijs et al., 1990; Visser et al., 1990, 1991). Similarly, it has become evident that the stem cells providing long-term chimerism are not responsible for the radioprotective effect of bone marrow transplantation. The production of mature offspring by stem cells is too slow to compensate the radiation induced leukopenia, and other cells than stem cells are needed for the short-term repopulation (Jones et al., 1990; Visser et al., 1990). These findings urge reconsideration and evaluation of experimental data, conclusions and theories about stem cells that were based on the CFU-S assay and on radioprotection or so-called 30-day survival tests. These findings also help to explain some of the failures in gene therapy protocols that were based on the infection of CFU-S. It has become clear that this test is not a measure of stem cell infection and therefore not predicting successful gene therapy. It has even been questioned whether stem cells from adult bone marrow could replicate without differentiation and it was hypothesized that they only are capable of selfrenewal during the fetal expansion of the hemopoietic system. This would be a compelling reason to use fetal liver as the source of stem cells. Gene therapy studies provided us with genetically marked, bone marrow derived stem cells and it was demonstrated that such stem cells with the marker at a unique insertion site, gave rise to extensive offspring with the same insertion site in secondary recipients of transplants (Beusechem et al., 1990; Bodine et al., 1990). This indicates that bone marrow stem cells are capable of selfrenewal, and can be used for gene therapy. It also indicates that there exist stem cells that do not differentiate during the culture needed to transfer the foreign gene.

There are other reasons to take fetal liver as a source of stem cells for retrovirus-mediated gene transfer. The most important one seems to be that it may be assumed that during the fetal expansion of the hemopoietic organ the stem cells are naturally proliferating, whereas they are mostly quiescent in the adult bone marrow. This is of importance, because gene transfer requires the proliferation of the target cells, and because the induction of proliferation of quiescent bone marrow stem cells in vitro results in differentiation and loss of pluripotency and selfrenewal capacity. Only during coculture or on stromal layers, conditions seem to induce and permit both proliferation and the maintainance of selfrenewal capacity in vitro.

The stem cells are rare and there seems to be little differences between stem cells and their committed daughter cells. Therefore, they are difficult to study directly and their isolation requires combinations of cell separation techniques. In spite of this, procedures have been described which may yield in between 100 and 1000 fold enrichment of stem cells. The efficiency of the protocols depends on the test system employed and according to Van Bekkum (personal communication) the most predominant property of the stem cell these days is its elusiveness: every attempt to purify this cell type resulted in the discovery of new heterogeneities, and in more questions about the assay systems. The gene therapy protocol provides its own test system, viz. the genetically marked stem cells, and the combination of gene therapy protocols with stem cell purification studies seems to be most useful to study the regulation of hemopoiesis (Jordan et al., 1990). On the other hand we would like to argue in this contribution that purification of stem cells is also of use for the development and application of gene therapy protocols. We list four reasons for this.

FOUR REASONS FOR PURIFYING STEM CELLS FOR GENE THERAPY

One: Growth factors produced during coculture cause differentiation.

Culture of unfractionated bone marrow cells not only induces proliferation, differentiation and maturation of different stages of progenitor cells and of hemopoietic stem cells, it also induces the production and release of growth factors from the monocytes and lymphocytes which are present in the bone marrow (e.g. Bot et al., 1987). These growth factors may act directly and in synergy with other regulatory factors to induce stem cell differentiation. Such differentiation must be avoided, since the aim of gene therapy is the infection of long-term repopulating stem cells with selfrenewal capacity. Therefore, monocytes, lymphocytes and all other cells which produce differentiation inducing factors have to be separated from the stem cells. Ikehara and coworkers (Miyaba-Inaba et al., 1987; Sugiura et al., 1988) reported the production of growth factors by cells with a similar phenotype as early myeloid cells and stem cells. Such cells would be difficult to remove from a stem cell suspension. The factors are not further analysed yet, and the investigators assume that the stem cells produce these regulatory factors themselves. The factors are thought to control quiescence and proliferation, but not differentiation. If that is the case, removal of such cells would not be of importance to prevent differentiation

Two: Improved Multiplicity of Infection.

In order to efficiently infect target cells with retroviral vectors, which are commonly used in the development of gene therapy protocols, the virus titer has to be above a certain threshold, and preferably as high as possible. Successful infections of stem cells were performed with titers of 10^5 viruses/ml and higher. The titer that can be obtained with a retroviral construct depends amongst others on the inserted gene, and for very large genes it is as yet not possible to reach titers above 10^6 viruses/ml. For retroviral constructs containing the beta-globin gene it is difficult to obtain higher virus titers than 10^5 viruses/ml, which is not optimal for the infection of stem cells. The infection of stem cells with such virus titers might be improved when the virus to cell ratio is raised by purifying the stem cells from the bone marrow.

Three: Quality control of gene transfer.

The clinical application of gene therapy will require quality assurance and the verification of each of the steps in the gene therapy protocol. The success rate of the first steps in the protocols, viz. the infection of stem cells, and the insertion of the foreign genes into their genome, can be directly analysed and controled if the stem cells are purified. Alternatively, a specific staining for the detection of stem cells may be developed that allows the direct examination of these cells within a heterogeneous suspension. Such a staining can be developed using purified stem cells. The procedure would enable the assessment of the infection efficiency of stem cells in the graft prior to its transplantation.

Four: Direct examination of stem cells.

In order to optimize gene transfer protocols and to evaluate different retroviral and other constructs with respect to their gene delivery and expression capability, it is of interest to be able to examine the target cells by a direct method at different time points during and shortly after coculture. Due to the low frequency of stem cells in the bone marrow, direct examination is as yet only possible by purification of the stem cells. By plating virus infected purified cells, single cell per well one can quantify both the infection efficiency and the expression capability of retroviral vectors in the cultured progeny of individual stem cells. In addition, purification of stem cells is of use in studying the regulation of differentiation and proliferation of these cells. The development of gene therapy protocols would profit from a better understanding of this regulation about which is still much unknown in spite of many years of research in the field of experimental hematology.

PURIFICATION OF STEM CELLS

There are several protocols to enrich for and purify pluripotent hemopoietic stem cells from mouse (Bertoncello et al., 1989, 1991; Lord and Spooncer, 1986; Muller-Sieburg et al., 1986; Spangrude et al., 1988; Spangrude and Johnson 1990; Jones et al., 1990; Jordan et al., 1990; Visser et al., 1984, 1990, 1991; Visser and de Vries, 1988, 1990), rat (Goldschneider et al., 1980; McCarthy et al., 1987), monkey (Berenson et al., 1988,) and man (Andrews et al., 1990; Civin and Loken, 1987; Szilvassy et al., 1989, Sutherland et al., 1989, 1990). These protocols consist of combinations of physical cell separation methods. Pretreatment of the donor or the cells using 5-fluorouracil or 4HC helps to pre-enrich the samples for stem cells (Bertoncello et al., 1986; Gordon et al., 1985; Sutherland et al., 1990; Yeager et al., 1986).

The performance of the various protocols depends strongly on the assay system used to enumerate the enrichment and the absolute purity. Since the CFU-S assay can not be used to count the stem cells, there is no clonal test and, therefore, no absolute quantitation of stem cells. Quantitation of the enrichment of stem cells can be done by titration of the graft size to obtain long-term repopulation (examined with genetic markers, the Y-chromosome probe, or surface antigen markers). The marrow-repopulating ability (MRA) assay gives similar results as the long-term repopulation tests until now, and so does the long-term, not the short-term, Cobblestone Area Formation on stromal layers (Sluijs et al., 1990; Visser et al., 1990, 1991).

It is not necessary to purify the stem cells to 100% homogeneity for each of the above mentioned applications. The removal of growth factor producing cells and the improvement of the multiplicity of infection can be obtained with partly purified suspensions. Although it seems obvious to employ only the CD34 antigen to partly enrich for human stem cells, it must be mentioned here that this is not sufficient to remove growth factor producing cells (Bot et al., 1987).

Partial enrichment of large numbers of mouse stem cells can be obtained efficiently using a combination of equilibrium density centrifugation and immunomagnetic bead separation (Table 1). The combination of the three antibodies 45D8, 6A2 and 15-1.1 removed 98% of low density bone marrow cells, and the enrichment for CFU-S was 40 to 80 fold. It was found, however, that the MRA was not equally enriched. Closer examination revealed that the antibody 6A2 removed MRA cells. Therefore, this antibody does

Table 1. ENRICHMENT OF MOUSE HEMOPOIETIC STEM CELLS USING IMMUNOMAGNETIC BEADS

number of CFU-S per 10^5 bone marrow cells

	day 8	day 12
unfractionated bone marrow cells	40 ± 5	41 ± 5
low density cells*	150 ± 16	174 ± 20
45D8-, 6A2-, 15-1.1-** low density cells	3083 ± 300	2867 ± 300

* metrizamide gradient as described (Visser et al., 1984).
**low density cells incubated with a cocktail of antibodies against mature cell types: 15-1.1 binds monocytes and granulocytes and their precursors, 6A2 erythroid cells, 45D8 lymphocytes and erythroid mature and immature cells. The labeled cells were removed using anti-rat antibody coated immunomagnetic beads (Dynabeads M-450; Dynal, Oslo).

not make part of the cocktail any more. Enrichments of 30 to 60 fold for MRA are obtained with only 15-1.1 and 45D8 which remove all growth factor producing lymphocytes and monocytes. The combination of methods can process large numbers of cells, so that subsequent more detailed cell sorting using flow cytometry yields sufficient numbers of highly purified stem cells for further experimentation within a reasonable time. The flow cytometry should include the use of the supravital dye Rhodamine 123 (Rh123). It has been demonstrated that the long-term repopulating stem cells are Rh123 dull (Visser et al., 1990, 1991). Rh123 dull cells contain the MRA and only part of the day 12-CFU-S (Bertoncello et al., 1985), the thymus repopulating cells, and no day 8-CFU-S (Mulder and Visser, 1987).
In pre-enriched suspensions, two populations of primitive cells can be distinguished by Rh123 (Visser and de Vries, 1988), and it can be argued that the Rh123 dull cells contain the quiescent stem cells, whereas the Rh123 bright population consists of predominantly committed progenitor cells and only a very small number, if any, of activated pluripotent stem cells (Visser et al., 1990, 1991; Ploemacher and Brons, 1988; Spangrude and Johnson, 1990).

CULTURE OF STEM CELLS.

The Rh123 dull sorted stem cells could not be cultured efficiently. Maximally 15 % could be induced to colony formation with combinations of growth factors (Visser and de Vries, 1988; Visser et al.,1990, 1991). The Rh123 bright sorted cells which contain most of the CFU-S but virtually no stem cells, can be cultured with a high plating efficiency (up to 50 %), and even with only IL-3 present an efficiency of 20 % can be obtained.
The stem cells appear to grow better on stromal layers. The production of Cobblestone Areas (CA) within long-term stromal

cell cultures by the Rh123 dull sorted stem cells is sustained, and so is the production of CFU-GM in such cultures (Visser et al., 1990, 1991; Sluijs et al., 1990). It is not known whether the stem cells selfrenew in the stromal layers, causing long-term CA and CFU-GM production. It may be that they are quiescent and that the stroma only serves to keep them alive, and that some of them at some random time after inoculation are triggered to differentiate. On the other hand, gene therapy studies have shown that stem cells can be co-cultured and infected without the loss of pluripotency and selfrenewal capability. It may well be that this success is due to the special characteristics of the cell lines used for co-culture in the sense that such cell lines were probably not only suitable for packaging and virus production but also for maintaining hemopoiesis.

REFERENCES

Andrews, R.G., Singer, J.W., and Bernstein, I.D. (1989): Precursors of colony-forming cells in humans can be distinguished from colony-forming cells by expression of the CD33 and CD34 antigens and light scatter properties. *J. Exp. Med.* 169, 1721-1731.
Baines, P., and Visser, J.W.M. (1983): Analysis and separation of murine bone marrow stem cells by H33342 fluorescence-activated cell sorting. *Exp. Hematol.* 11, 701-708.
Belmont, J.W., MacGregor, G.R., Wager-Smith, K., Fletcher, F.A., Moore, K.A., Hawkins, D., Villalon, D., Chang, S.M.W., and Caskey, C.T. (1988): Expression of human adenosine deaminase in murine hematopoietic cells. *Mol. Cell. Biol.* 8, 5116-5125.
Berenson, R.J., Andrews, R.G., Bensinger, W.I., Kalamaz, D., Knitter, G., Buckner, C.D., and Bernstein, D.(1988): Antigen CD34+ marrow cells engraft lethally irradiated baboons. *J. Clin. Invest.* 81, 951-955.
Bertoncello, I., Hodgson, G.S., and Bradley, T.R. (1985): Multiparameter analysis of transplantable hemopoietic stem cells.I. The separation and enrichment of stem cells homing to marrow and spleen on the basis of rhodamine-123 fluorescence. *Exp. Hematol.* 13, 999-1006.
Bertoncello,I., Bartelmez, S.H., Bradley, T.R., Stanley, E.R., Harris, R. A., Sandrin, M.S., Kriegler, A.B., McNiece, I.K., Hunter, S.D., and Hodgson, G.S. (1986): Isolation and analysis of primitive hemopoietic progenitor cells on the basis of differential expression of Qa-m7 antigen. *J. Immunol.* 136, 3219-3224.
Bertoncello, I., Bradley, T.R., and Hodgson, G.S. (1989): The concentration and resolution of primitive hemopoietic cells from normal mouse bone marrow by negative selection using monoclonal antibodies and dynabead monodisperse magnetic microspheres. *Exp. Hematol.* 17, 171-176.
Bertoncello, I., Bradley, T.R., and Watt, S.M. (1991): An improved negative immunomagnetic selection strategy for the purification of primitive hemopoietic cells from normal bone marrow. *Exp. Hematol.* 19, 95-100.
Beusechem, V.W. van, Kukler, A., Einerhand, M.P.W., Bakx, T.A., Eb, A.J. van der, Bekkum, D.W. van, and Valerio, D. (1990): Expression of human adenosine deaminase in mice transplanted

with hemopietic stem cells infected with amphotropic retroviruses. *J. Exp. Med.* 172, 729-736.

Bodine, D.M., Seidel, N, Karlsson, S., and Nienhuis, A.W. (1990): The combination of Il-3 and Il-6 enhances retrovirus mediated gene transfer into hematopoietic stem cells. In *The Biology of Hematopoiesis*, ed. N. Dainiak, E.P.Cronkite, R. McCaffrey, and R.K. Shadduck, pp. 287-299. New York: Wiley-Liss.

Bot, F.J., Dorssers, L., Wagemaker, G., and Löwenberg, B. (1988) Stimulating spectrum of human recombinant multi-CSF (IL-3) on human marrow precursors: Importance of accessory cells. *Blood* 71, 1609-1614.

Civin, C.I., and Loken, M.R. (1987): Cell surface antigens on human marrow cells: dissection of hematopoietic development using monoclonal antibodies and multiparameter flow cytometry. *Int. J. Cell Cloning* 5, 267-288.

Dick, J.E., Magli, M.C., Huszar, D., Phillips, R.A., and Bernstein, A. (1985): Introduction of a selectable gene into primitive stem cells capable of longterm reconstitution of the hemopoietic system of W/W^v mice. *Cell.* 42, 71-79.

Goldschneider, I., Metcalf, D., Battey, F., and Mandel, T. (1980): Analysis of rat hemopoietic cells on the fluorescence-activated cell sorter.I.Isolation of pluripotent hemopoietic stem cells and granulocyte-macrophage progenitor cells. *J. Exp. Med.* 152, 419-437.

Gordon, M.Y., Goldman, J.M., and Gordon-Smith, E.C. (1985): 4-Hydroperoxycyclophosphamide inhibits proliferation by human granulocyte-macrophage colony-forming cells (GM-CFC) but spares more primitive progenitor cells. *Leuk. Res.* 9, 1017-1021.

Jones, R.J., Wagner, J.E., Celano, P., Zicha, M.S., and Sharkis, S.J. (1990): Separation of pluripotent haemopoietic stem cells from spleen colony-forming cells. *Nature* 347, 188-189.

Jordan, C.T., McKearn, J.P., and Lemischka, I.R. (1990): Cellular and developmental properties of fetal hematopoietic stem cells. *Cell* 61, 953-963.

Keller, G., and Snodgrass, R. (1990): Life span of multipotential hematopoietic stem cells in vivo. *J. Exp. Med.* 171, 1407-1418.

Lim, B., Williams, D.A., and Orkin, S.H. (1987): Retrovirus-mediated gene transfer of human adenosine deaminase: expression of functional enzyme in murine hematopoietic stem cells in vivo. *Mol. Cell. Biol.* 7, 3459-3465

Lord, B.I., and Spooncer, E. (1986): Isolation of haemopoietic spleen colony forming cells. *Lymphokine Research* 5, 59-72.

Magli, M.C., Iscove, N.N., and Odartchenko, N. (1982): Transient nature of early haematopoietic spleen colonies. *Nature* 295, 527-529.

Magli, M.C., Dick, J.E., Huszar, D., Bernstein, A., and Phillips, R.A. (1987): Modulation of gene expression in multiple hematopoietic cell lineages following retrovirus vector gene transfer. *Proc. Natl. Acad. Sci. U.S.A.* 84, 789-793.

McCarthy, K.F., Hale, M.L., and Fehnel, P.L. (1987): Purification and analysis of rat hematopoietic stem cells by flow cytometry. *Cytometry* 8, 296-305.

Miyaba-Inaba, M., Ogata, H., Toki, J., Kuma, S., Sugiura, K., Yasumizu, R., and Ikehara, S. (1987): Isolation of murine hemopoietic stem cells in the Go phase. *Biochem. Biophys. Res. Comm.* 147, 687-694.

Mulder, A.H., and Visser, J.W.M. (1987): Separation and functional analysis of bone marrow cells separated by rhodamine-123 fluorescence. *Exp. Hematol.* 15, 99-104.

Mulder, A.H., Visser, J.W.M., and Engh, G.J. van den (1985): Thymus regeneration by bone marrow cell suspensions differing in the potential to form early and late spleen colonies. *Exp. Hematol.* 13, 768-775.

Muller-Sieburg, C.E., Townsend, K., Weissman, I.L., and Rennick, D. (1988): Proliferation and differentiation of highly enriched mouse hematopoietic stem cells and progenitor cells in response to defined growth factors. *J. Exp. Med.* 167, 1825-1840.

Ploemacher, R.E., and Brons N.H.C. (1988): Cells with marrow and spleen repopulating ability and forming spleen colonies on day 16, 12, and 8 are sequentially ordered on the basis of increasing rhodamine 123 retention. *J. Cell. Physiol.* 136, 531-536.

Ploemacher, R.E., and Brons, N.H.C. (1989): Separation of CFU-S from primitive cells responsible for reconstitution of the bone marrow hemopoietic stem cell compartment following irradiation: evidence for a pre-CFU-S cell. *Exp. Hematol.* 17, 263-266.

Szilvassy, S.J., Lansdorp, P.M., Humphries, R.K., Eaves, A.C., and Eaves, C.J. (1989): Isolation in a single step of a highly enriched murine hematopoietic stem cell population with competitive long-term repopulating ability. *Blood* 74, 930-939.

Sluijs, J.P. van der, Jong, J.P., Brons, N.H.C., and Ploemacher, R.E. (1990): Marrow repopulating cells, but not CFU-S, establish long-term in vitro hemopoiesis on a marrow-derived stromal layer. *Exp. Hematol.* 18, 893-896.

Spangrude, G.J., and Johnson, G.R. (1990): Resting and activated subsets of mouse multipotent hematopoietic stem cells. *Proc. Natl. Acad. Sci. U.S.A.* 87, 7433-7437.

Spangrude, G.J., Heimfeld, S., and Weissman, I.L. (1988): Purification and characterization of mouse hematopoietic stem cells. *Science* 241, 58-62.

Sugiura, K., Inaba, M., Ogata, H., Yasumizu, R., Inaba, K., Good, R.A., and Ikehara, S. (1988): Wheat germ agglutinin-positive cells in a stem cell-enriched fraction of mouse bone marrow have potent natural suppressor activity. *Proc. Natl. Acad. Sci. U.S.A.* 85, 4824 4826.

Sutherland, H.J., Eaves, C.J., Eaves, A.C., Dragowska, W., and Lansdorp, P.M. (1989): Characterization and partial purification of human marrow cells capable of initiating long-term hematopoiesis in vitro. *Blood* 74, 1563-1570.

Sutherland, H.J., Lansdorp, P.M., Henkelman, D.H., Eaves, A.C., and Eaves, C.J.(1990): Functional characterization of individual human hematopoietic stem cells cultured at limiting dilution on supportive marrow stromal layers. *Proc. Natl. Acad. Sci. U.S.A.* 87, 3584-3588.

Valerio, D., Einerhand, M.P.W., Wamsley, P.M., Bakx, T.A., Li, C.L., and Verma, I.M. (1989): Retrovirus-mediated gen transfer into embryonal carcinoma cells and hemopoietic stem cells: Expression from a hybrid long terminal repeat. *Gene* 84, 419-427.

Visser, J.W.M., and Vries, P. de (1988): Isolation of spleen-colony forming cells (CFU-s) using wheat germ agglutinin and rhodamine 123 labeling. *Blood Cells* 14, 369-384.

Visser, J.W.M., and Vries, P. de (1990): Identification and purification of murine hemopoietic stem cells by flow cytometry. In *Flow Cytometry*, ed. H. Crissman, and Z. Darzynkiewicz, pp. 451-468. Orlando: Academic Press.

Visser, J.W.M., Bauman, J. G. J., Mulder, A. H., Eliason, J. F., and Leeuw, A. M. de (1984): Isolation of murine pluripotent hemopoietic stem cells. *J. Exp. Med.* 59, 1576-1590.

Visser, J.W.M., Hogeweg-Platenburg, M.G.C., Vries, P. de, Bayer, J., and Ploemacher, R.E. (1990): Culture of purified pluripotent haemopoietic stem cells. In *The Biology of Hematopoiesis*, ed. N. Dainiak, E.P.Cronkite, R. McCaffrey, and R.K. Shadduck, pp.1-8. New York: Alan R. Liss, Inc.

Visser, J.W.M., Vries, P. de, Hogeweg-Platenburg, M.G.C., Bayer, J., Schoeters, G., Van Den Heuvel, R., and Mulder, D.H. (1991): Culture of hematopoietic stem cells purified from murine bone marrow. *Seminars in Hematology* 28, 117-125.

Yeager, A.M., Kaizer, H., Santos, G.W., et al. (1986): Autologous bone marrow transplantation in patients with acute nonlymphocytic leukemia, using ex vivo marrow treatment with 4-hydroperoxycyclophosphamide. *The New Engl. J. of Med.* 315,141-147.

RESUME : Les tests et modes de définition des cellules souches hématopoïétiques ont dû être modifiés avec le développement des protocoles de thérapie génique ; le test de CFU-S ne saurait être plus longtemps considéré comme un moyen d'identifier ces cellules souches. Le marquage génétique des cellules souches dérivées de la moelle osseuse indique avec certitude que celles-ci sont capables d'auto-renouvellement ; de plus, certaines ne subissent pas de différenciation pendant la culture nécessaire au transfert d'un gène exogène. Réciproquement, la purification de ces cellules souches serait extrêmement utile au développement et aux applications des protocoles de thérapie génique. On peut indiquer quatre raisons à cela : 1) Les facteurs de croissance produits pendant la co-culture par d'autres cellules que les cellules pluripotentes entrainent une différenciation non souhaitée ; 2) La purification de ces cellules permettrait d'améliorer le rapport multiplicité virale sur nombre de cellules à infecter ; 3) L'identification sélective des cellules souches permettrait de déterminer l'efficacité d'infection de ces cellules dans les greffons avant transplantation ; 4) L'examen direct des cellules souches contribuerait à pouvoir analyser celles-ci à intervalles réguliers pendant et peu après la co-culture. Un enrichissement partiel en cellules souches murines peut être obtenu en combinant une centrifugation par densité à l'équilibre, une séparation par des billes magnétiques chargées d'anticorps et une séparation par cytométrie de flux après coloration vitale avec la Rhodamine 123 (Rh123). Dans les suspensions pré-enrichies, deux populations de cellules primitives peuvent être distinguées : d'une part, les cellules ternes correspondant aux cellules souches quiescentes et d'autre part, une population cellulaire brillante avec la Rhodamine 123 constituée en majorité de progéniteurs engagés et peu ou pas du tout de cellules souches pluripotentes activées.

Hematopoietic stem and progenitor cells in human umbilical cord blood

Hal E. Broxmeyer [1-3]*, Cathy Carow [2, 3], Giao Hangoc [1, 3], Paul C. Hendrie [2, 3] and Scott Cooper [1, 3]

Departments of [1] Medicine (Hematology/Oncology), [2] Microbiology/Immunology, and the [3] Walther Oncology Center, Indiana University School of Medicine, 975 West Walnut Street, Room 501, Indianapolis, IN 46202-5121, USA

* Author for correspondence

Introduction

Hematopoietic cells circulating in the blood and found in other tissue areas are produced by stem and progenitor cells (Broxmeyer, 1982, 1983). Stem cells are pluripotent in that they can give rise to multiple lineages, lymphoid and myeloid or myeloid-restricted, but also have the very important characteristic of making more of their own kind (Williams et al. 1987). This latter capability has been termed self-renewal and is measured by transferring single colonies of hematopoietic cells from spleens in vivo or culture dishes in vitro into either secondary recipient mice or secondary culture dishes. A hierarchy of stem cells is considered to exist with greater to lesser capacity for "stemness" (Broxmeyer 1991). It would appear that stem cells, perhaps with less "stemness", move in catenated fashion into the multipotential progenitor cell compartment and then subsequently into the more lineage restricted progenitor cell compartments. Progenitor cells were considered to have little, or no capacity for self-renewal, although this concept, as mentioned below, has been re-evaluated. It is the stem and to a lesser extent the progenitor cells that are utilized as vehicles for recent studies in gene transfer/gene therapy.

In the adult, the primary source of hematopoietic stem and progenitor cells is the bone marrow, which is the usual cellular choice for hematopoietic reconstitution in an autologous or human leukocyte antigen (HLA)-matched allogeneic setting. Adult peripheral blood has had use in a strictly autologous setting but there is little information thus far to suggest that this source of cells may be useful in an allogeneic situation. There is also a concern that adult peripheral blood stem cells may have only a finite capacity for maintaining hematopoiesis.

Umbilical Cord Blood Stem and Progenitor Cells.

There are a number of clinical situations that can benefit from transplantation of the stem cells present in bone marrow. Registries exist for matching potential donors and recipients for such HLA-matched cells. However, many HLA types are not listed in the registry, especially those associated with minorities and various foreign groups, making the search for alternative sources of stem/progenitor cells an important one. In this context, hematopoietic stem and progenitor cells are ontologically found first in the yolk sac, next in the fetal liver and spleen and lastly in the fetal bone marrow (Tavassoli, 1991). Little is known regarding the mechanisms involved in this migratory pathway, but during this process fetal blood is highly enriched in stem/progenitor cells which are at a frequency equal to or greater than that found in adult bone marrow (Broxmeyer et al. 1989). This frequency decreases greatly after birth (Gabutti et al., 1975; Geissler et al., 1986). Clinical medicine is already the beneficiary of this fetal/neonatal phenomenon. Human umbilical cord and placental blood was used in an HLA-matched sibling setting to successfully reconstitute the hematopoietic system of a young boy with Fanconi anemia with his sister's normal cells (Gluckman et al., 1989). This treatment was based on laboratory studies assessing the content, collection, transplantation and cyropreservation of hematopoietic progenitor cells in such tissue (Broxmeyer et al., 1989). Cells were cryopreserved as reported by English et al., 1991. At present there have been four HLA-matched cord blood transplants done in Fanconi anemia (three by Dr. Eliane Gluckman's unit at the Hopital Saint Louis, Paris, France and one by Dr. Richard Harris, Children's Hospital, Cincinnati, Ohio, USA). Three of the 4 patients were successfully engrafted and at the time of this writing (April, 1991) are respectively 30, 17, and 10 months post transplant and are hematologically normal and clinically healthy (Broxmeyer et al., 1990, 1991b). There has also been a successful engraftment with HLA-matched female sibling cord blood in a male patient with juvenile chronic myelogenous leukemia (Wagner et al., 1991) done by Drs. John Wagner and George Santos, at Johns Hopkins, Baltimore, MD, USA, but it appears through the use of in situ Y-chromosome analysis and polymerase chain reaction studies of DNA polymorphism that the patient, now 9 months post-transplant, may be relapsing (Wagner, personal communication). All five of the above mentioned transplants were done with the cord and placental blood cells sent to the author's laboratory at the Indiana University School of Medicine for assessment of progenitor cell numbers, cryopreservation and storage. Upon need, the frozen samples were hand-delivered to the site of transplantation.

The encouraging results for cord blood engraftment have opened up the possibility of establishing cord blood banks for the storage of such cells for use in an autologous setting, but also for access to HLA-typed allogeneic cells (McGlave, 1991, Morris, 1991). The only perfectly matched set of cells is one's own, a point highlighted by a recent study which correlated rejection of an allogeneic marrow graft with a single amino acid substitution in an HLA class I-molecule (Fleischhauer et al., 1990, Parham, 1991). It is possible, and in the principal author's (HEB) estimation, highly likely that in the future each child born will have the capability of having their own cord blood cells stored in cyropreserved form for their own use should it be needed. Storage of cord blood for allogeneic transplant purposes offers the opportunity for access to HLA-types which are vastly under represented in the bone marrow registry.

Broadness of Applicability and Recent Information.

Still to be determined is the broadness of applicability of cord blood cells in terms of which diseases can be treated with these cells and whether or not there are enough cells in single cord blood collections for repopulation of the hematopoietic system of adults. It is considered likely by us that cord blood will have use in all disorders that currently or in the future can or will be treated by bone marrow transplantation. With regards to use in adults, it is certainly likely that in most cases there will be enough cells for autologous transplantation, a situation in which animal studies have already demonstrated the need for 10 fold fewer cells than in an allogeneic situation (Referenced in Broxmeyer et al., 1989, 1990, 1991b). It is also probable that a single collection of cord blood will successfully engraft an adult in an allogenic situation. This belief, not yet verified by clinical transplantation, is based on the in vitro assessment of hematopoietic progenitor cells in single collections. As seen in Table 1, there is a wide range of values in the 18 collections that were made with the knowledge that they may be used for sibling transplants. This table includes the 5 cases already transplanted. It is emphasized that the progenitor cell numbers found in the four successful engraftments were at or very close to the lower range of these values shown in Table 1. Moreover, it has recently become apparent that the numbers of progenitor cells shown in Table 1 are vast underestimates of the actual numbers of these cells (Broxmeyer et al., 1991c).

Table 1

Range of Pre-Freeze Values of Hematopoietic Progenitor Cells from Unfractionated Human Umbilical Cord Blood of Single Collections[a]

Progenitors No. x 10^{-5} in: Agar Culture	
Day 14 CFU-GM (Colonies)	0.4 - 21.9
Day 14 CFU-GM (Colonies + Clusters)	0.8 - 49.3
Methyl Cellulose	
Day 14 CFU-GM (Colonies)	0.7 - 108.5
Day 14 BFU-E (Colonies	2.5 - 38.1
Day 14 CFU-GEMM (Colonies)	0.4 - 12.8

[a] Progenitor cell assays performed as in Broxmeyer et al. 1989 (N=18 collections).

Mast cell growth factor (MGF), also termed stem cell factor or kit ligand (Williams et al., 1991, Zsebo, et al. 1991, Huang, et al. 1991) is a protein encoded by the murine steel locus and is a ligand for the receptor protein produced by the c-kit proto-oncogene. MGF has potent co-stimulating activity for multipotential (CFU-GEMM), erythroid (BFU-E) and granulocyte-macrophage (CFU-GM) progenitor cells when used in combination with hematopoietic colony stimulating factors (CSF) such as erythropoietin (Epo) and granulocyte-macrophage (GM)-CSF (Williams et al., 1991, Zsebo et al., 1991, Broxmeyer et al., 1991a) in terms of colony numbers and size. Moreover, MGF has analagous potent co-stimulating activity on a human factor-dependent cell line, MO7e (Hendrie et al., 1991) which opens up the possibility of evaluating MGF effects at the level of cellular and molecular biochemistry. When cultures of CFU-GM in human umbilical cord blood were stimulated by 100 U/ml recombinant human (rhu)GM-CSF plus 50 ng/ml rhu or rmurine (mu) MGF, on an average 8 to 10 fold more colonies were detected compared with cells grown in the presence of either 100 U/ml rhuGM-CSF or a 10% v/v of medium conditioned by the human urinary bladder carcinoma cell line, 5637 (= 5637 CM; a source of GM-CSF, G-CSF, interleukin (IL)-1, etc.). When cultures of CFU-GEMM in cord blood were stimulated by 1 U/ml rhuEpo, 100 U/ml rhuIL-3 and 50 ng/ml rhu or rmuMGF, on the average 13 to 14 fold more colonies were detected compared with cells grown in the presence of 1 U/ml Epo plus 100 U/ml rhuIL-3.

Interestingly, the increase in detection of CFU-GEMM colonies with MGF was associated with a decreased detection of BFU-E colonies noted when cord blood cells were stimulated with Epo, in the absence or presence of IL-3 (Broxmeyer et al., 1991c). This is in contrast with results using human bone marrow in which MGF enhanced detection of BFU-E-, CFU-GEMM- and CFU-GM-colonies (Broxmeyer et al., 1991a). These results were interpreted to suggest not only that we had underestimated by many fold the actual content for CFU-GEMM and BFU-E in cord blood, but that most cord blood colonies originally having been designated as being BFU-E-derived were in fact CFU-GEMM-derived (Broxmeyer et al., 1991c).

Expansion and Self-Renewal of Hematopoietic Progenitor Cells.

The characteristics that most distinguished hematopoietic stem from multipotential progenitor cells was the stem cell's characteristic of self-renewal. In vitro, self-renewal capacity is estimated by the replating capacity of single colonies. We used the experimental design diagrammed in Figure 1 to demonstrate that the presence of MGF in the primary cultures promoted the self-renewal of CFU-GEMM in umbilical cord blood and adult bone marrow (Carow et al., 1991). An average of approximately 30 colonies (CFU-GM, BFU-E and CFU-GEMM) per plate in secondary dishes formed from single CFU-GEMM replates. These results suggested a degree of self-renewal not previously attributed to CFU-GEMM and demonstrated the promoting activity of MGF for this effect.

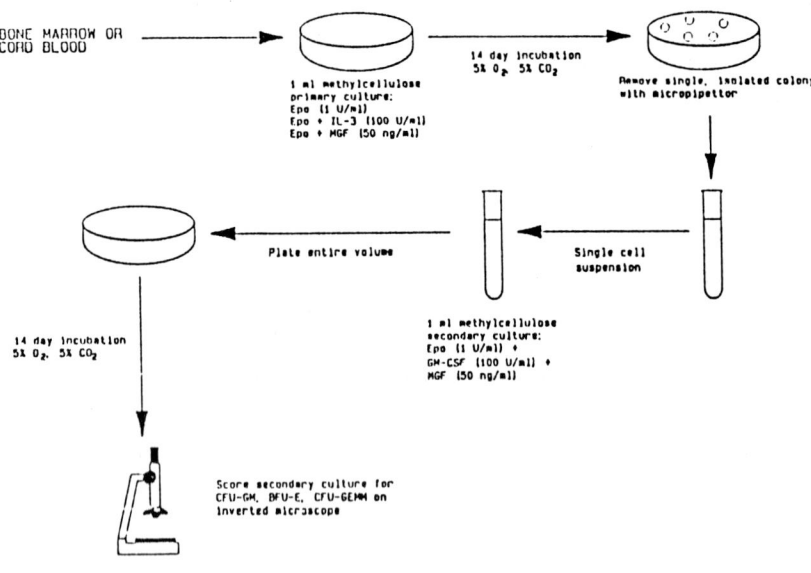

Figure 1

Growth of cells in suspension culture, as shown in Figure 2, has been used as a measure of self-renewal capacity by others, and as a means to evaluate expansion of cells by us and others. This system is not, in our opinion, conducive for evaluating self-renewal and in fact only experiments such as those shown in the design in Figure 1 are appropriate for assessment of this parameter. However, suspension culture assay is appropriate for evaluating expansion of stem and progenitor cells and we have used this methodology to show a 2-3 fold increase in output of hematopoietic progenitor cells compared to starting numbers when low density umbilical cord blood is cultured for 7 days in the presence of 50 ng/ml MGF (Hangoc, Broxmeyer, unpublished observations) as shown in Figure 2.

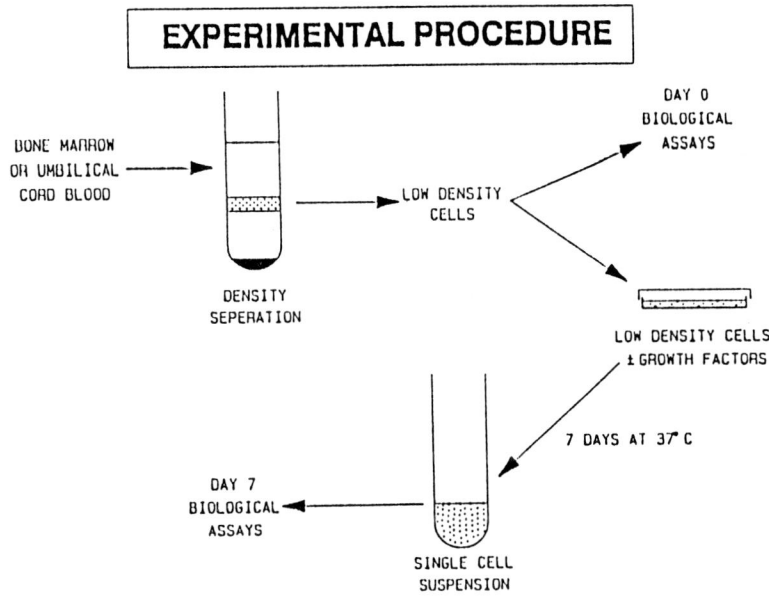

Figure 2

Summary and Conclusions

Umbilical cord blood and placental blood has already been used to successfully engraft 3 patients with Fanconi anemia and 1 patient with juvenile chronic myelogenous leukemia. There is optimism that this alternative source of hematopoietic stem and progenitor cells will be useful for autologous and HLA-matched allogeneic transplantation in a broader range of disorders. While there is a broad range of numbers of hematopoietic progenitor cells in single collections of cord blood, most collections contain numbers in a range well-above those in the collections already used for successful engraftment. This, plus the use of MGF to demonstrate that we had vastly underestimated progenitor cell numbers in cord blood, especially those for CFU-GEMM, and that CFU-GEMM can be replated and thus have a greater degree of self-renewal capacity than previously recognized, suggests that single collections of cord blood should be able to successfully engraft adults as well as children. This of course will need to be tested in a clinical setting. Umbilical cord and placental cells should be appropriate vehicles for future trials with gene transfer/gene therapy. Experiments to evaluate the comparative efficiency of infection by retroviral vectors of cord blood verses adult bone marrow, the current source of cells for such infections, is warranted.

Acknowledgments

These studies were supported by Public Health Service Grants R01 HL46549, R37 CA36464, R01 CA36740 and IT-AM-07519 to HEB. CC is supported by National Institutes of Health Training Grant IT-AM-07519. We thank Rebecca Robling for typing the manuscript.

References

Broxmeyer, H.E. (1982): Hematopoietic stem cells. In *Human Bone Marrow*, ed., S. Trubowitz, E. Davis, pp. 77-123. Boca Raton, Florida: CRC Press.

Broxmeyer, H.E. (1983): Colony assays of hematopoietic progenitor cells and correlations to clinical situations. *CRC Crit. Rev. Oncol/Hematol.* 1, 227-257.

Broxmeyer, H.E. (1991): Self-renewal and migration of stem cells during embryonic and fetal hematopoiesis: Important, but poorly understood events. *Blood Cells*, in press.

Broxmeyer, H.E. Douglas, G.W., Hangoc, G., Cooper, S., Bard, J., English, D., Arny, M., Thomas, L., & Boyse, EA. (1989): Human umbilical cord blood as a potential source of transplantable hematopoietic stem/progenitor cells. *Proc. Natl. Acad. Sci. USA* 86, 3828-3832.

Broxmeyer, H.E., Gluckman, E., Auerbach, A., Douglas, G.W., Friedman, H., Cooper, S., Hangoc, G., Kurtzberg, J., Bard, J., & Boyse, E.A. (1990a): Human umbilical cord blood: A clinically useful source of transplantable hematopoietic stem/progenitor cells. *Int. J. Cell Cloning* 8, 76-91.

Broxmeyer, H.E. Cooper, S., Lu, L., Hangoc, G., Anderson, D., Cosman, D., Lyman, S.D., & Williams, D.E. (1991a): Effect of murine mast cell growth factor (c-*kit* proto-oncogene ligand) on colony formation by human marrow hematopoietic progenitor cells. *Blood* 77, in press.

Broxmeyer, H.E. Kurtzberg, J., Gluckman, E., Auerbach, A.D., Douglas, G., Cooper, S., Falkenburg, J.H.F., Bard, J., & Boyse, E.A. (1991b): Umbilical cord blood hematopoietic stem and repopulating cells in human clinical transplantation. *Blood Cells*, in press.

Broxmeyer, H.E. Cooper, S., & Hangoc, G. (1991c): Growth and responsiveness of human umbilical cord blood myeloid progenitors to mast cell growth factor (MGF, a c-*kit* ligand). *Exp. Hematol.* (Abstract) in press.

Carow C., Hangoc, G., Cooper, S., Williams, D.E., & Broxmeyer, H.E. (1991): Murine mast cell growth factor promotes self-renewal of human myeloid progenitor cells *in vitro*. Exp Hematol (abstract) in press

English D., Cooper, S., Douglas, G., & Broxmeyer, H.E. (1991): Collection and processing cord blood for preservation and hematopoietic transplantation. In *Bone Marrow and Stem Cell Processing: A Manual of Current Techniques*, ed. E. Areman, R.A.S. Acher, H.J. Deeg, Philadelphia: FA Davis, in press.

Fleischhauer, K., Kernan, N.A., O'Reilly, R.J., Dupont, B., & Yang, S.Y. (1990): Bone marrow-allograft rejection by T-lymphocytes recognizing a single amino acid difference in HLA-B44. *New Engl. J. Med.* 323, 1818-1822.

Gabutti, V., Foa, R., Mussa, F., & Aglietta, M. (1975): Behavior of human haematopoietic stem cells in cord and neonatal blood. *Haematologica* 4,60.

Geissler, K., Geissler, W., Hinterberger, W., Lechner, K., & Wurnig, P. (1986): Circulating committed and pluripotential haemopoietic progenitor cells in infants. *Acta Haematol* 75,18-22.

Gluckman, E. Broxmeyer, H.E., Auerbach, A.D., Friedman, H.S., Douglas, G.W., Devergie, A., Esperou, H., Thierry, D., Socie, G., Lehn, P., Cooper, S., English, D., Kurtzberg, J., Bard, J., & Boyse, E.A. (1989): Hematopoietic reconstitution in a patient with Fanconi's anemia by means of umbilical cord blood from an HLA-identical sibling. *Proc. Natl. Acad. Sci. USA* 321,1174-1178.

Hendrie, P.C., Miyazawa, K., Yang, Y-C., Langefeld, C.D., & Broxmeyer, H.E. (1991): Mast cell growth factor (c-*kit* ligand) enhances cytokine stimulation of proliferation of human factor dependent cell line, M07e. *Exp. Hematol.*, in press.

Huang, E. Nocka, K., Beier, D.R., Chu, T.Y., Buck, J., Lahm, H.W., Wellner, D., Leder, P., & Besmer, P. (1991): The hematopoietic growth factor KL is encoded by the Sl locus and is the ligand of the c-*kit* receptor, the gene product of the W locus. *Cell* 63,225-233.

McGlave, P.B. (1991): An expanded role for cord blood transplantation. *Blood Cells*, in press.

Morris, G. (1991): Umbilical cord blood used for BMT. *Oncol. Times* 12(11), 1.

Parham, P. (1991): Making just the right match. *Nature* 350, 111-113.

Tavassoli, M. (1991): Embryonic and fetal hemopoiesis: An overview. *Blood Cells*, in press.

Wagner, J.E., Broxmeyer, H.E., Cooper, S., Zehnbauer, B., Emanuel, P., & Santos, G.W. (1991): Cord blood transplantation after myeloablative therapy in a patient with juvenile chronic myelogenous leukemia. *Exp. Hematol.* (abstract) in press.

Williams, D.E. Eisenman, J., Baird, A., Rauch, C., Van Ness, K., March, C.J., Park, L.S., Martin, U., Mochizuki, D.Y., Boswell, H.S., Burgess, G.S., Cosman, D., & Lyman, S.D. (1990): Identification of a ligand for the c-*kit* proto-oncogene. *Cell* 63, 167-174.

Williams, D.E., Lu, L., & Broxmeyer, H.E. (1987): Characterization of hematopoietic stem and progenitor cells. *Immunologic Res.* 6, 294-304.

Zsebo, K.M., Wypych, J., McNiece, I.K., Lu, H.S., Smith, K.A., Karkare, S.B., Sachdev, R.K., Yuschenkoff, V.N., Birkett, N.C., Williams, L.R., Satyagal, V.N., Tung, W., Bosselman, R.A., Mendiaz, E.A., & Langley, K.E. (1991): Identification, purification, and biological characterization of hematopoietic stem cell factor from buffalo rat liver-conditioned medium. *Cell* 63, 195-201.

RESUME : Le sang de cordon ombilical et le sang de placenta ont déjà été utilisés avec succès pour greffer trois patients avec une anémie de Fanconi et un patient atteint de leucémie myéloïde chronique juvénile. On peut raisonnablement espérer que cette source alternative de cellules souches hématopoïétiques et de cellules progénitrices puisse être utilisée pour des transplantations médullaires autologues ou allogéniques HLA compatibles dans un plus large éventail de pathologies. Si un large nombre de progéniteurs hématopoïétiques sont présents dans un seul prélèvement de sang de cordon, il est intéressant de noter que la plupart des prélèvements contient un nombre de ces progéniteurs largement plus élevé que les prélèvement déjà utilisés avec succès pour les greffes. L'utilisation du Mast Cell Growth Factor (MGF) a permis de démontrer que la quantité de progéniteurs présents dans un sang de cordon était jusqu'à présent très sous-estimée, en particulier pour ce qui concerne les CFU-GEMM ; Ces CFU-GEMM peuvent être repiqués, faisant ainsi preuve d'une capacité d'autorenouvellement d'un degré supérieur à ce qui avait été établi au préalable. Ces éléments suggèrent qu'un seul prélèvement de sang de cordon pourrait permettre de greffer avec succès tant les adultes que les enfants. Ceci devra bien-sûr être testé selon un protocole clinique. Les cellules de sang de cordon et de placenta pourraient constituer des cibles appropriées pour de futurs essais de transfert de gène et de thérapie génique. Des travaux en cours tentent d'évaluer l'efficacité comparative d'infection par les vecteurs rétroviraux des cellules de sang de cordon par rapport à des cellules de moelle adulte qui constituent actuellement le substratum de telles infections.

A human PBL/immunodeficient mouse model for *in vivo* preclinical studies of human gene therapy

Claudio Bordignon, Giuliana Ferrari, Silvano Rossini, Raffaella Giavazzi [1], Eli Gilboa [2] and Fulvio Mavilio

Istituto Scientifico H.S. Raffaele, Milano, Italy; [1] *Istituto di Ricerche Farmacologiche «Mario Negri» Bergamo, Italy;* [2] *Memorial Sloan-Kettering Cancer Center, New York, NY, USA*

INTRODUCTION

Gene therapy is based on the assumption that definitive cure for a genetic disease should be possible by directing treatment to the abnormal gene rather than to secondary effects of its products (Anderson, 1984; Parkman, 1986; Friedmann, 1989). Complementation of the altered gene can be obtained by introducing the normal gene into the cell genome by an appropriate vector. Several studies have demonstrated that retroviral vectors can be used successfully to introduce exogenous DNA sequences into hematopoietic progenitors and pluripotent stem cells. At least in the mouse model system, efficient gene transfer *in vitro* and *in vivo* has been reported (Keller, et al., 1985; Eglitis, et al., 1985; Bender, et al., 1989; Belmont, et al., 1986; Williams, et al., 1986; Belmont, et al., 1988; Wilson, et al., 1990). However, only low levels of gene transfer were achieved in cultured hematopoietic progenitors derived from dogs and primates (Kwok, et al., 1986; Wolfe, et al., 1990; Bodine, et al., 1990; Kantoff, et al. 1987). and only few studies have succeeded in demonstrating significant levels of expression of the transduced gene in cultured progenitor cells of human origin (Gruber, et al. 1985; Hock and Miller, 1986; Bordignon, et al., 1989).

Deficiency of the enzyme adenosine deaminase (ADA) results in a variant of severe combined immunodeficiency (SCID), a lethal disorder usually treated with allogeneic bone marrow transplantation (O'Reilly et al., 1989). This is the first genetic disorder considered for the clinical application of human somatic cell gene therapy (Anderson, 1984; Parkman, 1986; Friedmann, 1989; Gershon, 1990; Culliton, 1990). Although several studies in the murine model indicated that retroviral vectors can be used for the efficient gene transfer and expression of the ADA gene (Belmont, et al., 1986; Williams, et al.; 1986; Belmont, et al., 1988; Wilson, et al., 1990), no available data indicate that restoration of enzyme activity will result in reconstitution of immune functions. Recently, an alternative treatment, enzyme replacement with extracellular polyethylene glycol-conjugated bovine enzyme, has been tested in patients affected with this disease (Hershfield, et al., 1987). Although the therapeutic results of this treatment were variable, they supply a direct evidence that high levels of circulating enzyme can restore lymphocyte numbers and several immune functions (Levy, et al., 1988; Bordignon et al, in preparation).

A long term objective of our studies is to develop an efficient gene transfer system for the introduction of the human ADA gene into ADA deficient (ADA⁻) human cells. We previously showed that N2-based retroviral vectors were able to transduce the human ADA gene with high efficiency into established lymphoid cell lines derived from ADA⁻SCID patients (Kantoff, et al., 1986). On the other hand, only low levels of gene transfer and transient expression of the human enzyme were achieved when lethally irradiated *cynomolgus* monkeys were reconstituted with autologous marrow cells transduced with this vector (Kantoff, et al., 1987). Subsequently, the efficiency of progenitor cell transduction was improved *in vitro* in both short and long term culture, with expression of the newly introduced ADA enzyme occurring in both myeloid and lymphoid lineages (Bordignon, et al., 1989). However, in neither system direct evidence was available that expression of ADA activity in ADA⁻ cells would restore specific immune functions. To address this issue, ADA⁻PBL from SCID patients were infected with a retroviral vector expressing human ADA and subsequently injected into immunodeficient mice. Long term evaluation of the fate and function of the transduced cells is described in the following sections.

THE IN VIVO MODEL FOR ADA GENE TRANSFER INTO HUMAN CELLS

Recently, an animal model for functional *in vivo* analysis of the human immune system has been proposed, in which immunodeficient mice (SCID or BNX, i.e., homozygous $bg/nu/x^{id}$) were reconstituted with human peripheral blood lymphocytes (Mosier, et al., 1988; Kamel-Reid and Dick, 1988; Mc Cune et al. 1988). We have modified this model for application to gene transfer for ADA deficiency (Fig.1). A number of BNX mice were reconstituted with human ADA⁻PBL transduced with a human ADA gene containing retroviral vector (DCA: double-copy ADA) (Hantzopoulos, et al., 1989).

A total of twelve BNX mice were injected with either DCA-infected (eight) or mock-infected ADA⁻PBL (four). Twenty BNX mice were reconstituted with normal PBL as controls for the efficiency of reconstitution. Survival and function of human cells were monitored biweekly by assaying the level of human immunoglobulins (hu-IgG) in the recipients peripheral blood. Only one out of the 8 animals treated with DCA-infected ADA⁻PBL, showed no detectable level of hu-IgG. All others were positive, with values ranging from 3.7 to 672.1 mg/dl (median 48.0, control levels < 1 mg/dl). No hu-IgG were detected in peripheral blood of all recipients treated with mock-infected ADA⁻ PBL at 6-10 wks from injection. Low levels of hu-IgG were observed in only one of these animals, 2 wks after injection. Four out of the 20 animals reconstituted with normal adult PBL had no detectable levels of hu-IgG at 6 wks, whereas all others were positive, with values ranging from 3.1 to 429.0 mg/dl (median 29.8).

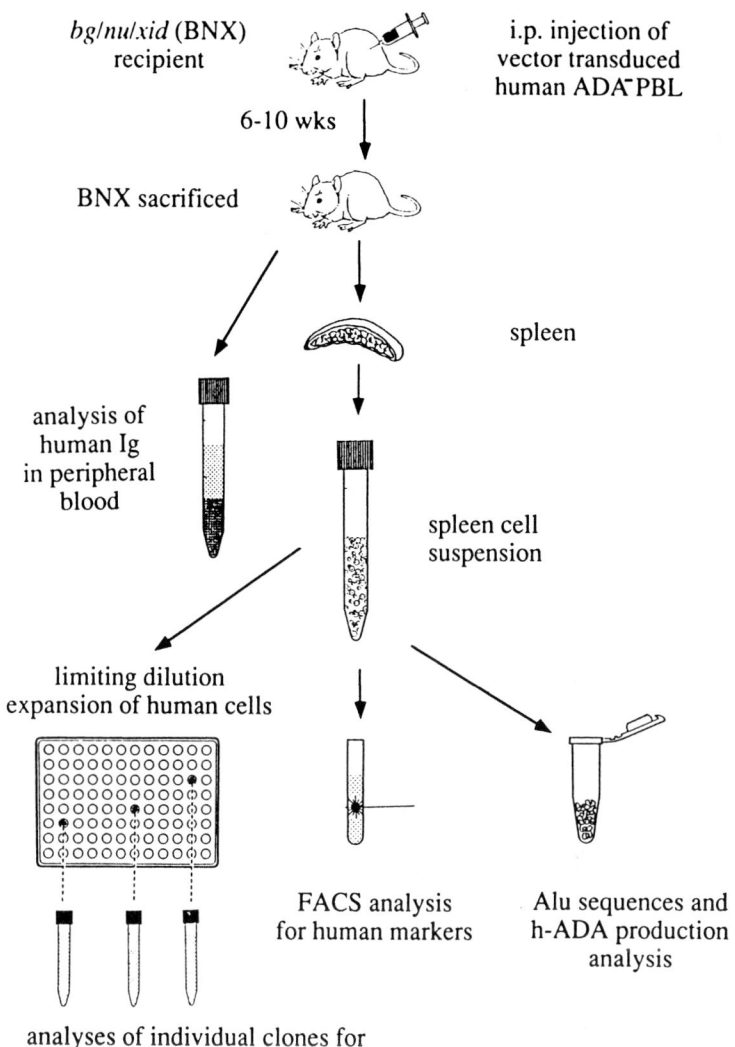

Fig.1 General outline of the model utilized in the study

All recipient animals were sacrificed 6 to 10 wks after treatment for analysis of human cell survival, hu-ADA activity, and immune functions.

IDENTIFICATION OF HUMAN CELLS AND HUMAN ADA IN BNX MICE

In vivo long term survival of human cells in the recipient BNX mice was demonstrated by the presence of human *Alu* sequences in the DNA extracted from the spleen of 3 animals reconstituted with vector-transduced ADA⁻PBL. Similar percentage of successful reconstitution at 6-10 wks was observed in the pool of control mice treated with normal adult PBL. Persistence of human cells was never observed in animals injected with mock-infected ADA⁻PBL, suggesting that intracellular expression of ADA is necessary for human cell survival. In a few cases, animals with detectable serum levels of hu-IgG showed no signal for *Alu* sequences in spleen DNA, suggesting that B and possibly T cells may either circulate or colonize different organs in BNX mice.

In the peripheral blood and spleen of BNX recipients, human cells were detected at very low frequency by FACS analysis with monoclonal antibodies against human cell surface markers. Detection of CD4+ human T cells in the spleen of a recipient BNX mouse, 6 wks after reconstitution was estimated at approximately 4%. In order to reduce artefacts due to non specific antibody binding, appropriate controls were included in the FACS analyses. The only other cell surface marker repeatedly detected at very low frequency (~2%) was the human CD20.

Production of human ADA in *Alu*-positive spleens from mice treated with DCA-infected cells was assayed by cellulose acetate (Cellogel) electrophoresis (Khan, 1971), followed by enzymatic staining. In this assay, human and mouse ADA enzymes can be distinguished by their different electrophoretic mobility. Human ADA activity was clearly detected in spleen samples of three recipients injected with DCA-infected ADA⁻ PBL. No human ADA band was observed in spleen lysates from animals treated with mock-infected ADA⁻ PBL, as well as from control untreated mice.

IN VIVO FREQUENCY OF HUMAN IYMPHOCYTES AND EX VIVO ANALYSES

In order to detect survival of human lymphocytes and further analyze the population of human cells surviving in BNX mice we attempted to expand both T and B human lymphocytes from spleens and peritoneal lavages of 5 animals reconstituted with DCA-infected ADA⁻PBL, and of 3 animals treated with mock-infected ADA⁻PBL. Human T cells were obtained from the spleens of BNX recipients reconstituted with DCA vector-transduced ADA⁻PBL, but never from animals treated with mock-infected ADA⁻PBL. These T cell clones were positive for human CD3 and CD4, confirming the human nature of the expanded cells. Furthermore, HLA typing confirmed the patient origin of the expanded cells. Frequency of human clonable T cells was variable in different reconstituted animals, spleens from 2 animals failed to give any clonable cells.

The availability of expanded populations of human cells from the spleens of repopulated BNX recipients enabled us to evaluate the frequency of clones positive for the presence of vector DNA. Only one clone (# 92) out of 58 clones obtained from the spleen of an animal reconstituted with DCA-infected ADA⁻ PBL tested negative for the presence of DCA vector, as analyzed by polymerase chain reaction (PCR) and vector-derived ADA activity. All other clones tested showed the expected 415 bp Neo-specific band, amplified by PCR. Control hybridization to a Neo radioactive probe confirmed the specificity of the amplified band. In addition, all PCR-positive clones showed high levels of vector-derived ADA activity, when compared to normal controls.

Ten clones were expanded for Southern blot analysis of the proviral sequences integrated in genomic DNA. Specifically, DNA from clones # 56, 70, 82, 52, 45, 89, 15, 76, 31, 94 were digested with the restriction enzyme *Xba I*, which cuts twice in the both 5' and 3' LTRs of the DCA provirus, and with *Hind III*, which does not cut in the proviral genome, and tested in Southern with a Neo-specific probe. A single 5.3 Kb band was observed when DNA was digested with *XbaI*, corresponding to the expected size for the intact integrated provirus. When DNA was digested with *Hind III*, a major band was obtained in clones # 56, 70, 82, 45 and 15, indicating the clonal nature of the cells expanded *in vitro*. Lane corresponding to clone # 89 showed two comparably intense bands. Lane corresponding to clones # 52, 76, 31 and 94 showed no prominent integration band, although they were all positive when digested with *Xba I*, indicating the presence of many independent integrations in these cells. This probably correlated with cell dilution in the cloning procedure since clones # 52, 76, 31 and 94 were obtained by plating 1,000 spleenocytes/well, while clones # 56, 70, 82, 45, 89 and 15 were obtained by plating 100 spleenocytes/well. Comparative analysis of the *Hind III* patterns showed the presence of bands with apparently the same molecular weight in different clones, suggesting that at least in some cases T cells may have originated from common progenitors.

11 attempts to establish EBV-transformed B-lymphoblastoid continuous cell lines from animals reconstituted with DCA-infected ADA⁻PBL were not successful. Positive proliferating foci were observed from cells obtained from peritoneal lavages. However, they failed to grow to continuous cell lines. Sufficient cell numbers, necessary for biochemical or molecular analyses were never obtained. Whether this was due to lack of DCA vector infection of ADA⁻B lymphocytes, or refractoriness of vector-transduced B cells to EBV transformation, could not be determined.

ANTIGEN-SPECIFIC IMMUNE RESPONSES IN RECONSTITUTED MICE.

We tested the capacity of vector-transduced ADA⁻PBL to express antigen-specific immune responses in our *in vivo* model. Vector-infected ADA⁻PBL used in the experiment of figure 8 were obtained from a patient undergoing enzyme-replacement treatment with PEG-ADA. The patient showed reconstitution of specific immune functions. In particular, after vaccination with tetanus toxoid (tt) both *in vivo* production of specific antibodies and *in vitro* proliferation of specific T cells were observed. Therefore, we reasoned that if human tt-specific precursor T cells from this patient had been successfully transduced with the vector, they could survive in the recipient animal and be expanded by specific stimulation with tt. A reconstituted mouse was immunized with tt plus tt-pulsed patient irradiated PBL (as antigen presenting cells). Two wks later, spleen cells were obtained and restimulated, with tt-pulsed irradiated PBL autologous to the patient. In this experiment limiting dilution was not performed because of the limited number of the patient PBL available as irradiated feeders. Thirty out of 33 T cell lines tested showed specific proliferative response to tt-pulsed, but not to unpulsed antigen presenting cells. All the tt-specific T cell lines showed high levels of vector-derived ADA activity as measured by adenosine to inosine conversion.

The capacity of the transduced human cells to produce specific immune responses was confirmed by the increased production of antigen-specific human IgG. In the animal reported above (#727) a three fold increase in the levels of circulating tt-specific human IgG was observed 2 wks after *in vivo* restimulation with tt and tt-pulsed PBL autologous to the patient.

CONCLUSIONS AND PROSPECTS.

Due to the absence of a suitable animal model, analyses of the effects of retroviral vector-mediated ADA gene transfer could not be performed in murine and primate models beyond the evaluation of the levels of gene expression (Belmont, et al., 1986; Williams et al., 1986; Belmont, et al., 1988; Wilson, et al., 1990; Know, et al, 1986; Wolfe, et al., 1990; Bodine, et al., 1990;;   Kantoff, et al, 1987; Bordignon, et al., 1989). We have described efficient retroviral vector based gene transfer systems for the introduction of the human ADA gene into bone marrow cells and peripheral blood lymphocytes derived from ADA deficient SCID patients (Bordignon, et al., 1989).

In the *in vivo* model described here, key evidence was obtained indicating that a gene therapy approach to ADA$^-$SCID could be potentially successful. First, ADA$^-$B and T lymphocytes transduced with an ADA-expressing retroviral vector are capable of relatively long survival *in vivo*. Proliferation and expansion of human lymphocytes in recipient animals could not be formally demonstrated. However, analysis of vector integration in the progeny of cells derived from the spleen of at least one reconstituted animal showed different clones sharing common integration sites. This suggests that cell proliferation may indeed have occurred *in vivo* in BNX mice, although the possibility that infected cells underwent clonal expansion during the infection procedure *in vitro*, before injection into recipient animals, cannot be formally ruled out. Second, correction of the ADA deficiency by expression of a functional, vector-derived enzyme, is apparently sufficient to restore normal T-cell functions, including antigen-specific immune response.

In this regard, previous clinical studies on the efficacy of PEG-ADA treatment have demonstrated that good levels of detoxification of the extracellular environment may produce reconstitution of the lymphocyte populations and of several immune functions (Hershfield, et al., 1987; Levy, et al., 1988; Bordignon, et al., in preparation). However, the intracellular presence of the enzyme confers to the positively transduced lymphocytes a significant advantage over non-transduced cells. In fact, in the mouse model, regardless of the presence of a detoxified environment, a strong selective advantage of vector-transduced cells, expressing intracellular ADA, over non-transduced cells was suggested by the analysis of clones obtained *ex-vivo*. Finally, although we were unable to grow and study human B lymphocytes from reconstituted mice, the available evidence indicates that B-cells from the patient survive *in vivo* where they can be stimulated to produce specific immunoglobulins.

In this study we have evaluated the therapeutic potential of vector transduced peripheral blood lymphocytes. If the strategy utilizing peripheral blood lymphocytes will be followed in the clinical application of the procedure, as already suggested by some authors (Gershon, 1990; Culliton, 1990; Kasid, et al., 1990), the possibility exists that the procedure will have to be repeated periodically. On the other hand, the chimeric status of non-conditioned ADA$^-$SCID patients treated with allogeneic bone marrow transplantation indicated that long-term immune reconstitution could by provided by donor T lymphocytes, while all other cell lineages, including B-lymphocytes were of host origin (7). The latter observation may suggest that long term reconstitution of T cells and T cell functions could come from either marrow or peripheral blood lymphocyte precursors.

Bone marrow cells and peripheral blood lymphocytes derived from ADA deficient SCID patients lack the ability to respond to non-specific proliferative stimuli such as IL-2 and PHA and to specific antigens. The restoration of PHA and IL-2 response, together with the *in vivo* production of human IgG and stimulation of antigen-specific T lymphocytes and IgG in immunodeficient recipient mice reconstituted with DCA-infected cells, present additional evidence as to the physiological relevance of this gene transfer system. For patients failing therapy with PEG-ADA the gene therapy approach may represent a safe an efficacious alternative of therapeutic potential.

ACKNOWLEDGMENTS

This work was supported by Grants awarded by the Italian National Council for Research (CNR: PF:Biotecnologie, PF:Ingegneria Genetica), by the Italian Association for Cancer Research (AIRC), and by the IV AIDS Project of the Istituto Superiore di Sanità.

REFERENCES

Anderson. W. F., Prospects for Human Gene Therapy, *Science*. 226, 401 (1984).

Belmont J.W., Henkel-Tigges J. Stephen M. W. Chang, Wager-Smith Karen, Rodney E. Kellems, Dick J. E., Magli M. C., Phillips R. A., Bernstein A. & Caskey C. T., Expression of human adenosine deaminase in murine haematopoietic progenitor cells following retroviral transfer, *Nature*. 322, 385 (1986).

Belmont J. W., MacGregor G., Wager-Smith K., Fletcher F. A., Moore K. A., Hawkins D., Villalon D., Chang S.M.W. and Caskey C. T., Expression of Human Adenosine Deaminase in Murine Hematopoietic Cells, *Mol. and Cel. Biol.* 8, 5116 (1988).

Bender M. A., Gelinas R.E., Miller A.D., A Majority of Mice Show Long-Term Expression of a Human ß-Globin Gene after Retrovirus Transfer into Hematopoietic Stem Cells,.*Mol. Cell. Biol.* 9, 1426 (1989).

Bodine M.B., Mc Donagh K.T., Brandt S.J., Ney P.A., Agricola B., Byrne E., Nienhuis A.W., Development of a high-titer retrovirus producer cell line capable of gene transfer into rhesus monkey hematopietic stem cells., *Proc. Natl. Acad. Sci USA..* 87, 3738 (1990).

Bordignon C., Yu S.F., Smith C.A., Hantzopoulos P., Ungers G.E., Keever C.A., O'Reilly R.J., Gilboa E., Retroviral vector-mediated high-efficiency expression of adenosine deaminase (ADA) in hematopoietic long-term cultures of ADA-deficient marrow cells, *Proc. Natl. Acad. Sci. USA.* 86, 6748 (1989).

Eglitis M. A., Kantoff P., Gilboa E., Anderson W.F., Gene Expression in Mice After High Efficiency Retroviral-Mediated Gene Transfer, *Science.* 230, 1395 (1985).

Friedmann.T., Progress Toward Human Gene Therapy, *Science* 244, 1275 (1989).

Gershon. D. (in: news) *Nature* 346, 402 (1990)

Culliton B.J.(in: news and comment) *Science* 246, 974 (1990).

Gruber H. E., Finley K.D., Hershberg R.M., Katzman S.S., Laikind P.K., Seegmiller J.E., Retroviral Vector-Mediated Gene Transfer into Hematopoietic Progenitor Cells. *Science.* 230, 1057 (1985).

Hantzopoulos P.A., Sullenger B.A., Ungers G., Gilboa. E., Improved gene expression upon transfer of the adenosine deaminase minigene outside the transcriptional unit of a retroviral vector, *Proc. Natl. Acad. Sci. USA* 86, 3519 (1989).

Hershfield M.S., Buckley R.H., Greenberg M.L., Melton A.L., Schiff R., Hatem C., Kurtzberg J., Markert M.L., Kobnayashi R.H., Kobayashi A.L., Abuchowski A., Treatment of adenosine deaminase deficiency with polyethylene glycol-modified adenosine deaminase, *N.Engl. J. Med.* 316, 589 (1987).

Hock R.A., Miller A.D., Retrovirus -mediated transfer and expression of drug resistance genes in human hematopoietic progenitor cells, *Nature.* 320, 275 (1986).

Kantoff P. W., Kohn D.K., Mitsuya H., Armentano D., Sieberg M.; Zwiebel J.A., Eglitis M.A., McLachlin J.R., Wiginton D.A., Hutton J.J., Horowitw S.D., Gilboa E., Blaese R.M., Anderson W.F., Correction of adenosine deaminase deficiency in cultured human T and B cells by retrovirus-mediated gene transfer, *Proc. Natl. Acad. Sci. USA.* 83, 6563 (1986).

Kantoff P. W., Gillio A.P., McLachlin J.R., Bordignon C., Eglitis M.A., Kernan N.A., Moen R.C., Kohn D.B., Yu S.F., Karson E, Karlsson S., Zwiebel J.A., Gilboa E., Blease R.M., Nienhuis A., O'Reilly R.J., Anderson W.F., Expression of uman adenosine deaminase in nonhuman primates after retrovirus-mediated gene transfer, *J. Exp. Med.* 166, 219 (1987).

Kasid A., Morecki S., Aebersold P., Cornetta K., Culver K., Freeman S., Director E., Lotze M.T., Blaese R.M., Anderson W.F., Rosenberg S.A., Human gene transfer: Characterization of human tumor-infiltrating lymphocytes as vehicles for retroviral-mediated gene transfer in man, *Proc. Natl. Acad. Sci. USA.* 87, 473 (1990).

Khan. P.M., Enzyme Electrophoresis on Cellulose Acetate Gel: Zymogram Patterns in Man-Mouse and Man-Chinese Hamster Somatic Cell Hybrids, *Arch. Biochem. Biophys* **145**, 470 (1971).

Keller G., Paige C., Gilboa E., Wagner E.S., Expression of a foreign gene in myeloid and lymphoid cells derived from multipotent haematopoietic precursors, *Nature* **318**, 149 (1985).

Kwok W. W., F. Schuening, R. B. Stead, A. D. Miller, Retroviral transfer of genes into canine hemopoietic progenitor cells in cultrure: A model for human gene therapy, *Proc. Natl. Acad. Sci. USA*. **83**, 4552 (1986).

Levy Y., Hershfield M.S., Fernandez-Mejia C., Polmar S.H., Scudiery D., Berger M., Soresen R.U, Adenosine deaminase deficiency with late onset of recurrent infections: Response to treatment with polyethylene glycol-modified adenosine deaminase, *J. Ped.* **113**, 312 (1988). C. Bordignon *et al.*, in preparation.

Mosier D.E., Gulizia R.G., Baird S.M., Wilson D.B., Transfer of a functional human immune system to mice with severe combined immunodeficiency, *Nature*. **335**, 256 (1988).

O'Reilly R.J., Keever C.A., Small T.N., Brochstein - J., The use of HLA-non-identical t-cell-depleted marrow transplants for correction of severe combined immunodeficiency disease, *Immunodef.Rev.* **1**, 273 (1989).

Parkman. R., The Application of Bone Marrow Transpantation to the Treatment of Genetic Disease, *Science* **232**, 1373 (1986).

Kamel-Reid S., Dick J.E., Engraftment of Immune-Deficient Mice with Human Hematopoietic Stem Cells, *Science*. **242**, 1706 (1988).

McCune J.M., Namikawa R., Kaneshima H., Shultz L.D., Lieberman M., Weissman I.L, The SCID-hu Mouse: Murine Model for the Analysis of Human Hematolymphoid Differentiation and Function, *Science* **241**, 1632 (1988).

Williams D. A., S.H. Orkin, R.C. Mulligan, Retrovirus-mediated transfer of human adenosine deaminase gene sequences into cells in culture and into murine hematopoietic cells in vivo, *Proc. Natl. Acad. Sci. USA*. **83**, 2566 (1986).

Wilson J. M., Danos O., Grossman M., Raulet D.H., Mulligan R.C., Expression of human adenosine deaminase in mice reconstituted with retrovirus-trasduced hematopoietic stem cells, *Proc. Natl. Acad. Sci. USA*. **87**, 439 (1990).

Wolfe J.H., Schuchman E.H., Stramm L.E., Concaugh E.A., Haskins M.E., Aguirre G.D., Patterson D.F., Desnick R.J., Gilboa E., Restoration of normal lysosomal function in mucopolysaccharidosis type VII cells by retroviral vector-mediated gene transfer, *Proc.Natl. Acad Sci. USA* **87**, 2877 (1990).

RESUME : L'objectif à long terme de nos travaux consiste à développer un système de transfert de gène efficace afin d'introduire le gène humain de l'ADA à l'intérieur de cellules humaines déficientes en ADA (ADA⁻). Nous avons déjà pu démontrer que des vecteurs rétroviraux basés sur la structure N2 étaient capables de transduire un gène humain d'ADA avec une grande efficacité dans des cellules lymphoides établies en lignées dérivées de patients ADA-SCID. D'autre part, l'efficacité de transduction de cellules progénitrices hématopoiétiques a pu être améliorée in-vitro sur des cultures à court et à long terme suivies de l'expression de l'enzyme nouvellement introduit à la fois dans les lignées myéloides et lymphoides. Cependant, dans aucun des systèmes une restauration des fonctions immunitaires consécutive au rétablissement de l'expression de l'activité ADA dans les cellules ADA⁻ n'a pu être démontrée. Afin de résoudre cette question, des lymphocytes du sang périphérique ADA⁻ issus de patients SCID ont été infectés avec un vecteur rétroviral exprimant l'ADA humaine puis injectés dans des souris immunodéficientes, dans le cas présent, il s'agit de souris BNX, homozygotes pour les mutations bg/nu/x^{id}. L'évaluation à long terme du devenir et de la fonction des cellules transduites est décrite en détail.

Expression of adenosine deaminase in genetically corrected T lymphocytes from an ADA⁻ SCID patient

Eric Braakman [1, 2*], Victor W. van Beusechem [2], Brigitte A. van Krimpen [1], Alain Fischer [3], Reinder L.H. Bolhuis [1, 4] and Dinko Valerio [2]

[1] *Department of Immunology of the Dr. Daniel den Hoed Clinic, Rotterdam, The Netherlands;* [2] *Gene Therapy section of the Institute of Applied Radiobiology and Immunology, Rijswijk, The Netherlands;* [3] *Département de Pédiatrie, Hôpital Necker-Enfants-Malades, Paris, France;* [4] *Institute of Applied Radiobiology and Immunology, Rijswijk, The Netherlands*
* Author for correspondence

SUMMARY

Mature T lymphocytes derived from the peripheral blood of a patient with documented severe combined immunodeficiency (SCID) resulting from adenosine deaminase (ADA) deficiency were expanded *in vitro*. The human ADA (hADA) gene was introduced in these replicating T lymphocytes with the use of an amphotropic recombinant retrovirus carrying the hADA gene. Subsequently, infected T lymphocytes were selected on basis of their ADA expression, by exposure to a combination of the toxic agent xylofuranosyl-adenine (Xyl-A) and the specific ADA inhibitor 2'-deoxycoformycin (dCF). Following two consecutive selection steps, the resulting population of T lymphocytes were shown to contain intact copies of the provirus, to express normal levels of hADA and to be resistant to the toxic effects of both 2'-deoxyadenosine (dAdo) and Xyl-A. On basis of these findings we estimate that 80-90% of the selected cells were succesfully transduced with the functional hADA gene.

INTRODUCTION

Adenosine deaminase (ADA) deficiency is an inherited condition that results in severe combined immunodeficiency (SCID) (Hirshhorn,1983; Thompson and Seegmiller, 1980). ADA is an enzym of the purine metabolism. Its catalytic activity drives the deamination of adenosine or deoxyadenosine (dAdo) to inosine or deoxyinosine, respectively. In the absence of ADA, dAdo accumulates and may be phosphorylated by adenosine kinases to deoxy ATP. It has been suggested that the intracellular accumulation of deoxy ATP results in inhibition of DNA synthesis and cell death (Thompson and Seegmiller, 1980; Carson et al., 1981) In comparison with other cell types, T lymphocytes express high concentrations of adenosine kinases and are therefore primarily affected. The humoral dysfunction in ADA⁻SCID is believed to be a secondary defect related to the absence of helper T cells necessary for an antibody response.

ADA⁻SCID patients usually die within the first years of life from recurrent opportunistic infections, unless immune functions are restored. Currently, ADA⁻SCID disease is treated with bone marrow transplantation (Wijnaendts et al., 1989). Complete immunologic reconstitution has been obtained in ADA⁻SCID patients by HLA-identical bone marrow transplantation (BMT)(Fischer et al., 1986; Silber et al., 1987). However, this treatment fails in 30-50 per cent of the cases because of graft failure or Graft versus Host (GvH) disease, after HLA non-identical BMT (Wijnaendts et al., 1989; O'Reilly et al., 1989). Recently, 19 ADA⁻SCID patients have been treated with an experimental enzym replacement therapy using bovine ADA coupled to polyethylene glycol (PEG-ADA) (Hershfield et al., 1987; levy et al., 1988). Because the toxic substrate dAdo is freely diffusible over cell membranes the infused PEG-ADA can detoxify the patients serum from the toxic dAdo without entering the patient's cells. The detoxification is accompanied by a gradual increase in the number of T lymphocytes in peripheral blood. Although partial restoration of immune functions have been observed, a significant problem appears to be the development of PEG-ADA neutralizing antibodies in some of the patients (Lee et al., 1990). Therefore, alternative or additional therapies for the treatment of ADA⁻SCID need to be developed.

For several reasons, gene therapy is considered to be an alternative therapy for ADA⁻SCID. Firstly, the possible risks of gene therapy protocols counterbalance the lethal nature of the disease and the inadequacy of the available therapies. Secondly, preclinical studies in mice and non-human primates demonstrated the feasibility to introduce and express the ADA gene in hemopoietic cells without any toxic side effects of the gene therapy protocol (Valerio et al., 1989; Van Beusechem et al., 1990; our own unpublished observations). Thirdly, precise and organ-specific control of ADA expression is probably not required for a curative effect, because large variation of ADA levels exist in healthy individuals (Thompson and Seegmiller, 1980).

The best gene therapy strategy would be to introduce the hADA gene into pluripotent hemopoietic stem cells residing in bone marrow. These hADA transduced stem cells would than continuously give rise to mature hemopoietic cells of all lineages that could repopulate the lymphoid compartments of the patient. Such a protocol would result in the permanent cure of the disease. However, retroviral gene transfer appears to occur only in cells that are activily replicating (Miller et al., 1990). Stem cells do not vigorously replicate and may lose (part of) their pluripotent nature once they start dividing.

One step removed from the ultimate gene therapy of stem cells is the introduction and expression of the hADA gene into mature T lymphocytes. The T lymphocytes that appear in the circulation of PEG-ADA treated ADA⁻SCID patients offers this possibility. Circulating T lymphocytes can be isolated, expanded to adequate numbers *in vitro*, infected with the recombinant ADA virus and selected on basis of their ADA expression. Reinfusion of such genetically corrected T lymphocytes into the patient can be expected to have a therapeutic effect either directly when enough different hADA-gene transduced T lymphocytes have been infused to

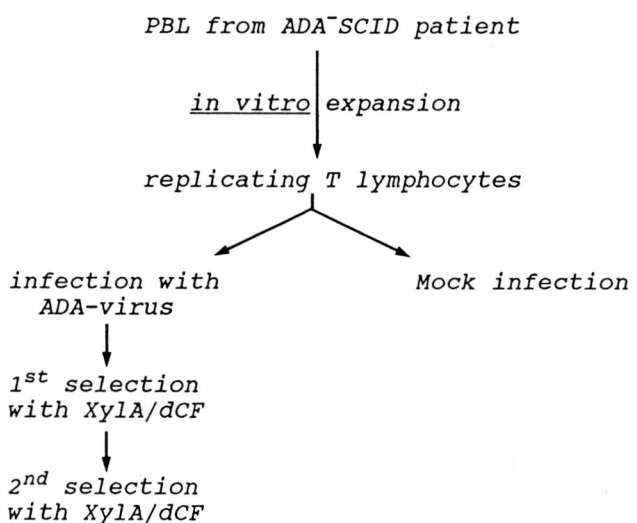

Fig. 1. Experimental approach to obtain genetically corrected T lymphocytes from an ADA⁻SCID patient.

restore some immunological functions or indirectly by detoxifying deoxyadenosine that diffuses from extracellular sites and thereby allowing endogenous hemopoiesis. The life span and homing of the reinfused, hADA-gene transduced T lymphocytes will determine the succes and duration of the therapeutic effect.

EXPERIMENTAL APPROACH

The experimental approach to obtain hADA gene transduced T lymphocytes from an ADA⁻SCID patient is schematically depicted in Fig.1. Peripheral blood leukocytes (PBL) were obtained from a two year old girl suffering from ADA⁻SCID. She had been treated with PEG-ADA for seven months at the time of blood collection, which resulted in an increase in her number of circulating $CD3^+$ T lymphocytes to $360/mm^3$. PBL were expanded in vitro under optimal culture conditions with the lectin phytohemagglutinin (PHA) and irradiated feeder cells as described earlier (Van de Griend et al., 1984a; Van de Griend et al., 1984b). Cells were harvested and replated with irradiated feeder cells and PHA-containing medium at weekly intervals. After two weeks of culture, cells had expanded over 3000-fold, yielding adequate numbers of exponentially growing cells. Virtually all of these cells were $CD3^+$/T cell receptor $(TCR)\alpha\beta^+$ T lymphocytes, half of them were $CD4^+CD8^-$, the other half $CD4^-CD8^+$. A small percentage of the cells were characterized to be $CD3^+/TCR\gamma\delta^+$.

The hADA gene was introduced in these rapidly replicating T cells with the use of our amphotropic recombinant virus carrying the

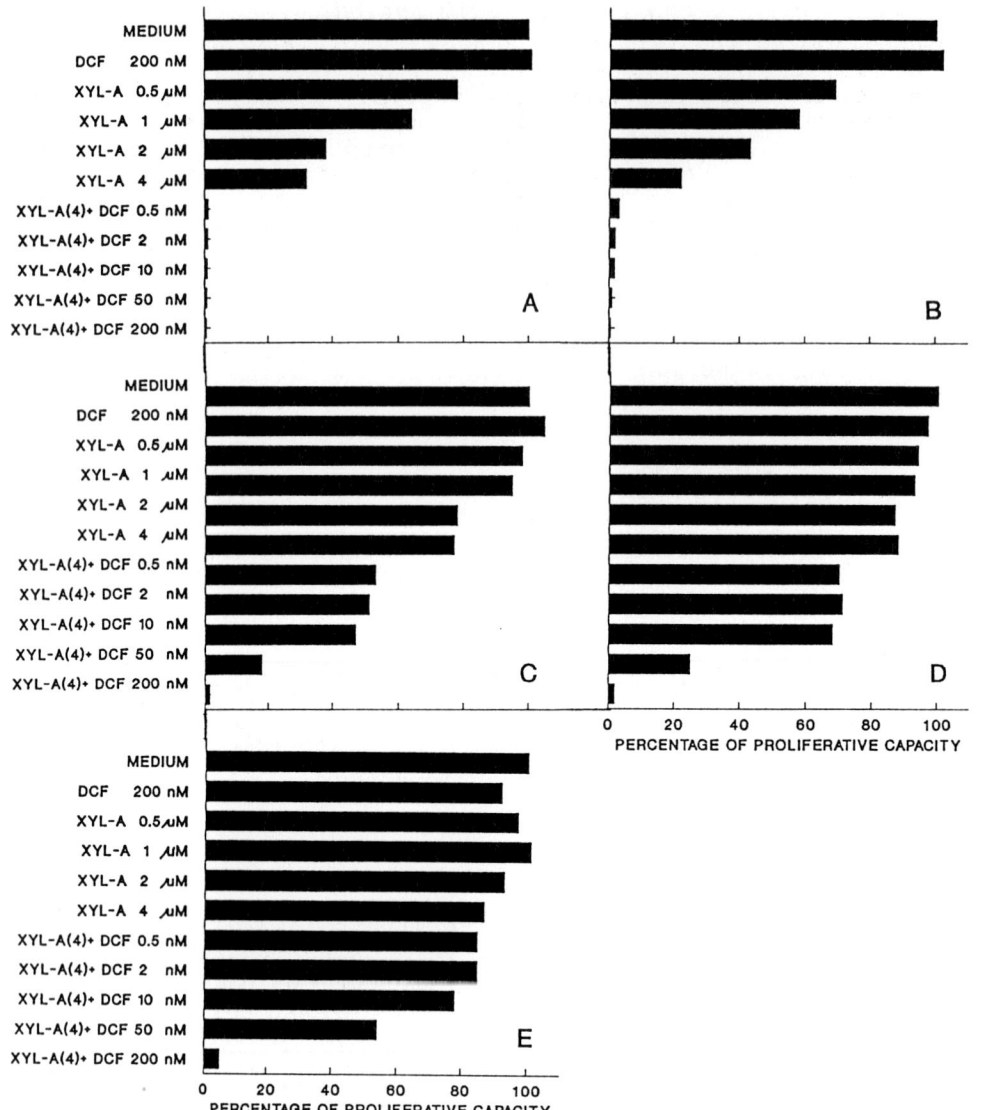

Fig. 2. Relative IL-2 induced proliferation in selective media. T lymphocytes were cultured at 4×10^4 cells per well in serum free medium + 50 U/ml r.IL-2 in the presence or absence of various concentrations Xyl-A and dCF. Cells were cultured for 48 hours, ^{3}H thymidine was added during the last 18 hr. of culture. Results are expressed as a mean value of quadruplicate cultures under selective pressure in comparison to the medium control. A-D; ADA$^-$ SCID T cells; A) mock-infected; B) ADA-virus-infected; C) ADA-virus-infected + selected; D) ADA-virus-infected + twice selected; E) T cell clone (D11) derived from a healthy individual.

hADA gene (LgAL(Δ Mo+PyF101; Van Beusechem et al., 1990). Transcription of the hADA gene in this virus is under control of a hybrid long terminal repeat (LTR) in which the enhancer from the Moloney murine leukemia virus was replaced by an enhancer from a host-range mutant polyoma virus (Linney et al., 1984; Valerio et al., 1989). This vector is being produced by a cell line designated POC-1. Sensitive helper virus assays showed that the POC-1 cell line produced recombinant viruses free of replication competent helper virus. This recombinant viral vector was previously shown to allow the expression of hADA in all hemopoietic lineages of the mouse (Van Beusechem et al., 1990). To introduce the hADA gene in the expanded T cells, 5×10^5 T cells were co-cultivated with a 70 per cent confluent irradiated monolayer of POC-1 cells in culture medium supplemented with 0.4 μg/ml polybrene. As a negative control, T cells were also co-cultivated with the ADA virus-negative parental packaging cell line ψCRIP (mock-infection).

Subsequently, hADA gene transduced T cells were selected on basis of their ADA expression by exposing them to the toxic selection agent xylofuranosyl-adenine (Xyl-A), which can be converted to the non-toxic Xyl-ionosine by ADA. The uninfected T cells retained some of their Il-2 induced proliferative capacity under a 4 μM Xyl-A selection pressure (Fig. 2A). To inhibit the low levels, (1-2 per cent of normal) of ADA activity in uninfected ADA⁻SCID T cells, low concentrations of the ADA inhibitor 2'-deoxycoformycin (dCF) were added. Addition of only 0.5 nM dCF completely abrogated the residual proliferative response of the uninfected ADA⁻SCID T cells under the 4 μM Xyl-A selection pressure (Fig. 2A). The proliferative capacity of T cells derived from healthy individuals was unaffected by selection pressures up to 4 μM Xyl-A + 10 nM dCF. In order to select for hADA-gene transduced T cells with at least normal expression levels of ADA activity, selection was performed under a pressure of 4 μM Xyl-A + 10 nM dCF.

To test the efficacy of the selection procedure, mixing experiments were performed in which 2 or 20 per cent of a T cell clone derived from a healthy individual were mixed with uninfected ADA⁻SCID T cells. By choosing a $CD3^+/TCR\gamma\delta^+$ T cell clone, which makes it phenotypically distinguisable from the $CD3^+/TCR\alpha\beta^+$ ADA⁻ SCID T cells, the effect of the selection procedure could be determined by FACS analysis. After selection of the mixed populations for 24 h.,the remaining cells were expanded for one week. Next, the fraction of $TCR\gamma\delta^+$ cells was determined in the various unselected and selected cell populations. Their proliferative capacity under the selection pressure was also determined. The fraction of $TCR\gamma\delta^+$ cells in the 2 and 20 per cent mixtures had increased to 30 and 90 per cent respectively after selection (Fig.3). The relative proliferation, i.e. Il-2 induced proliferation under Xyl-A/dCF selection pressure in comparison to no selection pressure, of the various cell populations correlated well with their fraction of $TCR\gamma\delta^+$ cells (Fig.3).

ADA⁻ SCID T cells that had been co-cultivated with POC-1 cells were subjected to two consecutive selection cycles. On the basis of their relative proliferative response under selection pressure (Fig.2) and their ADA activity (data not shown), we estimated that

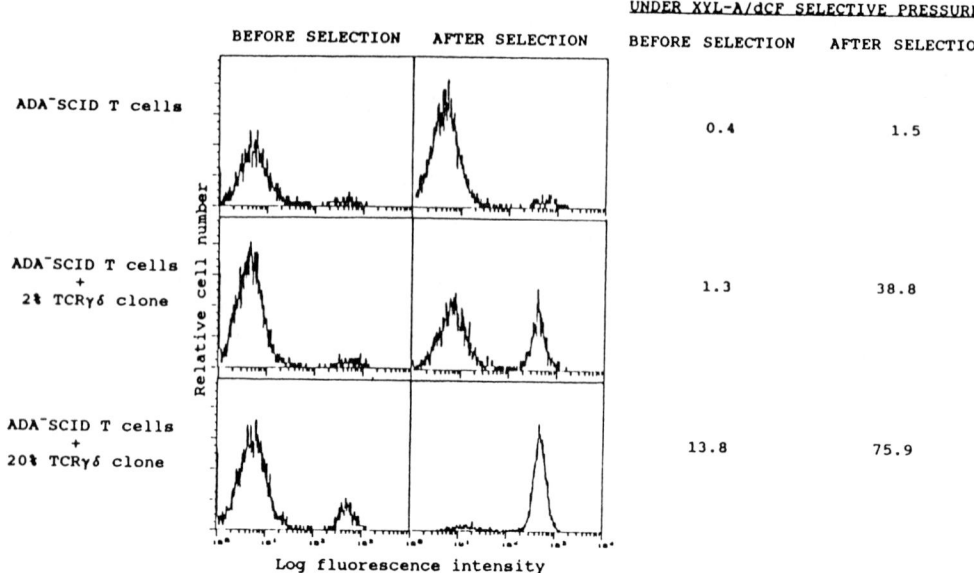

Fig. 3. Selection of T cells with normal ADA activity in 4μM Xyl-A + 10nM dCF selective medium. ADA⁻SCID T cells were mixed with either 0, 2 or 20 per cent TCRγδ T cell clone from a healthy donor before selection. Before and after selection, cell populations were stained with an anti-TCRγδ mAb (TCRγδ-1, Borst et al., 1988) and tested for their relative proliferation in 4μM Xyl-A + 10 nM dCF selective medium, as described in the legend to Fig. 2.

following infection 2-5 per cent of the cells had been succesfully transduced with a functional hADA gene. After one selection cycle the fraction of hADA-gene transduced T cells increased to approximately 40 per cent and after two selection cycles to 80-90 per cent. The efficacy of two consecutive selection steps of 24 h. is also obtained after a single selection step of 48 h. (data not shown). In the double selected T cells, the levels of ADA activity were found to be within the range of that of normal T cells. As expected, the high sensitivity of the uninfected ADA⁻SCID T cells to the toxic agent dAdo was also corrected in the hADA-gene transduced T cells. Since dAdo is believed to be the compound that is causitive for the absence of T cells in ADA⁻SCID patients, this finding is of importance for the possible use of such cells in gene therapy procedures.

At present, these cells have been maintained in culture for a period exceeding 4 months. The cells maintained their restored resistance to dAdo over this period. Optimal culture conditions allowed the hADA-gene transduced T lymphocytes to expand on average at least 500 fold per week. Thus, starting from a population of 1×10^6 transduced T lymphocytes, the number of T

lymphocytes required for therapy (estimated 10^{10-12} cells) can be obtained within 4 weeks.
A comparative functional analysis of the non-transduced and hADA gene-transduced T cells from this ADA⁻SCID patient and normal T cells is in progress.

This work was supported by the Praeventiefonds, grant no. 282020.

REFERENCES

Borst, J., Van Dongen, J.J.M., Bolhuis, R.L.H., Peters, P.J., Hafler, D.A., de Vries, E., and Van de Griend, R.J. (1988): Distinct molecular forms of human T cell receptor γ/δ detected on viable T cells by a monoclonal antibody. *J. Exp. Med.*, 167, 1625-1644.

Carson, D.A., Kaye, J., and Wasson, D.B. (1981): The potential importance of soluble deoxynucleotidase activity in mediating deoxyadenosine toxicity in human lymphocytes. *J. Immunol*, 126, 348-352.

Fisher, A., Durandy, A., de Villartay, J.P., Vilmer, E., Le Deist, F., Gerota, I., and Griscelli, C. (1986): HLA-haploidentical bone marrow transplantation for severe combined immunodeficiency using E rosette fractionation and cyclosporine. *Blood*, 67, 444-449.

Hershfield, M.S., Buckley, R.H., Greenberg, M.L., Melton, A.L., Schiff, R., Hatem, C., Kurtzberg, J., Markert, M.L., Kobayashi, R.H., Kobayashi, A.L., and Abuchowski, A. (1987): Treatment of adenosine deaminase deficiency with polyethylene glycol modified adenosine deaminase. *N. Engl. J. Med.*, 316, 589-596.

Hirshhorn, R. (1983): Genetic deficiencies of adenosine deaminase and purine nucleoside phosphorylase: overview, genetic heterogeneity and therapy. *Birth Defects.*, 19, 73-81.

Lee, N., Kobayashi, R.H., Chaffee, S., Hershfield, M.S., and Stiehm, E.R. (1990): Suppression of an inhibitory antibody to bovine adenosine-deaminase (ADA) and improved cellular immunity following intravenous gammaglobulin and prednisone in a SCID-ADA deficient child receiving Polyethylene-glycol-ADA (PEG-ADA). *Pediatric Research.*, 27, 158A.

Levy, Y., Hershfield, M.S., Fernandez Meija, C., Polmar, S.H. Scudiery, D., Berger, M., and Sorenson, R.U. (1988): Adenosine deaminase deficiency with late onset of recurrent infections: response to treatment with polyethylene glycol-modified adenosine deaminase. *J.Pediat.*, 113, 312-317.

Linney, E., Davis, B., Overhauser, J., Chao, E., and Fan, H. (1984): Non-function of a Moloney Murine Leukemia Virus regulatory sequence in F9 embryonal carcinoma cells. *Nature.*, 308, 470-472.

Miller, D.G., Adam, M.A., and Miller, A.D. (1990): Gene transfer by retrovirus vectors occurs only in cells that are actively replicating at the time of infection. *Mol. and Cell. Biol.*, 10, 4239-4242.

O'Reilly, R.J., Keever, C.A., Small, T.N., and Brochstein, J. (1989): The use of HLA-non-identical T-cell-depleted marrow transplants for the correction of severe combined

immunodeficiency disease. *Immunodeficiency Rev.*, 1, 273-309.
Silber, G.M., Winkelstein, J.A., Moen, R.C., Horowitz, S.D., Trigg, M., and Hong, R. (1987): Reconstitution of T- and B-cell function after T-lymphocyte-depleted haploidentical bone marrow transplantation in severe combined immunodeficiency due to adenosine deaminase deficiency. *Clin. Immunol. Immunopathol.*, 44, 317-320.
Thompson, L.F., and Seegmiller, J.E. (1980): Adenosine deaminase deficiency and severe combined immunodeficiency disease. In *Advances in enzymology*, ed. A. Meister, pp167-210. New York: Academic Press.
Valerio, D., Einerhand, M.P.W., Wamsley, P.M., Bakx, T.A., Li, C.L., and Verma, I.M. (1989): Retrovirus-mediated gene transfer into embryonal carcinoma cells and hemopoietic stem cells: Expression from a hybrid long terminal repeat. *Gene.*, 84, 419-427.
Van Beusechem, V.W., Kukler, A., Einerhand, M.P.W., Bakx, T.A., Van der Eb, A.J., Van Bekkum, D.W., and Valerio, D. (1990): Expression of human adenosine deaminase in mice transplanted with hemopoietic stem cells infected with amphotropic retroviruses. *J. Exp. Med.*, 172, 729-736.
Van de Griend, R.J., and Bolhuis, R.L.H. (1984a): Rapid expansion of allospecific cytotoxic T cell clones using nonspecific feeder cell lines without further addition of exogenous IL-2. *Transplantation.*, 38, 401-406.
Van de Griend, R.J., Van Krimpen, B.A., Bol, S.J.L., Thompson, A., and Bolhuis, R.L.H. (1984b): Rapid expansion of human cytotoxic T cell clones: Growth promotion by a heat labile serum component and by various feeder cells. *J. Immunol. Methods.*, 66, 285-298.
Wijnaendts, L., Le Deist, F., Griscelli, C., and Fischer, A. (1989): Development of immunologic functions after bone marrow transplantation in 33 patients with severe combined immunodeficiency. *Blood.*, 74, 2212-2219.

RESUME : Les lymphocytes T matures prélevés sur le sang périphérique d'un patient atteint de déficit immunitaire combiné sévère documenté (SCID) dû à un déficit en adénosine déaminase (ADA), ont été expandus in-vitro. Le gène ADA humain (hADA) a été introduit à l'intérieur de ces lymphocytes T en division à l'aide d'un rétrovirus recombinant amphotrope contenant le gène hADA. Les lymphocytes T infectés ont ensuite été sélectionnés sur la base de l'expression d'ADA par la mise en présence d'une combinaison de l'agent toxique xylofuranosyl-adénine (Xyl-A) et d'un inhibiteur spécifique de l'ADA la 2'-déoxycoformicine (dCF). Après deux étapes de sélection, la population de T-lymphocytes résultante contenait des copies intactes du provirus, exprimait des niveaux normaux de hADA et était résistante aux effets toxiques à la fois du 2'-déoxyadénosine (dAdo) et de Xyl-A. Sur la base de ces données, nous estimons que 80 à 90% des cellules sélectionnées ont été effectivement transduites avec le gène hADA fonctionel.

The regulation of human globin gene switching

Peter Fraser, Dale Talbot, Sjaak Philipsen, Sara Pruzina, Mike Antoniou, Mike Lindenbaum, Olivia Hanscombe, Niall Dillon and Frank Grosveld

Laboratory of Gene Structure and Expression, National Institute for Medical Research, The Ridgeway, Mill Hill, London NW7 1AA, UK

INTRODUCTION

The human β-globin gene cluster spans a region of 70kb containing five developmentally regulated genes in the order 5' $\epsilon, \gamma_G \gamma_A, \delta, \beta$ 3'. In the early stages of human development, the embryonic yolk sac is the haematopoietic tissue and expresses the ϵ-globin gene. This is followed by a switch to the γ-globin genes in the foetal liver and the δ- and ß-globin genes in adult bone marrow (for review, see Collins and Weissmann, 1984). These genes are expressed at exceptionally high levels giving rise to 90% of the total soluble protein in circulating red blood cells.

The entire β-like gene locus has been sequenced and a large number of structural defects collectively known as the β-thalassaemias, have been documented in and around the ß-globin gene (for review, see Collins and Weissman, 1984; Poncz et al., 1988). In a related condition, hereditary persistence of foetal haemoglobin (HPFH), γ-globin gene expression and hence HbF (foetal haemoglobin) production persist into adult life. These diseases are a prime target for gene therapy, since present treatment regimes are only partially succesful or involve non autologous bone marrow transplantation. However these mutations are not only clinically important, they also provide natural models for the study of transcriptional regulation during development, which would have to form the basis of any gene therapy protocol by DNA mediated gene addition.

The entire locus is regulated by the locus control region (LCR) which first became apparent from the study of a human γβ thalassaemia. This particular thalassaemia contained an intact β globin gene, but had a deletion of the upstream part of the locus which prevents activation of the β gene (Kioussis et al., 1983; Wright et al., 1984 Fig. 1, top). The LCR is located upstream of the ε-globin gene (Fig. 1) and is characterized by a set of developmentally stable, hypersensitive sites, 5' HS1, 2, 3 & 4 (Tuan et al., 1985; Grosveld et al., 1987; Forrester et al., 1987). The importance of these sites is confirmed by the deletion in Spanish γδβ thalassaemia (Driscoll, et al., 1989). Linkage of the LCR to a cloned β-globin gene resulted in high levels of erythroid specific expression of the transgene which was dependent on the copy number of the transgene and independent of the site of integration (Grosveld et al., 1987). It has since been shown that the LCR is required for high level position - independant expression of all the globin genes (Grosveld et al., 1987; Behringer et al., 1990; Dillon & Grosveld, 1991; Shih et al., 1990) and that its presence affects chromatin structure over a distance of at least 100kb (Forrester et al., 1990). This raises the questions of which sequences and factors are responsible for gene activation and how the genes are activated seperately. Both of those questions are important in light of any globin gene therapy; because the β-globin gene is expressed at a very high level in a erythroid specific manner.

To answer the question which sequences are responsible for β-globin activation we have mapped the minimal sequences in the LCR which are required for high level copy number dependent expression. Each of the hypersensitive regions was linked to the β-globin gene (Fig. 1) and tested in transgenic mice on MEL cells (Philipsen et al 1990, Talbot et al 1990,

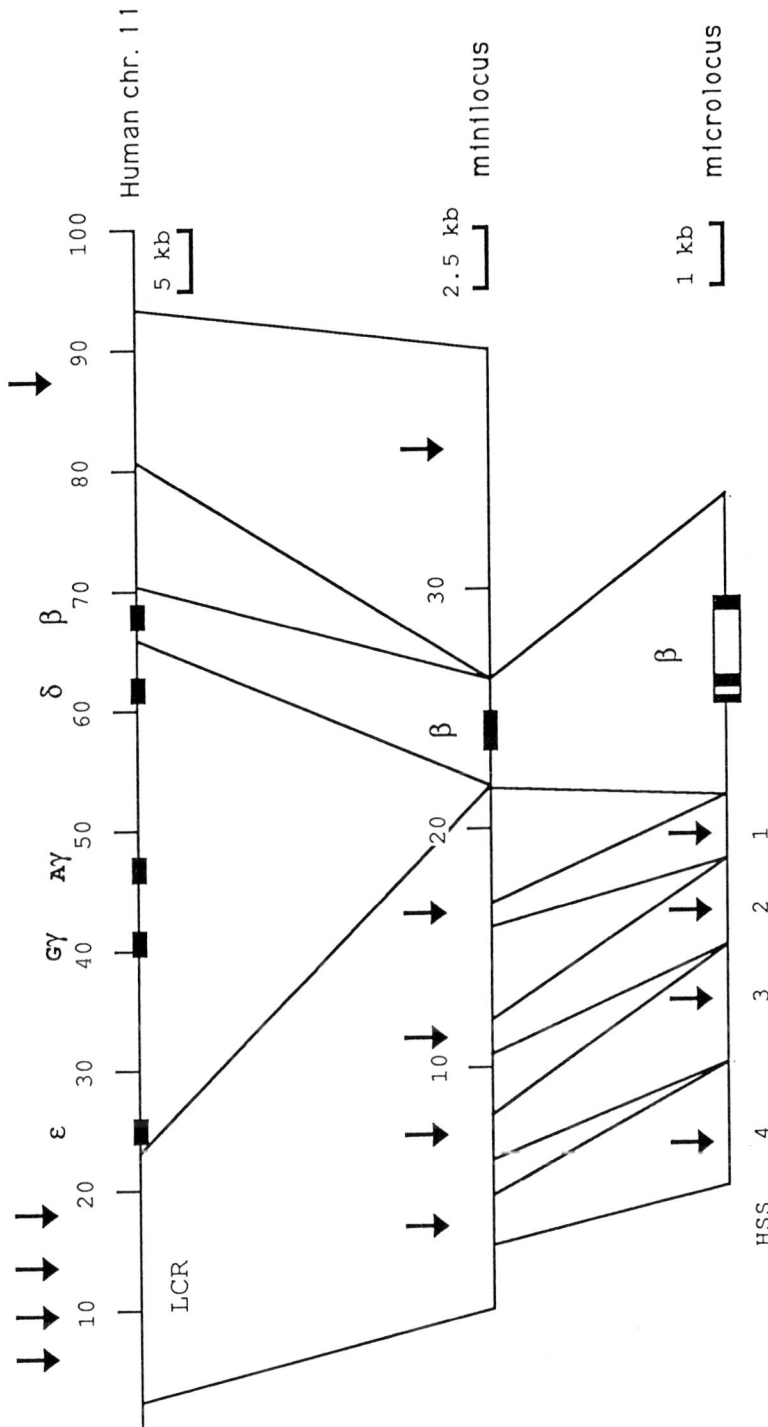

Figure 1. The human β globin locus.
The top line shows the human β-globin locus, the middle line the globin minilocus, that was used to show the functional significance of the LCR (Grosveld et al., 1987). The bottom line shows the constructs used to study individual hypersensitive regions.

Pruzina et al, 1991). In addition the in vitro binding sites of nuclear factors to these fragments were analysed by footprinting and gel shift assays. Fig. 2 shows a summary of these results. In agreement with the deletion found in Spanish δβ thalassimia (Driscoll et al, 1989). HS 2,3 and 4 are the active sites when tested in transgenic mice (Fraser et al, 1990). Each of these sites can be reduced to a core of 200-300 bp. which all contain at least one tandem binding site for the erythroid specific transcription factor GATA1. In addition they all contain a binding site for an unknown protein called J-BP (Fig. 2). HS2 also contains a tandem binding site for the erythroid specific factor NF-E2 (Talbot et al, 1990,

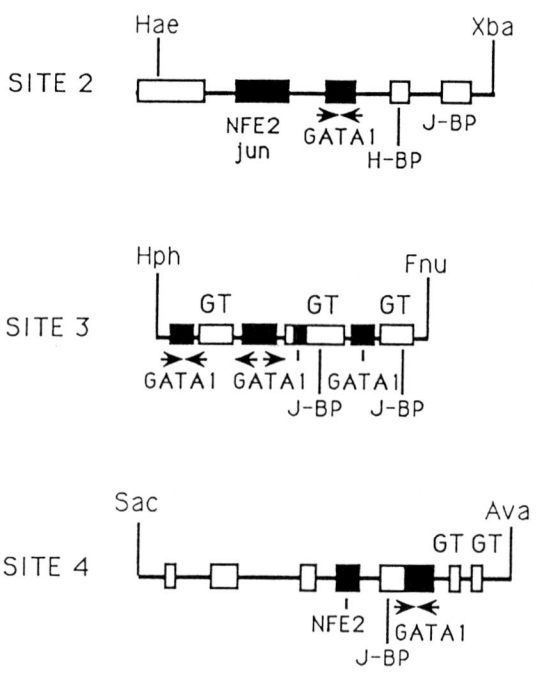

Figure 2. Summary of factor binding sites to the minimal fragment of 5'HS 2,3 and 4, which provide position independent expression in transgenic mice. Individual factors are described in the text. Black boxes indicate erythroid specific factors, open boxes indicate ubiquitous factors. GT indicates a GT rich motif (Philipsen et al., 1990).

Ney et al, 1990), which is essential for the enhancer activity that is observed only for HS2 in transient transcription assay.

Interestingly deletion of the NF-E2 or GATA1 binding sites show that neither of these activities is necessary for copy number dependent expression directed by HS2, although deletion of the NF-E2 sites leads to a severe reduction in transcription levels, (Caterina et al, 1991, Talbot & Grosveld 1991). A series of deletion/mutation experiments is in progress to determine whether the ubiquitiously expressed factor J-BP or any other factors (Fig. 2) are essential for this activity. Nevertheless the fact that the core activities have been reduced to 200-300 bp for HS2, 3 and 4 has allowed us to construct a very small LCR for retroviral constructs (Antoniou unpubl. results) which are presently under analysis (Mulligan unpubl.).

To address the question of how the different human globin genes are regulated we have also made use of transgenic mice. Without the LCR an embryonic human ϵ transgene is not expressed. Linkage to the LCR results in high level expression during the embryonic stage and the gene is switched off at the same time as the mouse embryonic genes and is completely silenced in the foetal liver and adult bone marrow (Shih et al., 1990; Raich et al., 1990; Lindenbaum et al., 1990; Fraser et al., 1991). Expression studies with deletion mutants in K562 cells have suggested that a region in the ϵ globin promoter, around -200 to -300, might play a role in such silencing (Cao et al., 1989). The positions of other supressor binding sequences are presently not known but a potential site is the CAAT box region in the promoter which shows good homology with the distal CAAT box region of the γ gene (see below).

Initial reports suggested that linkage of a γ gene to the LCR resulted in γ expression at all developmental stages (Enver et al., 1990, Behringer et al., 1990. However, experiments on only low copy nuclear mice showed that γ expression decreases during the foetal stage and is completely silenced at the adult stage, independant of the presence of the β gene or any of its 3' flanking region (Dillon and Grosveld, 1991). This result indicates that like the ε gene, transcription of the γ gene in the presence of the LCR can be completely blocked by the action of stage specific negative regulators binding to the sequences immediately flanking the gene. This removes the basis of the argument that the β gene is needed for γ silencing and invalidates a reciprocal competition model (Townes & Behringer, 1990). The available genetic data suggest that the sequences around the distal CAAT box are likely to be involved in this silencing. For example, a 13bp deletion which removes the distal CAAT box results in a very strong HPFH (30%) (Gilman et al., 1988). Two sub types can be distinguished; Japanese HPFH (11-14%) with a point mutation in the distal CAAT box which reduces affinity for the transcription factor CP1 (Fucharoen et al., 1990) and Greek HPFH (15-20%) with a mutation at -117 which has been suggested as causing reduced binding of an erythroid specific factor (NFE3) (Mantovani et al., 1989). These findings suggest that factors binding to the distal CAAT box could silence the γ gene by competing for interaction with factors bound to upstream promoter sequences and preventing the proximal CAAT box from forming such interactions. The distal CAAT box is located at -115 outside the normal optimal position for CAAT elements and this is likely to prevent it from functioning as an effective positive promoter element. One would expect this type of silencing mechanism to be very dependent on the topology of the promoter region and be partially bypassed by the creation of extra factor binding sites in the upstream sequences. The characterisation of the factors responsible for the suppression of the γ globin gene could be an important alternative approach to the treatment of thalassaemia, inhibition of such a factor (by pharmacological means) would lead to reactivation of the γ gene and alleviate the chain imbalance resulting in the thalassaemia.

Linkage of the adult β gene to the LCR results in inappropriate expression at the embryonic stage (Blom et al., 1989; Lindenbaum et al., 1990; Enver et al., 1990; Behringer et al., 1990; Hanscombe et al., 1991), albeit at a lower level than the mouse embryonic genes. This expression can be blocked by placing a γ gene or a human α globin gene between the β gene and the LCR (Behringer et al., 1990; Enver et al., 1990 Hanscombe et al., 1991), supporting the idea that competition plays a role in preventing premature β expression. However, when the order is reversed and the β gene is placed in the first position, both genes are expressed (Hanscombe et al., 1991). This is also observed in multicopy insertions which result in an LCR both upstream and downstream of the genes. Variation of the distances in such a situation showed that relative distance to an LCR is the important parameter. This indicates that the ability of the γ gene to block embryonic expression is not entirely a function of the γ promoter but is also dependent on it being closer to the LCR. The ability to compete effectively is apparently lost when the γ gene is further from the LCR. In the single copy situation in vivo this relative distance effect would appear as a polar effect of the LCR on the locus. (Hanscombe et al., 1991). The existence of polarity in the locus has long been suggested by the fact that the genes are arranged in the order of their expression during development and the discovery of the LCR 5' to the ϵ gene adds a further dimension to this. The observation that competition in the locus appears to be polar, together with the data showing that the ϵ and γ genes are silenced autonomously suggests a model of the type illustrated in Fig. 3. According to this model premature expression of late expressing genes is prevented by competition from the proximal genes while the early expressing genes are subject to promoter mediated silencing in the later stages.

Why would the expression of the upstream genes prevent premature expression of those located downstream but not vice versa? Existing competition models are based on the idea that the high level expression of

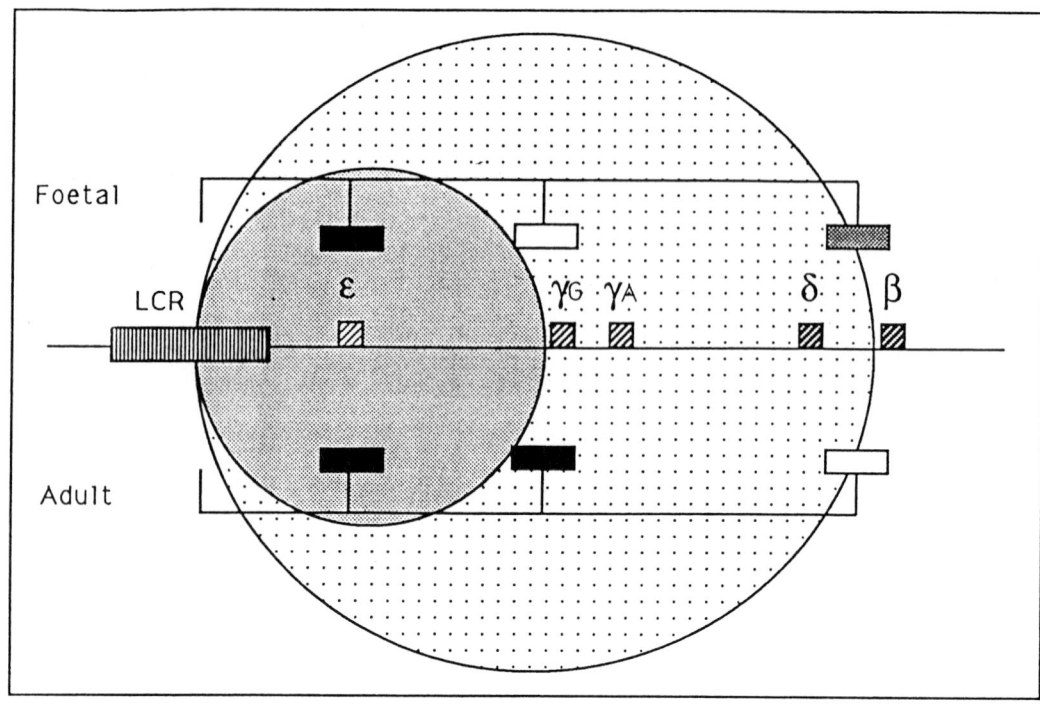

Figure 3. Regulation of the human β globin locus at the embryonic, foetal and adult stages of development.
An black bar indicates a blocked interaction between the promoter of the genes and the LCR, which is caused by stage specific repressors binding to the promoters. An open box indicates a productive interaction, a shaded box an intermediate interaction. The shaded circles indicate the relative volumes occupied by the Gγ and LCR or the β and the LCR.

the genes in the β globin locus is potentiated by direct interaction of each gene with the LCR. There is strong evidence that enhancers work through such interactions (Muller et al., 1989; Bickel and Pirotta, 1990 and references therein). Distance has also been established as a parameter using multiple linked genes in different systems, such as (non erythroid) transient assay systems (de Villiers et al., 1983; Wasylyk et al., 1983) or the transgenic mice discussed above (Hanscombe et al., 1991). The entire β globin locus has been shown to be part of a region of DNaseI sensitivity which extends at least 150kb downstream from the β globin gene in erythroid cells (Forrester et al., 1990 and references therein). This suggests that in an erythroid environment the locus and the LCR are part of a single large region of open chromatin. DNA which is part of an open loop will be free to move in three dimensions and the frequency with which contact will occur between two elements located on it will be determined by the volume they occupy relative to one another, i.e. their effective concentration. This will be restricted by their being held together by a tether. In an idealised situation the effective volume will be that of a sphere whose radius is the distance between the two elements (Fig. 3). This implies that the frequency of contact between two regulatory elements within the locus will be proportional to the cube of the distance between them. A difference in distance is therefore amplified into a much larger difference in effective concentration. Although the distance varies slightly, depending on which hypersensitive site in the LCR is used for the measurement, (Fig. 3), the β globin gene is approximately twice as far as the Gγ gene from the LCR and will, therefore, have an eight-fold lower frequency of interaction with the LCR.

It is a central proposition of any competition model that the competing genes each retain the capacity for significant interaction with the LCR. Stage specificity would be achieved by one gene gaining near total occupancy of the LCR and physically blocking out the other genes. In this type of situation, the frequency with which each gene comes into contact with the LCR will be a critical parameter in determining its ability to compete. During the foetal stage the interaction of the γ genes with the LCR would be much more frequent than that of the β gene and, owing to the action of stage specific factors, would also be stronger. The combination of these two parameters acting together would allow the γ genes to completely compete out β expression. In the adult stage, although the β gene would now have the stronger interaction with the LCR, its much lower frequency of contact would make it difficult for it to compete out a γ gene which retained a significant capability to form such interactions. To achieve this effect a very strong β interaction would be required and it seems unlikely that this would have evolved specifically to silence γ expression. The more likely alternative mechanism would be one of promoter mediated silencing of the early genes by stage specific factors and the transgenic mouse data indicate that this is the one which has in fact evolved.

The model described above would explain the fact that the order of the genes in the β globin locus is largely conserved among mammals. However it does not predict that the order of expression during development will follow that of the genes in the locus in all species. For example a gene located proximal to a Locus Control Region could be subject to factor mediated repression early in development and then activated at a later stage. This activation would bring competition into play and would result in a switch from a distal to a proximal gene. A change in the position of the LCR would also alter the parameters affecting competition. In the chicken β globin locus, for which competition was first proposed (Choi and Engel, 1988), there is evidence that part of the LCR lies between the β and ϵ genes (Reitman et al., 1990).

The model which we have proposed relating competition to effective volume makes specific predictions on the effect of relative distance on two equivalent genes competing for the LCR. The calculation that the frequency of interaction of two elements will decrease very rapidly with increasing distance has important implications for gene therapy. Any of the DNA mediated gene transfer techniques, except in the case of homologous recombination, positions the new gene in a more or less random position in the genome of the recipient cells. In addition to potential insertional mutagenesis by interrupting essential host genome sequences, the regulatory unit of the inserted sequences could also have a "position" effect on neighbouring host genes, disturbing their normal pattern of expressing, e.g. cellular oncogenes could be potentially be activated. Our model suggests that such deregulation may not be a problem and when the regulatory sequences on the inserted DNA are placed close to the promoter of the inserted gene and position effects could be prevented even further, by placing additional promoter(s) producing sterile transcripts on the border with the host DNA. Alternatively natural transcriptional domain borders may be included (Schedl et al 1991 and references therein), although it is unknown whether the inclusion of such sequences would be be deleterious to the production of recombinant viruses carrying these sequences incombination with the gene and control sequences. Experiments are presently in progress to test those possibilities.

Acknowledgements

We are grateful to all our colleagues for their discussions and helpful suggestions.

REFERENCES

Behringer, R. R., Ryan, T. M., Palmiter, R. D., Brinster, R. L. and Townes, T. M. (1990), Genes and Devel., 4, 380-389.

Blom van Assendelft, G., Hanscombe, O., Grosveld, F., Greaves, D. R. (1989), Cell, 56: 969-977.

Bickel, S. and Pirotta, V., (1990). EMBO J. 9, 2959-2967.

Cao, S., Gutman, P. D., Dave, H. P. G. and Schechter, A. J. (1989) Proc. Natl. Acad. Sci. USA, 86, 5306-5309.

Caterina, J., Ryan, T., Pawlik, K., Palmiter, R., Brinster, R., Behringer, R. and Townes T., (1991), Proc. Natl. Sci. USA, 88, 1626-1630.

Choi, O-R. and Engel, J. D. (1988), Cell, 55, 17-26.

Collins, F. S. and Weissman, S. M. (1984), Prog. Acid Res. Mol. Biol., 1984, 31, 315-462.

deVilliers, J., Olson, C., Banerji, J. and Schaffner, W. (1982) Cold Spring Harbor Symp. Quant. Biol., 47, 911-919.

Dillon, N. and Grosveld, F. (1991). Nature, 350, 252-254.

Driscoll, C., Dobkin, C. and Alter, B. (1989). Proc. Natl. Acad. Sci.USA 86, 7470-7474.

Enver, T., Raich, N., Ebens, A. J., Papayannopoulou, T., Costantini, F. and Stamatoyannopoulos, G. (1990), Nature, 344, 309-313.

Forrester, W., Takegawa, S., Papayannopoulou, T., Stamatoyannopoulos, G., and Groudine, M. (1987). Nucleic Acids Res. 15, 10159-10177.

Forrester, W., Epner, E., Driscoll, C., Enver, T., Brice, M., Papayannopoulou, Groudine, M.,(1990) Genes and Dev., 4, 1637-1649.

Fraser, P., Watt, P., Pruzina, S., Grosveld, F. and Proudfoot, N. (1991). submitted.

Fraser, P, Hurst J, Collis P, Grosveld F (1990), Nucleic Acids Res. 18, 3503-3508.

Fucharoen, S., Shimiza, K. and Fukumaki M. (1990), Nucl. Acid Res. 18, 5245.

Gilman J., Mishima, N., Wen, X., Stoming, T., Lobel, J. and Huisman T. (1988).Nucl. Acid Res., 18, 10635-10642.

Grosveld, F., Blom van Assendelft, G., Greaves, D. and Kollias, G. (1987). Cell, 51, 975-985.

Hanscombe, O., Whyatt, D., Fraser, P., Yannoutsos, N., Greaves, D. and Grosveld, F., (1991). Genes & Dev., 1991, submitted

Kioussis, D., Vanin, E., deLange, T., Flavell, R. A. and Grosveld, F. (1983). Nature, 306, 662-666.

Lindenbaum, M. and Grosveld, F. (1990). Genes and Dev., 4, 2075-2085.

Mantovani, R., Superti-Fuga, G., Gilman, J. and Ottolenghi, S. (1989), Nucl. Acids Res., 17, 6681-6691.

Martin, D., Tsai, S. and Orkin, S. (1989). Nature, 338, 435-438.

Muller, H., Sogo, J. and Schaffner, W. (1989). Cell 58, 767-777.

Ney PA, Sorrentino BP, Lowrey CH, Nienhuis AW (1990), Nucleic Acids Res. 18, 6011-6017.

Philipsen, S., Talbot, D., Fraser, P. and Grosveld, F., EMBO J., 1990, 9, 2159-2167.

Poncz, M., et al. (1989) Globin Gene Expression in Hereditary Persistence of Fetal Hemoglobin and $\delta\beta$ Thalassaemia, Oxford University Press.

Pruzina, S., Hanscombe, O., Whyatt, D., Grosveld, F. and Philipsen, S., (1991), Nucl. Acids Res., 19, 1413-1419.

Raich N., Enver T., Nakamoto B., Josephson B., Papayannopoulou T. and Stamatoyannopoulos G. (1990), Science 250, 1147-1149.

Reitman, M., Lee, E., Westphal, H. and Felsenfeld, G. (1990). Nature, 348, 749-752.

Shih, D., Wall R. and Shapiro, S. (1990), Nucl. Acids Res. 18, 5465-5472.

Talbot D, Philipsen S, Fraser P, Grosveld F (1990), EMBO J. 9, 2169-2178.

Talbot, D. and Grosveld, F., EMBO J., (1991), in press.

Townes, T.M. & Behringer, R.R. TIG. 6, 219-223 (1990).

Tuan, D., Solomon, W., Li, Q. and London, I. (1985), Proc. Natl. Acad. Sci. USA. 82, 6384-6388.

Wasylyk, B., Wasylyk, C., Augerean, P. and Chambon, P. (1983), Cell, 32, 503-514.

Wright, S., deBoer, E., Rosenthal, A., Flavell, R. A. and Grosveld, F. G., (1984). Phil. Trans. Royal Soc. London, B307, 271-282.

RESUME : Chez l'homme, le cluster des gènes codant pour la chaine bêta de la globine couvre une région de 70 kilobases contenant 5 gènes différents régulés dans le développement et positionnés dans l'ordre suivant de 5' en 3' : ε, γ_G, γ_A, δ et β. Dans les premières étapes du développement humain, le sac vitellin embryonnaire exprime le gène ε de la globine. Il est relayé par les gènes γ dans le foie foetal ; enfin les gènes δ et β de la globine sont exprimés dans la moelle osseuse adulte. La totalité du locus bêta a été séquencée et un large nombre de défauts moléculaires regroupés sous le nom de β-thalassémie ont été documentés. L'intégralité du locus est régulée par une région appelée "locus control region" (LCR). Le LCR est situé en amont du gène ε ; il est caractérisé par un ensemble de sites hyper-sensibles stables pendant le développement, avec respectivement de 5' en 3' HS1, 2, 3 et 4. Nous avons pu démontrer que le LCR est indispensable à un taux d'expression élevé indépendant de la position, pour tous les gènes de globine; sa présence affecte la structure de la chromatine sur une distance d'au moins 100 kilobases. Les questions actuellement posées sont relatives 1) à l'identification des séquences et des facteurs responsables de l'activation génique et 2) à la façon dont ces gènes peuvent être activés séparément et d'une manière parfaitement érythroïde spécifique. Afin de répondre à ces questions, nous avons localisé à l'intérieur du LCR des séquences minimales nécessaires à l'expression de ces gènes, et étudié l'importance du positionnement relatif des gènes du locus dans la régulation de leur expression. Un modèle rendant compte de cette régulation est proposé. Des expériences sont actuellement en cours afin de vérifier que des virus recombinants contenant l'ensemble des séquences régulatrices et bordantes nécessaires pourraient être construits sans interférences délétères à la production du virus. Une thérapie génique touchant ce locus ne saurait se concevoir sans avoir au préalable approfondi et solutionné l'ensemble de ces difficultés.

2. Other tissues

2. Autres tissus

Lymphocytes for gene therapy

R. Michael Blaese

Cellular Immunology Section, Metabolism Branch, National Cancer Institute, National Institutes of Health, Building 10, Room 6B05, Bethesda, Maryland 20892, USA

SUMMARY

The problem of stably introducing exogenous genes into stem cells is common to most of the current attempts to develop techniques for the clinical application of gene therapy. With most tissue types, self-renewal is critical if the gene transfer effect is to last beyond a relatively brief time. Retroviral-mediated gene transfer is the current method of choice for stably introducing genes into proliferating cells. This chapter explores the use of T lymphocytes as an alternative tissue for use in gene therapy. T cells lend themselves to three different general types of clinical application, two of which have already been initiated in ongoing clinical protocols. Some of the relative advantages and limitations of T lymphocytes as cellular vehicles for gene therapy are discussed.

EX VIVO THERAPY

The relatively inefficient, low titer gene transfer techniques available today coupled with concerns over the possible introduction of foreign genetic material into the patients' germ cells has limited early attempts at gene therapy to *"ex vivo"* treatment protocols. Thus candidate diseases are limited at present to those where diseased somatic cells can be removed from the body, treated by gene transfer *in vitro*, and then returned to the body where they must reestablish themselves and then provide the "corrected" normal function. Tissues or cell types which could be manipulated *ex vivo* and successfully return to normal function when reimplanted into the body are quite limited. Neurons, skeletal or cardiac muscle, or kidney for example do not readily lend themselves to such *ex vivo* treatment with our present technology. Bone marrow, vascular endothelial cells, keratinocytes, fibroblasts, and possibly hepatocytes are cell types which have been successfully manipulated *in vitro* and resume function upon return to the body.

Another problem in common to all approaches is the desire to stably insert corrective genes into self-renewing stem cell populations of the cell type/tissue under consideration, whether hematopoeitic, hepatic, endothelial or skin. Without the capacity for self-renewal, the gene transfer effect will last only as long as the individual genetically modified cell survives and will disappear when that cell reaches senescence and dies. Perhaps the best clinical example of transplantation of stem cells with prolonged survival and continued function is the experience with bone marrow transplantation.

A broad array of genetic diseases affecting various bone marrow derived cell lineages are curable by allogeneic bone marrow transplantation (Parkman, 1986). These include severe primary immunodeficiency disorders as well as the hemoglobinopathies, granulocyte defects, and several storage diseases. If these diseases are curable by providing normal allogeneic marrow stem cells, theoretically it should be possible to correct the genetic defect in the patient's own stem cells by gene transfer and similarly cure the disease without running the risk of graft versus host disease that is often associated with allogeneic bone marrow transplantation. Thus the bulk of the early work on the development of gene therapy for genetic diseases has focused on gene transfer into the bone marrow stem cell (Anderson,1984; Kohn et al.,1987). However, the somewhat unexpected and so far intractable problem of stably introducing genes into the totipotent bone marrow stem cells of large animals including primates has stalled progress (Kantoff et al.,1987; Williams,1990). Similarly, technical problems have limited the clinical application of gene-modified vascular endothelium, skin and liver.

LYMPHOCYTES FOR GENE INSERTION

Another tissue/cell type which has been successfully transplanted in both experimental and clinical applications is the lymphocyte. In experimental immunology, the transfer of lymphocytes to study the functional properties of these cells has been routinely employed for over a half century. Mature T cells and plasma cells as well as less differentiated immune precursor cells readily engraft and function well in their new host.

Lymphocytes have several attractive features for their use as cellular targets for gene transfer (Culver et al.,1988; Culver et al.,1990; Culver et al.,1991). They are readily available from peripheral blood where collection by apheresis can yield 10^9 or more cells at a single sitting without causing anemia often associated with the removal of whole blood. Processing of blood is a routine clinical procedure not requiring the development of new technologies or support systems. Even cryopreservation of lymphocytes is now a routine procedure so that the cells used for gene modification could be stored frozen for repeated treatments if desirable. Since lymphocytes are ordinarily a single cell suspension of blood cells, their administration by simple intravenous or intraperitoneal infusion is also a routine clinical procedure.

Another feature of lymphocytes which is particularly attractive for their use in gene therapy procedures is their adaptability to tissue culture. T cells can be readily grown in culture where the availability of several different recombinant growth factors (IL1, IL2, IL4, IL6, etc.) and monoclonal antibodies to specific populations permits the selective expansion of different functional subsets of cells. The capacity to induce polyclonal or oligoclonal cellular proliferation of T cells with mitogens or antigens is a critical advantage since successful retroviral-mediated gene transfer resulting in stable gene integration only occurs when the target cells are actively synthesizing DNA. Our inability to induce bone marrow stem cell proliferation without also inducing differentiation is one of the principal factors currently restricting the clinical application of bone marrow gene therapy.

Although T cells may not seem to be as long lived or self-renewing as hematopoeitic stem cells, in fact antigen primed T cells and their progeny can survive for decades *in vivo*. Most adults have not been actively immunized with common antigens such as tetanus toxoid since childhood and yet they remain immune to tetanus. The T cells which were primed to the tetanus antigen in childhood remain in the lymphoid tissues and blood well into adult life and continue to be able to respond specifically to rechallenge with tetanus toxoid. If a gene had been inserted into such a tetanus a responsive T cell in childhood, its continued presence and expression into adult life is very possible. Further, simple reimmunization with the specific antigen to which that T cell is immune could result in *in vivo* proliferation and expansion of the gene-modified T cell population without needing to repeat gene transfer into a new cellular cohort. Another feature of antigen specific T cells is their capacity to home or target to deposits of antigen in the body. The use of such "homing" lymphocytes modified with inserted genes would potentially provide a "magic bullet" for delivery and localized production of specific gene products.

T lymphocytes adapt extremely well to tissue culture and yet retain the ability to reestablish themselves when returned to the body. This capacity for prolonged culture provides time for repeated attempts at gene insertion, time to test for expression of the inserted genes, time for selection of those gene-expressing cells, and perhaps most importantly provides time for safety testing of the gene-modified cells. For the first application of retroviral-mediated gene transfer in man, our ability to demonstrate that the gene-modified cells had not acquired a malignant phenotype *in vitro* and that they were not producing contaminating recombinant helper virus was essential before we could reintroduce the modified cells into patients. (Culver et al., 1991; Cornetta et al.,1990)

T CELLS IN GENE THERAPY

T lymphocytes could be used in at least three distinct therapeutic gene insertion scenarios. One setting in which T cells could be used for gene therapy would be the situation where a long-lived cell is needed for the continuous production of a missing gene product which is ordinarily found in the circulation or as a cellular source for an enzyme needed to catabolize a freely diffusible potentially toxic substrate. There is no reason in principle that a serum protein ordinarily produced by the liver could not be produced by a T cell, provided that the T cell contained (or was engineered to contain) all the accessory machinery needed for the synthesis, post translational processing and secretion of that protein. In such a setting the immune specificity of the T cell is not critical since the cell is not performing an immune function but rather acting as a circulating protein factory. Antigen specific T cells could be used in this situation if it was desirable to have a mechanism to boost the number of gene-modified cells by immunization of the host with the antigen to which the T cells were immune. It may well turn out that periodic antigen stimulation will be required for gene-modified T cells to persist for long periods.

T cells engineered to produce adenosine deaminase (ADA) or purine nucleoside phosphorylase (PNP) could be useful in the treatment of the associated immunodeficiency diseases by providing intracellular enzyme which would degrade the potentially toxic substrates which accumulate in the tissues of these patients (Kantoff et al., 1986). Since deoxyadenosine and deoxyquanosine are freely diffusible across cell membranes, their intracellular catabolism would result in the formation of a concentration gradient followed by the diffusion of additional toxic substrate into the ADA or PNP expressing cells to also be degraded. T cells modified by gene insertion to secrete clotting factors VIII or IX could potentially be used to treat patients with hemophilia. Gene-modified T cells might be used for the degradation of excess serum phenylalanine in young adult females with PKU, permitting them to become pregnant without fear that the developing central nervous systems of their fetuses will be adversely affected.

A second potential use for T cells in gene therapy would be in the setting of immunity to a specific antigen where gene-modification of specific antigen reactive cells could be used to augment host defense. For example, tumor immune lymphocytes are now used in the immunotherapy of human cancer (Rosenberg et al.,1988). Our initial experiments with gene transfer in man were carried out in a system in which tumor infiltrating lymphocytes (TIL), grown *in vitro* from tumor deposits surgically obtained from patients with malignant melanoma, were returned to the patient to treat his malignancy. Using an inserted bacterial neomycin resistance gene (neoR) to provide a unique nucleotide sequence to "label" the TIL (Culver et al.,1991; Kasid et al., 1990), we showed that these tumor immune T cells "home" preferentially to deposits of tumor in these patients. (Rosenberg et al.,1990). As a strategy for therapy, the insertion of a gene encoding the production of a tumoricidal product such as tumor necrosis factor (TNF) into the TIL which would then target or home to the tumor deposit, would provide for local delivery of a gene product which might be too toxic for systemic administration. Our colleague Steven Rosenberg has recently started exactly such a clinical protocol in patients with malignant melanoma. Fox and Culver have also shown that the cytolytic capacity of tumor specific T cells can be significantly augmented by inserting cytokine genes into these TIL. Perhaps other functional properties of antigen specific T cells can also be enhanced by gene insertion. It may also become possible to produce hybrid cellular receptors (eg., immunoglobulin variable region genes from tumor reactive murine hybridomas coupled with T cell receptor constant region peptides) on cytolytic T cells which will direct their immune attack on determinants which are ordinarily nonimmunogenic in man. It is even possible to visualize a scenario in which gene-modified antigen specific T cells might be used to augment the therapy of refractory infections with organisms such as the atypical mycobacteria, certain parasites or even perhaps leprosy.

Finally, polyclonal T cell populations could be gene-modified and then used for general immune reconstitution in disorders such as ADA or PNP deficiency or AIDS (Blaese et al.,1990). In this setting the strategy would be to "gene-correct" as broad a sample of the T cell immune repertoire as possible. Therefore, broad spectrum polyclonal T cell stimulants such as phytohemagglutinin or anti-CD3 would be used to induce proliferation permitting retroviral-mediated gene insertion. Because some T cell specificities may be lost with prolonged culture by dilution with more rapidly dividing cells, maintenance of the cells in culture for only a brief period would be most desirable. This general approach would only be useful in those clinical situations where a broad spectrum T cell repertoire exists. Several strategies for introducing resistance genes into T cells of patients infected with HIV are under study. For those HIV infected patients already experiencing CD4 T lymphopenia, peripheral blood lymphocyte gene-modification might well occur too late for significant clinical benefit since a polyclonal T cell repertoire may no longer be available.

A number of fundamental questions concerning the actual utility of T cells for gene therapy remain to be answered. It is still not clear just how long these cells will persist and whether inserted genes will continue to be expressed throughout the lifetime of the cell. Lymphocytes are a heterogeneous population of cells with distinct functional subpopulations. In addition to the well recognized CD4 and CD8 subpopulations, additional subgroups of each phenotype also exist. Some T cells are clearly long lived and recirculate continuously from blood to lymph to blood. Included in this population are memory cells. Other T cells reside in the blood only briefly and then migrate to various tissues and do not recirculate. Included with these are "inflammatory lymphocytes" which participate in effector immune functions and are apparently short lived.

Our studies in monkeys have demonstrated that gene-modified blood and lymphnode T cells could be regrown from the peripheral blood of recipient animals as long as 2 years after receiving just a single intravenous or intraperitoneal infusion of cells (Culver et al.,1990). These gene-modified cells also continued to express the introduced NeoR gene which conferred resistance to the neomycin analogue G418. In mice transplanted with antigen specific CD4 cells carrying an inserted hADA gene, cells expressing hADA could be recovered from the spleens of recipients of the gene-modified T cells for at least 3 months after injection of just a few million cells. In addition, these cells retained their immune specificity and were able to provide specific helper function for antibody production to "their" antigen (Culver et al.,1991).

Gene containing T cells could be detected in the blood of cancer patients receiving infusions of 10^{10} NeoR gene-transduced TIL, a tissue derived T cell population, for about 3 weeks after infusion. Additionally, gene-marked TIL could be recovered from tumor deposits in these patients for as long as 2 months after treatment (Rosenberg et al.,1990). By contrast, our children with ADA deficiency SCID treated with only about 10^8 gene-corrected blood derived T cells have maintained these gene modified cells in their blood for a much longer period of time.

It is yet to be determined whether this difference observed in the survival of TIL and blood T cells represents a distinct difference in the intrinsic lifespans of these different T cell populations or if other factors may significantly impact on *in vivo* survival. TIL are grown in high concentrations of IL2 for 6-8 weeks while the ADA deficient T cells are exposed to IL2 for only 9-12 days of culture. It is possible that *in vitro* "addiction to IL2" might occur that limits the survival of cells grown for longer periods with this cytokine when they are finally removed from the growth factor and reinjected. It is clear, however, that one to two weeks of IL2 supported growth does not prevent the cells from long survival and continued function *in vivo*.

The ongoing clinical gene therapy protocols using lymphocytes modified with either a "corrective gene" for ADA deficiency or with a gene introducing a "new functional property" as with the TNF gene-modified TIL will provide the ultimate answer as to the clinical utility of T cells as cellular vehicles for gene therapy. Preliminary findings in the patients treated on the ADA gene therapy protocol are very encouraging and suggest that polyclonal T cells can be genetically corrected and used successfully in the therapy of an inherited severe immunodeficiency disease.

REFERENCES

Anderson, W.F. (1984): Prospects for human gene therapy. *Science* 226,401-409.

Blaese, R.M., Anderson, W.F., & Culver, K.W.(1990): The ADA gene therapy protocol. *Hum. Gene Therapy* 1, 327-62.

Cornetta, K., Moen, R.C., Culver, K.W., Morgan, R.A., McLachlin, J.R., Sterm, S., Silegue, J., London, W., Blaese, R.M. & Anderson, W.F. (1990): Amphotropic murine leukemia retrovirus iis not an acute pathogen for porimates. *Hum. Gene Therapy* 1, 15-30.

Culver, K.W., Freeman, S.F., Kohn, D., Wood, M., Anderson, W., Berzofsky, J.A, & Blaese, R.M. (1988): Retroviral-mediated gene transfer into cultured lymphoid cells as a vehicle for gene therapy, *J. Cell Biochem.* Suppl. 12B,171.

Culver, K.C., Morgan, R.A., Osborne, W.R.A., Lee, T. T., Lenschow, D., Able, C., Cornetta, K., Anderson, W.F. and Blaese, R.M. (1990): *In vivo* expression and survival of gene-modified T lymphocytes in Rhesus monkeys. *Hum. Gene Therapy*, 1:399-410.

Culver, K.W., Cornetta, K., Morgan, R., Morecki, S., Aebersold, P., Kasid, A., Lotze, M., Rosenberg, S.A., Anderson, W.F., & Blaese, R.M. (1991): Lymphocytes as cellular vehicles for gene therapy in mouse and man. *Proc. Natl. Acad. Sci.* 88, 3155-59.

Kantoff, P.W., Kohn, D.B., Mitsuya, H., Armentano, D., Sieberg, M., Zwiebel, J.A., Eglitis, M.A., McLachlin, J.R., Wiginton, D.A., Hutton, J.J., Horowitz, S.D., Gilboa, E., Blaese, R.M., & Anderson, W.F. (1986): Correction of adenosine deaminase deficiency in cultured human T and B cells by retrovirus-mediated gene transfer. *Proc. Natl. Acad. Sci.* 83, 6563-6567.

Kantoff, P.W., Gillio, A., McLachlin, J.R., Bordignon, C., Eglitis, M.A., Kernan, N.A., Moen, R.C., Kohn, D.B., Yu, S.F., Karson, E., Karlsson, S., Zwiebel, J.A., Gilboa, E., Blaese, R.M., Nienhuis, A.W., O'Reilly, R., & Anderson, W.F. (1987): Expression of human adenosine deaminase in nonhuman primates after retrovirus-mediated gene transfer. *J. Exp. Med.* 166, 219-234.

Kasid, A., Morecki, S., Aebersold, P., Cornetta, K., Culver, K., Freeman, S., Director, E., Lotze, M.T., Blaese, R.M., Anderson, W.F., & Rosenberg, S.A. (1990): Human gene transfer: characterization of human tumor-infiltrating lymphocytes as vehicles for retroviral-mediated gene transfer in man. *Proc. National Acad. Sci.* 87, 473-477.

Kohn, D.B., Kantoff, P.W., Eglitis, M.A., McLachlin, J.R., Moen, R.C., Karson, E., Zwiebel, J.A., Nienhuis, A.W., Karlsson, S., O'Reilly, R., Gillio, A., Bordignon, C., Gilboa, E., Zanjani, I.D., Anderson, W.F. & Blaese, R.M. (1987): Retroviral-mediated gene transfer into mammalian cells. *Blood Cells* 13, 285-298.

Parkman, R. (1986): The application of bone marrow transplantation to the treatment of genetic diseases. *Science* 232, 1373-1378.

Rosenberg, S.A., Packard, B.S., Aebersold, P.M., Topalian, S.L., Toy, S.T., Simon, P., Lotze, M.T., Yang, J.C., Seipp, C.A., Simpson, C., Carter, C., Bock, S., Schwartzentruber, D., Wei, J.P., & White, D.E. (1988): Use of tumor infiltrating lymphocytes and interleukin-2 in the immunotherapy of patients with metastatic melanoma. *N. Engl. J. Med.* 319, 1676-1680.

Rosenberg, S.A., Aebersold, P., Cornetta, K., Kasid, A., Morgan, R.A., Karson, E., Lotze, M.T., Yang, J.C., Topalian, S., Moen, R., Culver, K., Blaese, M., and Anderson, W.F. (1990): Gene transfer into humans-immunotherapy of patients with advanced melanoma using tumor-infiltrating lymphocytes modified by retroviral gene transduction. *N. Engl. J. Med.* 323, 570-578.

Williams, D.A. (1990): Expression of Introduced Genetic Sequences in Hematopoietic Cells Following Retroviral-mediated Gene Transfer, *Hum. Gene Therapy* 1, 229-239.

RESUME : L'introduction stable de gènes étrangers à l'intérieur de cellules souches est un problème commun à la plupart des tentatives actuelles de développement de techniques destinées aux applications cliniques de la thérapie génique. Quelque soit le type de tissu concerné, la question de l'autorenouvellement des cellules cibles est cruciale lorsque l'effet du transfert de gène est destiné à durer au-delà d'un temps relativement bref. Le transfert de gène médié par les rétrovirus est actuellement la méthode de choix pour introduire de façon stable des gènes à l'intérieur de cellules en prolifération. Dans ce chapitre, l'utilisation des lymphocytes T comme autre cible potentielle pour la thérapie génique est envisagée. Les cellules T se prêtent à trois types différents d'applications cliniques dont deux sont déjà explorés dans des protocoles actuellement en développement. Certains des avantages relatifs et des limites des lymphocytes T comme véhicule cellulaire de thérapie génique sont discutés.

Gene therapy of the respiratory tract

Steven L. Brody and Ronald G. Crystal

Pulmonary Branch, National Heart, Lung and Blood Institute, National Institutes of Health, Bethesda, Maryland, USA

INTRODUCTION

As the technology of gene transfer has matured and the concepts regarding sites for gene therapy have expanded beyond that of bone marrow cells, the lung has emerged as a primary target. The lung is the major site of disease for cystic fibrosis (CF) and α1-antitrypsin (α1AT) deficiency, two of the most common fatal hereditary disorders in the United States and Europe (Rommens et al., 1989; Crystal, 1990). Further, the lung has a unique anatomy that permits delivery of gene therapy vectors directly to its parenchyma. The tracheobronchial tree and the pulmonary vascular tree both have the potential to deliver vectors to >95% of the cellular mass of the tissue, and the pleural cavity has the potential to deliver vectors to the entire outer surface of the organ.

The purpose of this review is to summarize these concepts and to detail the current progress in making respiratory tract gene therapy a reality. To do so, we will review the potential respiratory tract cell targets for gene therapy, the diseases that are relevant objectives for this approach, and three vectors systems with the capacity to modify the gene program of cells in the respiratory tract.

AVAILABLE CELL TARGETS

The overall goal of organ-specific gene therapy is quite different from approaches being considered to treat diseases manifesting primarily in the blood, in which it is preferable that the genetically altered cells circulate throughout the body. For organ-specific gene therapy, the strategy is to have the altered gene program manifest only in one, or a limited number of organs. There are several approaches to accomplishing this goal, including: (1) modifying a specific cell type in vitro and capitalizing on the inherent (or engineered) properties of the cell to direct it to a specific organ; (2) modifying a specific cell type in vitro and transplanting the modified cells to a specific organ; (3) exploiting cell-specific promoters, thus limiting expression of the gene of interest to one or a few cell types; and (4) delivering the gene directly to the organ either by using vectors that are organ or cell-specific or delivering the vector directly to the organ of interest.

In the lung, the available cell targets for gene therapy include the parenchymal cells, the alveoli and the tracheobronchial tree, normal resident host defense cells, and cells that may be abnormal residents of the lung or abnormally modified as a consequence of disease e.g., tumor cells or cells chronically infected with microorganisms.

To appreciate the normal lung cell targets, the unique structure of the lung must be considered. From the point of view of gene transfer, the normal lung can be thought of as comprised of five "compartments"; the epithelium lining the air side, the endothelium lining the vascular tree, the interstitium including mesenchymal cells, the mesothelium covering the surface of the lung and the interior of the chest wall, and an inflammatory cell host defense system comprised of macrophages and lymphocytes.

The appeal of the lung as a unique organ for organ-specific gene therapy is that the cellular components of each of these major compartments are easily accessible using commonly used clinical techniques which have little risk and minimal patient discomfort. Fiberoptic bronchoscopy, a technique in which a flexible scope is passed into the trachea, can be used to sample inflammatory cells on the epithelial surface by bronchoalveolar lavage, bronchial epithelial cells by brushing, and small pieces of bronchi and alveoli by biopsy. Further, the bronchoscope can potentially be used to direct gene vectors to specific epithelial sites or neoplastic lesions. For more diffuse delivery, aerosol systems can deliver vectors to the epithelial surface of the respiratory tree, including distal bronchi and alveoli. The vascular bed of the lung is accessible by using available catheters to cannulate the pulmonary artery. Angioscopes are available for visualization and potentially sampling cells from the pulmonary artery. Cells of the pleural space, including mesothelial cells and inflammatory cells, can be targeted by use of thoracentesis, in which a small catheter is introduced into the pleural space. Lastly, techniques of cell culture have made it possible to culture in vitro many of the pulmonary resident inflammatory cells, epithelial, or endothelial cells, providing the possibility to recover autologous cells that could be modified in vitro and reintroduced into the affected individual.

<u>Considerations Relevant to Cell Proliferation</u>
An important cell characteristic to consider when choosing targets for gene therapy in the lung is the rate of cell turnover. Rapid cell turnover is an essential feature for integration of retroviral vectors (Miller et al., 1990), whereas lung parenchymal cells replicate slowly. This may obviate the use of retroviral vectors for in vitro use, since lung parenchymal cells proliferate slowly, at most, with 1-2% of the cells proliferating daily (Evans & Shami,1989). Further, the ciliated cell, the major epithelial cell of the airways, is terminally differentiated, as is the type I epithelial cell, the cell covering 95% of the surface area of the alveoli. These biologic facts present a major hurdle for retroviral vectors; if they will be useful, it likely will be by targeting parenchymal stem cells, a cell population as yet unidentified. The feasibility of this strategy is being investigated by directly transferring genes with retroviral vectors to fetal cells in utero, an approach that potentially could be used for treating lung hereditary diseases (Sanes et al., 1986).

One strategy around the problem of slow proliferation is to use what is now the "classic" strategy for gene therapy: remove cells from the affected individual, grow the cells in culture in the presence of appropriate growth factors, introduce the gene of interest (e.g., with a retroviral vector) and reintroduce the modified cells back into the lung. For the lung, this approach may be adaptable for T-lymphocytes and endothelial cells, since the techniques for growing these cells in culture are well established.

One class of cells that do proliferate rapidly in vivo and thus is an attractive target for retroviral gene therapy in the lung, is the neoplastic cell. Included in this group are the highly lethal, rapidly growing bronchogenic carcinomas and pleural mesothelioma. Theoretically, these cells could be infected in vivo via the aerosol route or by direct injection via bronchoscopy or thoracoscopy, with retroviral vectors carrying therapeutic genes that lead to cell death directly, or by eliciting antitumor immunity.

Some lung diseases, such as α1AT deficiency (see below), do not require that the therapeutic protein be produced in the lung. A gene therapy strategy relevant to these diseases is to modify cells in vitro, and transplant the modified cells to an extrapulmonary site. Finally, it is possible to use the matrix of the highly vascular and well oxygenated pulmonary parenchyma as an ectopic site or reservoir for foreign (non-lung) cells which produce a deficient protein or fulfill an extra-pulmonary organ function. While major safety issues would have to be overcome to use this approach, the latter strategy has been use in experimental animals for the implantation of isolated liver cells as a therapy for hepatic failure. In a liver failure rat model, hepatocytes delivered to the lung by transcutaneous injection survived for up to 6 months and dramatically rescued animals from fulminant hepatic failure (Then et al., 1991).

THE DISEASES

Several lung diseases may be amenable to gene therapy. The most obvious of these are the hereditary diseases manifest primarily in the lung, α1AT and CF. Although rare, there are a variety of other hereditary diseases that affect the lung including immunodeficiency diseases (e.g. chronic granulomatous disease), inborn errors of metabolism, and ciliary dysmotility syndromes.

Acquired lung diseases represent a second major area for gene therapy, including chronic persistent infectious diseases, acute infections in immunodeficient hosts, and pulmonary neoplastic diseases such as bronchogenic carcinoma and mesothelioma, tumors which are rarely cured by currently available therapies. Other lung diseases that may be considered for gene therapy include acquired disorders that are associated with inflammatory states (e.g., interstitial lung disease, emphysema, chronic bronchitis, adult respiratory distress syndrome), and chronic thromboembolic disease.

α1-Antitrypsin Deficiency
α1-Antitrypsin deficiency is an autosomal hereditary disorders characterized by a low serum level of α1AT and emphysema by ages 30 to 40 years. A subgroup of affected individuals develop hepatitis and cirrhosis. The α1AT gene is comprised of 7 exons spread over 12.2 kb, on chromosome 14 at q31-32.3. A variety of mutations have been identified which result in decreased or absent levels of the α1AT in the blood and the lung (Crystal, 1990). α1AT is a 52 kDa glycoprotein that is produced mostly in hepatocytes. It functions in the lung to inhibit neutrophil elastase, a potent proteolytic enzyme capable of causing lung destruction. The pathogenesis of α1AT deficiency is directly linked to this fact; without α1AT to protect the lung, neutrophil elastase chronically deposited by neutrophils in the lower respiratory tract slowly destroys the lung over a period of many years. α1AT deficiency is associated with a shortened life span; in the USA only 52% of affected 18-year-olds live to age 50 (compared to 93% in the general population) and 16% survive to age 60, compared to 85% of the general population. Individuals with α1AT deficiency who smoke cigarettes have a life span shortened by 10 years more than non-smokers.

Currently, intravenous α1AT augmentation therapy is the therapy for this disease.

Conventionally, the therapy is started only after the disease is clinically apparent. Human plasma αlAT is administer once weekly or once monthly for the life of the patient, a therapy that is inconvenient and expensive, making gene therapy an attractive alternative. Further, αlAT deficiency is theoretically the easiest and most feasible of lung diseases to treat with gene therapy. A wide variety of approaches are possible because high levels of αlAT are not toxic, eliminating the need to tightly control the expression of gene.

Cystic Fibrosis
CF is an autosomal recessive disorder characterized by lung, liver, pancreatic, and intestinal disease. The pancreatic and intestinal manifestation of CF can be adequately treated with available therapy, but the respiratory disease is invariable fatal. Beginning early in childhood, CF is associated with mucus abnormalities, chronic airway infection and chronic neutrophil-dominated airway inflammation. The typical course involves chronic suppurative airway infections, mucus impaction, and recurrent pneumonia. There is progressive airway and alveolar destruction. Despite advances in antibiotic therapy and techniques to help clear respiratory secretions, the disease is usually fatal by ages 25 to 30 years.

The gene associated with CF, a 250 kb, 27 exon segment of chromosome 7 at q31, controls the production of the "cystic fibrosis transmembrane regulator" (CFTR) protein (Rommens et al., 1989). The most common (approximately 70%) mutation responsible for the CF phenotype is an in-phase deletion of 3 bases at position 508, with the loss of a phenylalanine residue (F508). The available evidence suggests that CFTR protein is a cAMP regulable chloride channel (Anderson et al., 1991). Importantly, transfer of the normal CF cDNA into immortalized epithelial cells from CF patients, using vaccinia virus or retroviral vectors, reverses the defect in chloride secretion (Drumm et al., 1990; Rich et al., 1990). The precise link between chloride channel dysfunction and the pathophysiology of lung disease remains to be determined.

There are currently no specific therapies for the respiratory manifestations of CF other than supportive therapy such as antibiotics to treat chronic lung infections and pneumonia, and chest physiotherapy to aid drainage of thick mucus. Experimental therapies under investigation include: (1) aerosolized amiloride to alter airway sodium transport and decrease the accumulation of mucous (Knowles et al., 1990); (2) aerosolized DNAse to cleave the DNA in purulent airway mucus, and thus reduce obstruction (Hubbard et al., 1991); and (3) aerosolized αl AT protect the airways from its high burden of neutrophil elastase resulting from the massive influx of neutrophils in the chronically infected lung (McElvaney et al., 1991). It is unlikely that any of these therapies will correct the primary disorder and thus, gene therapy is an attractive approach to cure the disease.

Other Lung Diseases
Lung cancer is one of the leading causes of cancer deaths in the world. The major forms of bronchogenic carcinoma are all epithelial cell tumors. Most are highly metastatic, and thus curative therapy has to be early (e.g., prior to metastases) or designed to eliminate the tumor cells throughout the body. In this context, the strategies (and problems) for gene therapy of bronchogenic carcinoma are similar to those for other neoplasms. However, mesothelioma, a uniformity fatal neoplastic disease of the pleura (and less commonly, the peritoneum), remains confined to the pleural space, offering the possibility of using therapeutic genes delivered via cells placed in the pleural space (e.g., modified lymphocytes) or by exposing the tumor to the vector in vivo by placing the vector in the pleural space or into the tumor itself.

Chronic thromboembolism, a pulmonary diseases characterized by clot in the pulmonary vasculature, results in disabling chronic respiratory limitation, right-sided heart failure and early death. Currently, the primary therapy for this disorder is chronic systemic anticoagulation to prevent recurrent clot, a therapy with a high complication rate. One approach to gene therapy for this disease similar to that being considered for coronary artery and arterial disease, in which vascular grafts seeded with genetically modified endothelial cells produce anticoagulants/fibrinolytics such as tissue plasminogen activating factor (TPA) (Dichek et al., 1989). Alternatively, it is possible that vectors containing genes for TPA, or anticoagulants (e.g., protein C, antithrombin III, or modified forms of α1AT with anticoagulant activity), could be introduced into the pulmonary artery for direct infection of the pulmonary endothelium.

Surfactant deficiency is a life threatening problem of premature neonates in which the lungs cannot inflate normally due to a deficiency in surface active material on the epithelial surface of the lower respiratory tract. The major problem in this disorder is an inability of the type II epithelial cells of the immature lung to express the genes for the apoproteins of surfactant (Weaver & Whitsett, 1991). Although there are therapies available in the form of intratracheal administration of surfactant, it is feasible that neonates (or in utero for at risk neonates) could be treated with gene transfer of the surfactant apoproteins.

There is a significant incidence of pulmonary infections in individuals with chronic granulomatous disease (CGD). The cytokine interferon-γ administered intravenously decreases the rate of infections in CGD (The International CGD Study Group, 1991). It is possible that vectors containing the interferon-γ gene could be introduced into the lung of CGD patients, rather than to be treated with weekly or monthly interferon-γ injections. Further, this cytokine enhances host defense in animal models of other chronic diseases such as tuberculosis (Rook et al., 1986), suggesting a possibility for enhancing respiratory tract host defenses in infections refractory to current antimicrobial therapy or in the immunosuppressed host. Once the infection was overcome, interferon-γ would no longer be needed, and thus a vector associated with transient expression may be ideal for such disorders.

VECTORS AND THEIR POTENTIAL USE

Three major vectors have been used in experimental models of gene transfer for lung targets: plasmids complexed with liposomes, retroviruses, and adenoviruses. Each vector system has advantages for different aspects of gene therapy in the lung. The plasmid systems generally exhibit transient expression, an advantage for potentially toxic genes or acquired lung disease. In contrast, retroviral vectors are useful for integrating genes into cells in vitro that can be subsequently transferred to the respiratory epithelial surface. Adenoviral vectors afford the advantage of respiratory tract-specific epithelial cell tropism, an important target cell for gene therapy.

Liposome-Plasmid Complexes
Plasmids have been used in a "naked" form to transfer genes in vivo to mouse skeletal muscle and heart, but to date, transfer to lung tissue has not been successful using this technique (Felgner and Rhodes, 1991). Instead, the cationic lipid reagent, lipofectin, has been used to facilitate in vivo uptake and expression (Felgner et al., 1987). In either case, the plasmid does not permanently integrate into the host genome. Liposome-plasmid complexes are easier to construct than viral vectors. The scale-up of plasmids can be done in conventional fermentation facilities and the liposome itself can be customized to bind to specific protein targets in the lung and can be designed to withstand aerosoliza-

tion (Mannino & Gould-Fogerite, 1988)).

The most dramatic demonstration of plasmid transfer has been into muscle, where expression is extensive and prolonged (Wolff et al., 1990). Of more relevance to the lung is the studies in which liposomes containing the E. coli lacZ gene was transferred in vivo to the iliofemoral artery endothelium (Nabel et al., 1990). Strikingly, β-galactosidase (the lacZ product) expression was observed for up to 42 days. While this approach has not been adapted to the lung, Brigham et al. (1989a) have transfected cultured bovine pulmonary artery endothelial cells with liposomes complexed with the Rous sarcoma virus promoter-chloramphenicol acetyltransferase (CAT) fusion gene and observed CAT expression for up to 14 days, suggesting that pulmonary endothelium may be modified in vivo with similar constructs.

The feasibility of respiratory tract genetic modification by introducing liposome-DNA complexes into the trachea was demonstrated by Hazinski et al. (1990), by injecting a liposome complex comprised of a plasmid containing the CAT gene driven by the Rous sarcoma virus promoter, into the trachea of rats. CAT expression was detected for up to 48 hours. Brigham et al. (1989b), using a similar construct, injected liposome-plasmid complexes into the lungs of mice and found in vivo CAT expression for 48 hours. In our laboratory, K. Yoshimura has demonstrated longer term expression of liposome facilitated gene transfer to the lung. In these studies, a plasmid containing the firefly luciferase DNA driven by the Rous sarcoma virus promoter was complexed with cationic liposomes and instilled intratracheally into mice. Efficacy of gene transfer was determined by resection of the lungs, homogenizing to lyse cells and evaluation using the luciferase assay. Increasing doses of plasmid (1-1500 μg/animal) resulted in a dose dependant increase in luciferase activity. Serial evaluation of animals revealed luciferase activity detected up to 2 weeks after intratracheal delivery (unpublished observations).

From these studies, it appears that liposome-mediated plasmid transfer appears to be feasible. However, the in vivo studies have not specifically identified the target cell infected by the vector. The amount of DNA required is large and further studies need to be done to determine the efficiency of respiratory cells gene transfer. In addition, transfer by this strategy is limited by a short expression period. This may be used to an advantage in some pulmonary diseases, particularly acquired infections, or to minimize undesirable adverse effects. Alternatively, because the liposome-plasmid vehicles are simple to prepare, and safety of the liposome-plasmid complex itself is not a major problem, repeated therapy by aerosolization of the vector to the lung might circumvent the transient nature of the expression.

Retroviral Vectors
Several types of viral vectors have been developed for gene transfer from a variety of RNA viruses including retroviruses and simian virus 40 (SV40) (McLachlin et al., 1990). The retroviral vector used in the Pulmonary Branch is based on the constructs developed from the Moloney murine leukemia virus by Gilboa (Gilboa et al., 1982) and Miller (Miller & Rosman, 1989).

There are a number of advantages of using retrovirus for gene therapy. First, the structure of the retrovirus allows modification so that large cDNA sequences can be inserted, including the gene of interest and a selectable marker gene, allowing for in vitro, and potentially in vivo, cell selection. Second, the gene to be transferred is integrated into the host genome, enhancing the possibility that the target cell will retain the altered genotype. Finally, modified retrovirus have been used for human gene therapy with no adverse effects associated with the vector (Rosenberg et al., 1990).

The initial strategy to adapt retroviral vectors for gene therapy relevant to the lung was to transfer a SV40 promoter-human α1AT cDNA recombinant gene into murine fibroblasts to mimic liver production of α1AT. Garver et al. (1987) implanted modified murine 3T3 cells producing human α1AT into the peritoneum of mice as a "factory" for α1AT production. When animals were evaluated after 4 weeks, human α1AT was detected in the blood and lung epithelial lining fluid of the animals. When the fibroblasts were recovered after 4 weeks, they contained the integrated gene, suggesting this strategy is associated with long term expression.

There are two problems with this approach. First, fibroblasts are not an appropriate cell target, since there is a risk of developing fibrosis at the site of transplantation. Second, whatever cell target might be used, α1AT would have to be produced to provide sufficient amounts of α1AT to protect the lung, a daunting prospect given the amounts required and the limitations of protein production and secretion of most cell types (other than hepatocyte, the natural source of α1AT). Both problems might be circumvented by using lymphocytes as targets and directly transplanting the modified lymphocytes to the lungs. The concept of repopulating the lung with genetically modified autologous lymphocytes has a clinical basis in that mild, sub-clinical cases of pulmonary diseases such as sarcoidosis and hypersensitivity pneumonitis are associated with large numbers of lymphocytes on the respiratory epithelial surface without associated abnormalities in lung function or other evidence of disease. Using animal models, we have demonstrated that genetically modified lymphocytes can be safely introduced into the respiratory tract, that these modified cells can survive and continue to express the new gene in the lungs for a significant period of time.

In the initial studies, Fukayama et al. (1991) used CTLL2 cells, a murine cytotoxic interleukin-2 (IL-2) dependent T-cell line, derived from C57Bl/6 mice. These cells were modified in vitro with a retroviral vector continuing cDNA for the E. coli marker gene lacZ and the Neo^R selectable gene. The modified, selected CTLL2 cells were transplanted via the trachea to the respiratory tract of syngeneic mice and flow cytometry was used to quantify the β-galactosidase containing cells. The CTLL2/lacZ cells remained in the lung for up to one week. Importantly, only a small percentage of modified cells could be detected in the spleen, suggesting that transplantation of the modified lymphocytes was lung specific. Further, when the transplanted animals were treated with intraperitoneal IL-2, there was a marked increase in numbers of modified lymphocytes in the lung.

Kanno et al. (1991) demonstrated that genetically modified T-cells transplanted to the respiratory tract can produce a therapeutic protein to potentially treat human disease. CTLL2 cells were genetically modified by a variety of different retroviral constructs and different promoters, each containing human α1AT cDNA and Neo^R resistance gene. Following selection, the modified cells were delivered by intratracheal transplantation to the respiratory epithelial surface. Evaluation of respiratory epithelial lining fluid demonstrated human α1AT 3 days later.

Finally, using primates, we have transplanted modified autologous T-lymphocytes to the respiratory epithelial surface and demonstrated the modified T-lymphocytes remain in the lung and continue to express a marker gene over several months. Autologous rhesus monkey T-lymphocytes where modified in culture by a retroviral vector containing the Neo^R gene. The cells were delivered to the lung via a fiberoptic bronchoscope, and the animals were evaluated serially by bronchoalveolar lavage and in blood for the T-cells containing the Neo^R gene. The modified cells gene could be detected post-transplantation in the lung and blood for at least 6 months. Further, no adverse effects have been associated with the transplantation or modification of the lymphocytes (unpublished observations).

Together, these studies suggest the feasibility of the use of transplanted genetically modified autologous lymphocytes for a variety of gene therapy applications in the lung. In addition to α1AT deficiency, cytokines such as interferon-γ could be delivered to the lung for use in host defense, as could genes coding for proteins relevant to treating lung tumors, and molecules such as DNase to help clear purulent mucus.

It is conceivable that retroviral vectors may be delivered directly to the respiratory epithelial cells by the aerosol route. As discussed above, the major problem with this strategy is the slow rate of proliferation of the target cells. It is certainly feasible in vitro, as Chytil et al. (1988) using an α1AT cDNA, have shown that human epithelial cells can be modified in culture using retroviral vectors. Currently, experiments are underway to attempt to infect the pulmonary epithelial cell with retrovirus in vivo by stimulating tracheobronchial epithelial cell turnover prior to instilling the vector. This approach is feasible, although there are several safety parameters that need to be evaluated before human studies are considered.

Finally, retroviruses have been used to transfer genes to hepatocytes (Friedmann et al., 1989), although the efficiency of this process is limited by the difficulties in having primary hepatocytes proliferate in vitro. For α1AT deficiency, the hepatocyte is an obvious target because it is the natural site of expression of the gene. S. Woo and his colleagues (Ponder et al., 1991) have developed the strategy of modifying hepatocytes with a retroviral vector in vitro and then infusing the modified hepatocytes into the spleen or liver. The results are encouraging in that animal studies demonstrate the modified cells are implanted in the liver, remain viable and express the newly introduced gene.

Adenoviral Vectors
Adenoviral vectors represent a third, and especially attractive vector for gene transfer to the lung. Adenoviral vectors are derived from disabled adenoviruses, double-stranded DNA viruses that are trophic for respiratory epithelium and responsible for acute respiratory tract infections. Unlike retroviruses, the adenovirus does not require host cell proliferation for gene transfer, making it an ideal vector for cell targets that have been difficult to approach with retroviral vectors because of their slow rate of proliferation. Furthermore, in contrast to liposome-mediated gene transfer, expression of genes transferred by the adenoviral vectors hold the promise of long term expression, despite the fact that it is not clear that the adenovirus transferred genes are integrated into the genome. For example, transfer of ornithine transcarbamylase (OTC) using an adenoviral vector to OTC deficient mice (Spf-ash) have demonstrated correction of the deficiency for over one year (Stratford-Perricaudet et al., 1990).

Rosenfeld et al. (1991) used a recombinant adenoviral vector (derived from wild type 5 adenovirus), made replication deficient by the deletion of a portion of the viral Ela coding sequence. Studies with a vector containing the human α1AT cDNA driven by the powerful major late promoter have demonstrated the feasibility of infecting a variety of rat and human lung epithelial cell lines and directing the synthesis and secretion of human α1AT by the modified cells. The vector has also been used to infect freshly obtained and human lung epithelial cells from individuals with α1AT deficiency and demonstrated successful in vitro production of human α1AT.

In vivo gene transfer has also been successfully carried out using this adenoviral vector. When instilled into the airways of cotton rats, functional human α1AT protein could be detected in the lung for at least one week. In situ hybridization studies revealed mRNA transcripts present in the respiratory epithelium. Adenoviral vectors may be the ideal approach for gene therapy of the respiratory manifestations of CF. By the nature of the disease, the strategy for gene therapy of CF must be quite different from that for disease due to a deficiency of secreted proteins such as α1AT, i.e, the use of genetically modified cell vehicles transplanted to the lung will not be useful. Instead, the most logical approach would be to integrate the normal gene into the cell that is the site of disease - the respiratory epithelial apical membrane that contains the defective chloride channel. It is known that individuals heterozygous for the CF gene have normal cell function, and thus the goal for gene therapy would be, at a minimum, to have expression of the normal newly introduced gene to be equivalent to expression of the endogenous gene. In this regard, Trapnell et al. (1991) have shown that the CF gene is normally expressed in airway epithelial cells at low levels (1-2 mRNA transcripts/cell) as is the mutated gene. Further, studies by Yoshimura et al. (1991) have shown that the promoter of the CF gene has features typical of a "housekeeping" gene, with low level expression. Thus, to correct the genetic defect in the respiratory tract of individuals with CF, the major problem is not level of expression (as it is with α1AT) but rather the ability to get the normal gene transferred to the respiratory epithelium. In this regard, using an adenoviral vector constructed in a fashion similar for the α1AT cDNA, the normal CF cDNA has been inserted under the control of the adenovirus major late promoter and used to transfer the recombinant CF gene to respiratory epithelial cells of cotton rats in vivo and freshly isolated epithelial cells from individuals with CF in vitro (Rosenfeld et al. 1991b).

Adenoviral vectors can be used for gene transfer to several other targets relevant to human lung disease. Studies in the Pulmonary Branch have demonstrated that human endothelial cells and fibroblasts can be modified to produce human α1AT, reflecting the versatility of this vector. Jaffe et al. (1991) have used the adenoviral vector containing human α1AT to infect primary hepatocytes in vitro. Expression of the α1AT protein was detected for up to 1 month after gene transfer. Further, in vivo studies of vector delivery into the portal vein have demonstrated α1AT synthesis and secretion in liver cells for at least 1 week after infection.

HURDLES

Several major hurdles must be overcome before lung-specific gene therapy can be used in humans. These can be put into three categories: (1) technical aspects of gene transfer; (2) creating animal models for gene transfer; and (3) demonstrating the safety of gene therapy in animal models and humans.

Technical problems of gene transfer to the lung include improving the efficiency of gene transfer and increasing the expression of transferred genes. For most pulmonary diseases being considered for this approach, a high percentage of target cells must be infected. This could be done by using unique receptor molecules to enhance targeting (Roux et al., 1989) and by increasing viral vector titers. To improve gene expression, stronger promoters or promoters turned off or on by specific proteins present in the respiratory tract may be used. It has been hypothesized that specific microorganisms could be combated by using retroviral vectors that contained toxin-inducible promoters, leading to the expression of a gene coding for a protein capable of killing a microorganism (Goldsmith, 1990).

The lack of animal models of CF and α1AT have limited the evaluation of gene therapy for these pulmonary diseases, so that extrapolation to human therapies is difficult. Another problem with lung-related animal models of gene therapy is that when the cells of a normal host animal are modified with a human cDNA, the animal may develop immunity to the newly produced human protein causing difficulties in the evaluation of efficacy of therapy. We and others have attempted to circumvent this problem by using genes that produce non-secreted proteins such as reporter genes β-galactosidase and neomycin phosphotransferase (Neo^R). Recently, Bennett and Chang (1990) have demonstrated the feasibility of using cyclosporin A pretreatment of animals or immunologically immature neonatal rats as recipients to delay antibody production after delivering in vivo human growth factor by using genetically modified fibroblasts implanted in the peritoneum.

Finally, safety issues must be addressed before viral vectors can be used for human diseases. Unlike currently approved retroviral gene transfer experiments in humans, treatment of respiratory disease would often be by the aerosol rather than the intravenous route. This mandates that studies be performed to prevent the infection of unintended targets by vector that could escape into the local environment. Another issue unique to use of replication defective adenoviral vector is that recipients may harbor wild type adenovirus which, if recombined into the defective vector in a precise location, could re-enable defective adenovirus making it replication competent. This and other biosafety issues will have to be investigated to ensure that the benefit to risk ratio is sufficiently high to proceed with human trials.

REFERENCES

Anderson, M.P., Rich, D.P. et al.(1991): Expression of cAMP-activated choride currents by expression of CFTR. Science 251, 679-682.
Bennett, V.J. & Chang, P.L. (1990): Supression of immunological response against a novel gene product delivered by implants of genetically modified fibroblasts Mol. Biol. Med. 7, 471-477.
Brigham, K.L., Meyrick, B. et al. (1989a): Expression of a prokaryotic gene in cultured lung endothelial cells after lipofection with a plasmid vector. Am. J. Resp. Cell. Mol. Biol. 1, 95-100.
Brigham, K.L., Meyrick, B. et al. (1989b): In vivo transfection of murine lungs with a functioning prokaryotic gene using a liposome vehicle. Am. J. Med. Sci. 298, 278-281.
Chytil, A., Garver, R. & Crystal, R. (1988): Human α1-antitrypsin production by human epithelial cells infected with a retroviral vector containing the human α1-antitrypsin gene. Am. Rev. Respir. Dis. 137, A371.
Crystal, R.G. (1990). α1-Antitrypsin deficiency, emphysema, and liver disease-genetic basis and strategies for therapy. J. Clin. Invest. 85, 1343-1352.
Dichek, D.A., Neville, R.F. et al. (1989): Seeding of intravascular stents with genetically engineered endothelial cells. Circulation 80, 1347-1353.
Drumm, M.L., Pope, H.A. et al. (1990): Correction of the cystic fibrosis defect in vitro by retrovirus-medicated gene transfer. Cell 62, 1227-1233.
Evans, M.J. & Shami, S.G. (1989): Lung cell kinetics. In: Lung Cell Biology, ed C. Lenfant & G.D.C. Massaro, pp. 1-36, New York: Marcel Dekker.
Felgner, P.L. & Rhodes, G. (1991): Gene therapeutics. Nature 349, 351-2.
Felgner, P.L., Gadek, T.R. et al. (1987) Lipofection: A highly efficient, lipid-mediated DNA-transfection procedure. Proc. Natl. Acad. Sci. USA 84, 7413-7417.
Friedmann, T., Xu, L. et al. (1989): Retrovirus vector-mediated gene transfer into hepatocytes. Mol. Biol. Med. 6, 117-125.
Fukayama, M., Kanno, T. et al. (1991): Respiratory tract "organ specific" gene therapy: Transplantation of genetically modified T-lymphocytes directly to the respiratory epithelial surface. Am. Rev. Respir. Dis. Abstr. (In press).
Garver Jr., R.I., Chytil, A. et al. (1987): Clonal gene therapy: Transplanted mouse fibroblast clones express human α-1 antitrypsin gene in vivo. Science

237, 762-764.
Goldsmith, M.A. (1990): From molecular biology to "genetic antibiotics". Prospect. Biol. Med. 34, 99-108.
Gilboa, E., Kolbe, M. et al. (1982): Construction of a mammalian transducing vector from the genome of a Moloney murine leukemia virus. J. Virol. 44, 845-851.
Hazinski, T.A., Magnunson, A. et al. (1990): Liposome-mediated insertion and regulated expression of fusion genes into the intact Lung. Am. Rev. Respir. Dis., 141, A354.
Hubbard, R.C., McElvaney et al. (1991):Aerolsolized recombinant DNase therapy for cystic fibrosis. Am. Rev. Respir. Dis. Abstr., (In press).
Jaffe, H.A., Longenecker, G. et al.(1991): Adenoviral mediated transfer and expression of a normal human α1-antitrypsin cDNA in primary rat hepatocytes. Clin. Res. Abstr., (In press).
Kanno, T., Fukayama, M. et al. (1991): Retroviral transfer of the human α1-antitrypsin gene to T-lymphocytes for in vivo gene therapy. Am. Rev. Respir. Dis., Abstr., (in press).
Knowles, M.R., Church, N.L. et al.(1990): A pilot study of aerosolized amiloride for the treatment of lung disease in cystic fibrosis. N. Engl. J. Med. 322, 1189-1194.
Mannino, R.J. & Gould-Fogerite, S. (1988): Liposome mediated gene transfer. Biotechniques 7, 682-690.
McElvaney, N.G., Hubbard, R.C. et al. (1991): Aerosol α1-antitrypsin treatment for cystic fibrosis. Lancet 337, 392-394.
McLachlin, J.R., Cornetta, K. et al. (1990):Retroviral-mediated gene transfer. Prog. Nucleic Acid Res. Mol. 38:91-135.
Miller, A.D. & Rosman, G.J. (1989): Improved retroviral vectors for gene transfer and expression. Biotechniques 7, 980-990
Miller, D.G., Adam, M.A. & Miller, A.D. (1990): Gene transfer by retrovirus vectors occurs only in cells that are actively replicating at the time of infection. Mol. Cell. Biol. 10, 4239-4242.
Nabel, E.G., Plautz, G. & Nabel, G.J. (1990): Site-specific gene expression in vivo by direct gene transfer into the arterial wall. Science 249, 1285-1288.
Ponder, K.P., Gupta, S. et al. (1991): Mouse hepatocytes migrate to liver parenchyma and function indefinetely after intrasplenic transplantation. Proc. Natl. Acad. Sci. USA 88, 1217-1221.
Rich, D.P., Anderson, M.P. et al. (1990): Expression of cystic fibrosis transmembrane conductance regulator corrects defective chloride channel regulation in cystic fibrosis airway epithelial cells. Nature 347, 358-363.
Rommens, J.M., Iannuzzi, M.C. et al. (1989): Identification of the cystic fibrosis gene: Chromosome walking and jumping. Science 245, 1059-1065.
Rook, C.A.W., Steele, J. et al (1986): Activation of macrophages to inhibit proliferation of Mycobacterium tuberculosis: comparison of the effects of recombinant gamma-interferon on human monocytes and murine peritoneal macrophages. Immunology 59, 333-338.
Rosenberg, S.A., Aebersold et al. (1990): Gene transfer into humans-immunotherapy of patients with advanced melanoma, using tumor-infiltrating lymphocytes modified by retroviral gene transduction. N. Engl. J. Med. 323, 570-578.
Rosenfeld, M.A., Siegfried et al. (1991a): In vivo transfer of a functional human α-1 antitrypsin cDNA directly to the respiratory epithelium with a recombinant adenoviral vector. Science (in press).
Rosenfeld, M.A., Yoshimura, K. et al. (1991b): In vivo transfer of the human cystic fibrosis gene to the respiratory epithelium. Clin. Res. Abstr., (In press).
Roux, P., Janteur, P. & Piechaczyk (1989): A versatile and potentially general approach to the targeting of specific cell types by retroviruses: Application to the infection of human cells by means of major histocompatibility complex

class I and class II antigens by mouse ecotropic murine leukemia virus-derived viruses. Proc. Natl. Acad. Sci. USA 86, 9079-9083.

Sanes, J.R., Rubenstein, J.L.R. & Nicholas, J-F. (1986): Use of a recombinant retrovirus to study post-implantation cell lineage in mouse embryos. EMBO J. 5,3133-3142.

Selden, C., Gupta, S. et al. (1984): The pulmonary vascular bed as a site for implantation of isolated liver cells in inbred rats. Transplantation 38, 81-83.

Stratford-Perricaudet, L.D., Lervero, M. et al. (1990): Evaluation of the transfer and expression in mice of an enzyme-encoding gene using a human adenovirus. Human Gene Therapy 1, 241-256.

The International Chronic Granulomatous Disease Cooperative Study Group (1991): A controlled trial of interferon gamma to prevent infection in chronic granulomatous disease. New Engl. J. Med. 324, 509-516.

Then, P., Sandbichler, P. et al. (1991): Hepatocyte transplantation into the lung for treatment of acute hepatic failure in the rat. Transplant. Proceed. 23, 892-893.

Trapnell, B.C., Chu, C-S. et al. (1991): Expression of the cystic fibrosis transmembrane conductance regulator gene in the respiratory tract of normals and individuals with cystic fibrosis. Proc. Natl. Acad. Sci. USA (In press)

Weaver, T.E. & Whitsett, J.A. (1991): Function and regulation of expression of surfactant-associated proteins. Biochem. J.15, 249-64.

Wolff, J.A., Malone, R.W. et al (1990): Direct gene transfer into mouse muscle in vivo. Science 247, 1465-1468.

Yoshimura, K. Nakamura, et al. (1991): The cystic fibrosis gene has a "housekeeping"-type promoter and is expressed at low levels in cells of epithelial origin. J. Biol. Chem. (In press).

RESUME : Au fur et à mesure de l'évolution à la fois de la technologie du transfert de gène et des concepts relatifs aux sites de la thérapie génique qui s'est élargie au delà des cellules de la moelle osseuse, le poumon est apparu comme une cible de choix. Cet organe est le site principal de maladies comme la mucoviscidose ou fibrose kystique du pancréas (CF), et du déficit en alpha1-antitrypsine (alpha1AT), deux maladies parmi les plus fréquentes des désordres héréditaires mortels, aux Etats-Unis et en Europe. De plus, le poumon a une anatomie particulière qui permet de délivrer des vecteurs de thérapie génique directement à son parenchyme. L'arbre trachéobronchique et l'arbre vasculaire pulmonaire cumulent à eux deux un potentiel supérieur à 95% pour distribuer des vecteurs à l'ensemble de la masse cellulaire de ce tissu ; enfin la cavité pleurale représente une possibilité d'accès à la surface externe de l'organe. L'objet de cette revue consiste à résumer l'ensemble de ces concepts et à détailler les progrès actuels faisant de la thérapie génique du tractus respiratoire une réalité. Dans ce but, nous envisagerons l'ensemble des cibles cellulaires possibles pour une thérapie génique du tractus respiratoire, ainsi que les maladies qui relèvent de cette approche ; et enfin, les trois systèmes de vectorisation de l'ADN capables de modifier le programme génétique des cellules de ce tractus.

# Germinal and somatic gene therapy of a liver enzymatic defect in mouse

Pascale Briand [1], Catherine Cavard [1], Leslie D. Stratford-Perricaudet [2], Massimo Levrero [3], Iman Makeh [1], Gisèle Grimber [4], Jean-François Chasse [4], Michel Perricaudet [2]

[1] Laboratoire de génétique et pathologie expérimentales, Institut Cochin de Génétique Moléculaire INSERM CJF 90-03, 22, rue Méchain, 75014 Paris, France; [2] Laboratoire de génétique des virus oncogènes, Institut Gustave Roussy, 94805 Villejuif Cedex, France; [3] Clinica Medica, Universita di Roma and Fondazione A. Cesalpino, Rome, Italy; [4] Laboratoire de biochimie génétique URA CNRS 1335, Hôpital Necker, 149, rue de Sèvres, 75743 Paris, France

Introduction

Impressive progress has been made in the understanding of pathogenesis of human genetic diseases and in the isolation of disease-related genes. The preparation of a physical map along with the sequencing of the entire human genome will undoubtedly contribute to these advances. Nevertheless, current therapies for most human genetic diseases remain inadequate and this discrepancy between diagnosis and treatment potentials leads to major ethical problems. Thus, to any new approaches to diagnosis must be added new approaches to disease treatment. With the development of molecular genetics, the concept of gene therapy has progressively emerged, setting a cohort of technical and ethical problems. First, it was necessary to demonstrate that the addition of a normal gene to the genome was able to compensate the deficiency of the corresponding endogenous sequence. This was rapidly performed on several models using the transgenic mice technology (Hammer *et al* 1984; Le Meur *et al* 1985; Yamamura *et al* 1985; Mason *et al* 1987; Pinkert *et al* 1985; Readhead *et al* 1987; Cavard *et al* 1988; Costantini *et al* 1986; Jones *et al* 1990). As an example, we describe in this paper, the experiments we carried out to demonstrate that it is possible to correct an enzymatic defect, the ornithine transcarbamylase (OTC) deficiency, by gene transfer of the rat OTC cDNA into the mouse germ line (Cavard *et al* 1988). This was the first step toward an elaboration of human OTC deficiency treatment by gene transfer. Nevertheless, such an approach is irrelevant to the human species since germinal gene therapy would require the selection of normal embryos among abnormal ones, opening the possibility for their reintroduction. In contrast to this, somatic gene therapy rapidly emerged as a potential therapeutic method suitable for humans, its principle being very close to the more classic organ transplantations. Most of the work in the development of techniques for clinically applicable gene transfer had centered around the addition of genes to target cells, *in vitro*, followed by the reimplantation *in vivo* of the genetically modified cells (Friedmann *et al* 1989, Briand & Kahn 1990). For this purpose, the target cells must be able to produce the lacking protein in such a way that the impaired function can be restored. Such targeted cells should be manipulable with ease *in vitro* and should of course be reimplantable. If the appropriate stem cells can be reached, stability of correction may then be ensured. In contrast to bone marrow cells which satisfy most of these criteria, many tissues in which it may prove necessary to target a normal gene are not so easy to manipulate. Such is the case for hepatocytes, the preferred target for gene therapy due to many inborn errors of metabolism and for which transplantation is currently warranted. Despite, and paradoxically because of, the important progress made in this field, liver transplantation is first limited by the number of available organs, and secondly because it remains a surgical procedure with high mortality and continues to require life-long immunosuppressive therapy. For the special case discussed here however, the OTC deficiencies, liver transplantations have been successfully applied to cure heterozygous females. Concerning hemizygous males exhibiting a severe deficiency with a neonatal onset of symtoms, therapy has to be administered rapidly. With this in mind, we designed an approach involving the direct *in vivo* introduction of a gene transfer vector carrying the normal OTC sequence. This method was tested on the mouse model for OTC deficiency previously used to assess the efficiency of germinal gene therapy (Stratford-Perricaudet *et al* , 1990).

Ornithine transcarbamylase deficiencies in mouse and human species.
OTC is a mitochondrial enzyme that catalyses the synthesis of citrulline from ornithine and carbamylphosphate in the mammalian urea cycle. The enzyme is encoded by an X-linked gene and is expressed in the liver and small intestine . Human OTC deficiency is one of the most frequent hereditary hyperammonemias (Brusilow, S. & Horwich A.L. 1989). This X-linked inherited disease leads to the death of 75% of affected males. Positive diagnosis is based on a rapid clinical deterioration after a short normal period ranging from one to several days after birth. Lethargy, vomiting and coma are typical symptoms. Biochemical markers including elevated level of blood ammonia, hyperglutaminemia and hypocitrullinemia, and orotic aciduria are the hallmarks of this disorder. The diagnosis can be confirmed by measuring the OTC activity in a liver biopsy. Besides the neonatal forms, milder enzymatic defects are also found in males; some heterozygous females also express some features of

the disease (Briand et al, 1982). Even in these cases, an irreversible hyperammonemic coma can never be excluded. Despite restricted protein intake and improved pharmaceutical therapy which includes administration of sodium benzoate, phenylacetate or butyrate to reduce the nitrogen load, many patients die or are mentally retarded. The only real therapy is liver transplantation, but it cannot be readily applied before the first deterioration which is induced by the severe hyperammonemia developed by severely affected males. Furthermore, for heterozygous females or males with a late onset of symptoms, donor livers are not always available. These factors make this monogenic hereditary metabolic disease a good candidate for somatic gene therapy. In addition, elaboration of somatic gene therapy is highly facilitated by the availability of the spf and spf-ash murine models of OTC deficiency (Doolittle et al, 1974; Qureshi et al, 1979). These mutants are due to point mutations either in the coding sequence thus altering the pH optimum of the enzyme (mutation spf : 117 his asp), or in the splicing (mutation spf-ash : G A at the last base pair of the exon 4) (Veres et al, 1987; Hodges & Rosenberg, 1989). Both spf and spf-ash strains of mice exhibit the classic symptoms of human OTC deficiency, and in addition, they are hypotrophic and their fur is sparse at least until weaning. We have used the spf-ash mice to determine whether gene transfer of a normal OTC sequence could correct this inborn error of the metabolism (Cavard et al 1988).

Germinal gene therapy of the spf-ash mutation.

The rat OTC cDNA coupled to the SV40 large T antigen promoter region was microinjected into fertilized eggs obtained from homozygous Spf-ash females mated with C57BL males. One transgenic male was obtained. When compared with the other male of the same litter, the transgenic animal had a normal fur, a quite normal orotic aciduria and a normal weight. The OTC expression analysed in F1 transgenic spf-ash animals was quite normalised in the liver and small intestine (80 to 90% of control values). We also detected a low level of transgene expression in the spleen and lungs where endogenous activity has never been found. Analysis of the progeny of the corrected animal mated with homozygous spf-ash females allowed us to assert that the mutation was still present in the transgenic animal and that corrected phenotypes were clearly due to transgene expression. Thus, it was demonstrated that gene transfer of a normal OTC sequence could correct the inborn spf-ash OTC deficiency. Recently, M. Grompe et al have also corrected the spf mutation by transfer of the human OTC cDNA put under the transcriptional control of the mouse OTC promoter in spf embryos (Grompe et al 1990).

Altogether these results demonstrate that the mouse OTC deficiencies can be corrected by gene transfer.

Somatic gene therapy of the mouse spf-ash OTC deficiency
A second step in the elaboration of somatic gene therapy in humans is to test its feasibility on animal models. We tried to perform somatic gene transfer on the spf-ash strain of mice previously used to assess germinal gene transfer efficiency. As previously mentioned, ornithine transcarbamylase deficiency is a monogenic disease exhibiting specific problems with regard to gene therapy. The first problem is linked to the fact that the therapy has to be engaged very rapidly after birth. The second problem concerns the tissue in which this enzyme is mainly found.

In contrast to skeletal myofibers and myocardial cells, hepatocytes do not appear to efficiently take up DNA, thus eliminating direct delivery of DNA by injection into the liver. Several groups have described the transduction of cultured hepatocytes with retroviruses (Ledley et al 1987, Wolff et al 1987, Wilson et al, 1988 a and 1988b, Anderson et al 1989, Friedman et al 1989) the current vectors in the limelight for gene therapy, but concerning *in vivo* delivery, previous studies have demonstrated that hepatocytes are refractory to Moloney murine leukemia virus infection (Jaenish 1976, Jaenish and Hoffmann 1979, Jaenish 1980). This could impede the application of retroviruses to gene transfer into fully differenciated hepatic tissue *in vivo*. It has also been reported that retroviruses might be unstable and can provide inefficient gene expression. Their low titers are also a problem for direct delivery. Increasing interest is emerging in other expression vectors such as vaccinia, herpes, adeno-associated, bovine papilloma and adenovirus. For the numerous reasons described by Michel PERRICAUDET in this issue, we chose to evaluate the feasibility of adenovirus to directly provide spf-ash mutant mice after birth with the lacking functional gene. A recombinant adenovirus harboring the rat OTC cDNA under the control of the viral major late promoter (MLP) was constructed and injected into Spf-ash mutant mice which exhibit a reduction to 5% of the wild-type level of functional OTC protein. The recombinant adenovirus designated AdMLP-OTC is defective for the E1A gene, but can be efficiently propagated on 293 cells that complement this defect. The Ad MLP-OTC recombinant virus is able to express the OTC gene after infection of HeLa and 293 cells, as well as primary rat hepatocytes.

<u>Biological activity of the recombinant Ad MLP-OTC Spf-ash mice.</u>
The virus was inoculated intravenously into neonatal Spf-ash mice obtained by mating hemizygous males with homozygous females for the spf-ash mutation, and OTC activity was assayed in the liver. An evaluation of the expression of the OTC sequence carried by the

injected virus was made by monitoring the hepatic OTC activity at 1, 2 and 15 months post injection. A wide spectrum of values ranging from those observed in mutant animals, to those found in normal mice was obtained. The mice displaying the highest OTC activity no longer presented the visual phenotype of Spf-ash animals. Nevertheless, a number of mice had an intermediate phenotype. The recombinant virus was also injected directly into the peritoneal cavity or in the liver of older animals leading to variable levls of expression in the liver (data not shown).

As indirect evidence of the biological action of the gene introduced, it was found that the orotic aciduria assayed in urine samples collected until 15 months post injection was reduced to quite normal values.

DISCUSSION , CONCLUDING REMARKS AND PERSPECTIVES

Our results confirm the ability of adenovirus to act as a high-performance tool for the expression of genes in cells and demonstrate that it could be considered as a potential vector for direct delivery of functional transcriptional information *in vivo*.

Nevertheless, it is clear that many questions are still open:

1- What are the levels of OTC activity that are necessary to correct the impaired metabolism in humans? It seems that in the mouse, 20 % of OTC activity could be sufficient. Nevertheless, if in spf or spf-ash mice 5% OTC activity is compatible with a quite normal life, this residual activity is most often not compatible with a prolonged life in humans. Furthermore, even with higher OTC residual levels late irreversible hyperammonaemia might occur on the occasion of an infection or other hypercatabolic situation leading to the death of the individual (Brusilow & Horwich 1989). Thus, it will be difficult to precisely estimate the minimal OTC level in the mouse animal models without extensive experiments including evaluation of the responses to hypercatabolic stress and hyperproteinic diets after somatic gene therapy.

2 Is an ectopic or over-expression susceptible to be deleterious? The use of appropriate regulatory regions to target and control the OTC transgene expression would resolve this problem. Naturally, the OTC regulatory sequences would appear to be the best. Part of the upstream enhancer elements of rat and mouse OTC have been identified but more has to be done before their use in a perfectly regulated OTC corrector minigene. Another way could be to limit the integration of the recombinant DNA to the liver.

3-What are the reasons behind the variability of the correction from one animal to another? Are they related to immunological reactions or to great variations in the virus uptake by hepatocytes ? Experiments are now in progress with a recombinant adenovirus carrying the reporter gene *LacZ* controlled by the RSV LTR, to more precisely evaluate the number and localization of hepatocytes expressing the recombinant adenovirus as well as the stability of the transgene expression. Preliminary results show that 15 days after intravenous introduction of the recombinant adenovirus, many pulmonary cells and hepatocytes strongly express the reporter gene. In the spleen, the kidney, and the heart some positive cells were also detected. The use of the LacZ reporter gene will allow comprehensive studies concerning the virus uptake and the expression stability of adenoviral vectors.

4-Are hepatocytes the unique cellular targets for OTC deficiency gene therapy? In fact, if OTC is mainly found in the liver, the enzyme activity is also present in the intestine where it reaches 20% of the hepatic level. Jones *et al* (Jones *et al*, 1990) have recently demonstrated by transgenesis that a slight increase in OTC expression in the small intestine was sufficient to restore a normal ammoniac elimination in spf mice. Consequently, repeated oral delivery of recombinant OTC adenovirus could be considered as an alternative approach for the treatment of OTC deficiencies.

5- Finally, what are the risks of using recombinant adenoviruses in humans, and is it time to perform such a therapy in humans? The general risks of defective recombinant adenoviral-based therapy would be mainly linked to their propagation following an opportunistic wild-type Ad infection. However, such a production can be severely hampered by the use of a vector harboring a mutated packaging sequence. Experiments are now in progress in the Michel PERRICAUDET's laboratory to demonstrate this hypothesis. Once this point confirmed, taking into account the severity of the disease and the positive results obtained with the spf-ash animal model, it would seem reasonable to submit the project for ethical evaluation.

In conclusion, this work shows the usefulness of appropriate animal models to rapidly elaborate gene therapy potentially applicable to the human species.

References

Anderson, K.D., Thompson, J.A., Di Pietro, J.M., Montgomery, K.T., Reid, L.M., and Anderson, W.F., (1989) Gene expression in implanted hepatocytes following retroviral-mediated gene transfer. Somat. Cell. Mol. Genet. 15, 215-227.

Briand, P. et Kahn, A. (1990) Nouvelles orientations pour la thérapie génique. médecine/sciences 2, 144-149.

Briand, P., Baudoin, F., Rabier, D., and Cathelineau, L. (1982): Ornithine transcarbamylase deficiencies in human males. Kinetic and immunological classification. Biochim. Biophys. Acta. 704, 100-106.

Brusilow, S. & Horwich, A. L. (1989): Urea cycle disorders. In The metabolic basis of inherited diseases, 6th edn, ed Scriver, C. R., Beaudet, A. L., Sly, W. S., & Valle, D., pp 629-663, New-York: Mc Graw-Hill.
Cavard, C., Grimber, G., Dubois, N., Chasse J.F., Bennoun, M., Minet-Thurriaux, M., Kamoun, P., and Briand P. (1988): Correction of mouse ornithine transcarbamylase deficiency by gene transfer into the germ line. Nucleic Acids Res. 16, 2099-2110.
Costantini, F., Chada, K., and Magram, J. (1986): Correction of murine b-thalassemia by gene transfer into the germ line. Science. 233, 1192-1194.
Doolittle, D. P., Hulbert, L. L., and Cordy, C. A. (1974): A new allele of the sparse fur gene in the mouse. J. Hered. 65, 194-195.
Friedmann, T., (1989) Progress toward human gene therapy Science. 244, 1275-1281.
Friedmann, T., Li, X., Wolff, J.,Yee, J.K., and Miyanohara, A. (1989) Retrovirus vector mediated gene transfer into hepatocytes. Mol. Biol. Med. 6, 117-125.
Grompe, M., Jones, S.N., and Caskey, C.T. (1990): Molecular detection and correction of ornithine transcarbamylase deficiency. Trends. Genet. 6, 335-339.
Hammer, R.E., Palmiter, R.D., and Brinster, R.L. (1984) Partial correction of murine hereditary growth disorder by germ-line incorporation of a new gene. Nature. 311, 65-67.
Hodges, P. E. and Rosenberg, L. E. (1989): The spf-ash mouse: a missense mutation in the ornithine transcarbamylase gene also causes aberrant mRNA splicing. Proc. Natl. Acad. Sci. USA. 86, 4142-4146.
Jaenisch, R. (1976) Germ line integration and mendelian transmission of the exogeneous Moloney leukemia virus. Proc. Natl. Acad. Sci. USA. 73, 1260-1264.
Jaenisch, R., (1980) Retroviruses and embryogenesis: microinjection of Moloney leukemia virus into midgestationmouse embryos. Cell. 19, 181-188.
Jaenisch and Hoffmann.(1979) Transcription of endogeneous C-type viruses in resting and proliferating tissues of Balb/Mo mice. Virology 98, 289- 297.
Jones, S.N., Grompe, M., Munir, M.I., Veres, G., Craigen, W.J. and Caskey, C.T. (1990) : Ectopic correction of ornithine transcarbamylase deficiency in sparse fur mice. J. Biol. Chem. 265, 14684-14690.
Ledley, F., Darlington, G., Tahn, T., and woo,S. (1987) Retroviral geen transfer into primary hepatocytes: implications for genetic therapy of liver specific functions. Proc. Natl. Acad. Sci. USA 84, 5335-5339.
Le Meur, M., Gerlinger P., Benoist C., and Mathis D. (1985): Correcting an immune-response deficiency by creating E gene transgenic mice. Nature. 316, 38-41.

Mason, A.J. Pitts, S.H., Nikolics, K., Szonyi, E., Wilcox, J.N., Seeburg, P.H., and Stewart, T.A. (1987): The hypogonadal mouse: reproductive functions restored by gene therapy. Science. 234, 1372-1377.
Pinkert, C.A. Widera, G., Cowing, C., Heber-Katz, E., Palmiter, R.D., Flavell, R.A., and Brinster, R.L. (1985): Tissue-specific, inducible and functinal expression of the E MHC class II gene in transgenic mice. EMBO J. 4, 2225-2230.
Qureshi, I. A., Letarte, J., and Ouellet, R. (1979): Ornithine transcarbamylase deficiency in mutant mice: studies on the characterization of enzyme defect and suitability as animal models of human disease. Pediatr. Res. 13, 807-811.
Readhead, C., Popko, B., Takahashi,N., Shine, H.D., Saavedra, R.A., Sidman, R.L., and Hood, L. (1987): Expression of a myelin basic protein gene in transgenic shiverer mice: correction of the dysmyelinating phenotype. Cell. 48, 703-712.
Stratford-Perricaudet ,L., and Perricaudet M. (1991) Gene transfer into animals: the promise of adenovirus. In this issue.
Stratford-Perricaudet, L.D., Levrero, M., Chasse, J.F., Perricaudet, M., and Briand, P (1990): Evaluation of the transfer and expression in mice of an enzyme-encoding gene using a human adenovirus vector. Human Gene Therapy 1, 241-256.
Veres, G., Gibb, R. A., Scherer, S. E., and Caskey, C. T. (1987): The molecular basis of the sparse fur mouse mutation. Science. 237, 415-420.
Wilson, J.M., Jefferson, D., Chowdhury, J., Novikoff, P., Johnston, D., and Mulligan, R. (1988a) Retrovirus-mediated transduction of adult hepatocytes. Proc.Natl. Acad. Sci. USA 85, 3014-3018.
Wilson, J.M., Johnston, D., Jefferson, D.,and Mulligan, R. (1988b) Correction of genetic defect in hepatocytes from the watanabe heritable hyperlipidemic rabbit. Proc. Natl Acad. Sci. USA 85, 4421 4425.
Wilson, J.M., Yee, J.K., Skelly, H., Moores, J., Respess, J., Friedmann, T., and Leffert, H., (1987) Expression of retrovirally-transduced genes in primary cultures of adult rat hepatocytes. Proc. Natl. Acad. Sci. USA 84, 3344-3348.
Yamamura, K., Kikutani, H., Folsom. V., Clayton, L.K., Kimoto, M., Akira, S., Kashiwamura, S., Tonegawa, S., and Kishimoto,T. (1985): Functional expression of a microinjected E gene in C57BL/6 transgenic mice. Nature. 316, 67-69.

RESUME : Afin de faire progresser le concept de thérapie génique, il semblait nécessaire dans un premier temps de démontrer que l'addition d'un gène normal était capable de compenser la déficience des séquences endogènes correspondantes ; ceci a effectivement été réalisé dans des modèles de souris transgéniques. Nous avons ainsi pu démontrer qu'il était possible de corriger un défaut enzymatique, le déficit en ornithine transcarbamylase (OTC), par transfert du cDNA d'OTC du rat dans la lignée germinale de la souris. Ceci a constitué notre premier pas vers l'élaboration d'un traitement du déficit en OTC par transfert de gène. Compte-tenu de la précocité d'apparition des symptomes dans la période néo-natale et dans le but de développer un protocole de thérapie génique somatique, notre approche a consisté à l'introduction directe du vecteur portant la séquence d'OTC normale in-vivo. Cette méthodologie basée sur l'utilisation d'un adénovirus recombinant a été testée sur le modèle murin de la souris `spf-ash` préalablement normalisée par transfert de gène à la lignée germinale.

A procedure for stable gene transfer into the liver

Nicolas Ferry [1], Olivier Duplessis [2], Denis Calise [3], Didier Houssin [2], Jean-Michel Heard [1] and Olivier Danos [1]*

[1] Laboratoire Rétrovirus et Transfert Génétique, Institut Pasteur, 28, rue du Docteur Roux, 75015 Paris; [2] Laboratoire de Recherche Chirurgicale, UER Cochin-Port Royal, 27, rue du Faubourg Saint-Jacques, 75014 Paris; [3] Laboratoire de Chirurgie Expérimentale, CHU Necker-Enfants-Malades, 156, rue de Vaugirard, 75015 Paris, France

* Author for correspondence

SUMMARY

Stable gene transfer into hepatocytes might be used to compensate for a genetic deficiency affecting liver function or to deliver diffusible factors into the blood stream. In rats, we have combined retroviral-mediated gene transfer with a surgical procedure in which the liver is temporarily excluded from the circulation and infected in vivo. Partial hepatectomy was performed 24 to 48 hours before perfusion with virus in order to induce hepatocyte division and facilitate viral integration. A helper-free recombinant retrovirus coding for ß-galactosidase with nuclear localization was used to score cells that expressed the transgene. For at least three months following gene transfer, up to five percent of hepatocytes expressed nuclear ß-galactosidase. Whereas in vitro reimplantation of genetically modified hepatocytes has proven inefficient in stably transferring genes into the liver, our approach provides a feasible alternative.

The liver plays a central role in intermediary metabolism and supplies the organism with most of the serum proteins. Stable gene transfer into the liver may be considered for the treatment of numerous inherited liver diseases where either a metabolic function or the secretion of a serum protein is affected. A gene introduced in the liver parenchymal cells could also direct the synthesis of a therapeutic protein secreted into the blood stream. This protein could complement a genetic defect or display a curative function at remote sites in the organism.

The liver also stands out as a suitable target for gene transfer because following partial hepatectomy, intense cell proliferation is observed (Higgins and Anderson, 1931). During the regeneration where the partially ablated liver returns to its original mass, hepatocytes, which are normally quiescent, enter the cell cycle. Up to 30 % of the parenchymal cells reach the S phase within the first 24 hours (Fabrikant, 1968). As a rule, the mitotic state is required for stable integration of foreign genetic material. During the regeneration phase, hepatocytes would therefore be susceptible to stable gene transfer. Hepatocytes can also be triggered into cell cycle when explanted and cultivated in vitro. Stable gene transfer can be achieved under these conditions(Ledley et al., 1987; Wilson et al., 1988). Explanted hepatocytes can be stably engrafted back in the liver, or in the spleen where they form functional hepatic nodules(Mito et al., 1979; Ponder et al., 1991; Woods et al., 1982).

Two different approaches for stable gene transfer into the liver can therefore be imagined: a) *in vitro* transfer to explanted hepatocytes, followed by reimplantation, or b) direct transfer into the regenarating organ. In this communication, we describe our studies on rats where a retroviral vector carrying a marker gene was used to document the utility of the two strategies.

1) Retroviral vector and ex vivo gene transfer:

We have used retroviral vectors because the *in vivo* stability and long term expression of transgenes introduced in somatic cells by this means have been well documented(Flowers et al., 1990; Nabel et al., 1989; Wilson et al., 1989). We have constructed a vector containing a modified E. coli ß-galactosidase gene (nlslac Z)(Flowers et al., 1990; Nabel et al., 1989; Wilson et al., 1989). Histochemical X-gal staining of cells expressing the transgene is easy and allows to directly quantify gene transfer efficiency. The acquired ß-galactosidase activity being localized at the periphery of the cell nucleus, it is possible to perform double stainings in order to reveal specific cytoplasmic markers and to unambiguously characterize the nature of the target cell. In addition, the transgene activity is easily distinguished from an eventual endogenous signal from lysosomal enzymes.

The ß galactosidase gene was inserted in a Moloney murine leukemia virus-derived vector as shown in Fig. 1.

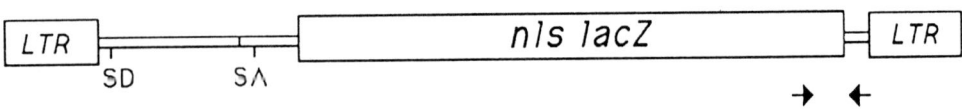

Fig. 1. Structure of the MFG-NB retroviral vector. Localizations of the oligodeoxynucleotide primers used for PCR are indicated by arrows.

High titer helper-free amphotropic recombinant retroviruses were generated in the ΨCRIP packaging cell line(Danos and Mulligan, 1988). The titers of individual producer clones ranged between 1 and 5×10^5 cfu / ml. Retroviral supernatants were used to infect primary rat hepatocytes in culture. Cells were plated and grown for three days before overnight incubation with retrovirus containing supernatant. Under these conditions, transgene expression could be detected in about 15% of the cells.

Growth of freshly explanted hepatocytes after injection in the spleen or in the liver of syngeneic animals has been documented(Mito et al., 1979; Ponder et al., 1991; Woods et al., 1982). In order to assess the possibility of stably grafting genetically modified hepatocytes, we injected our nlslacZ marked cells into the spleen of recipient rats. The spleens were analysed after 15 days for the presence of hepatic nodules and for ß-galactosidase activity. Although engrafment was observed when freshly explanted hepatocytes were injected, previously cultivated cells were unable to colonize the spleen.

2) In situ gene transfer to the regenarating liver:

We reasoned that a more efficient approach to transfer genes to the liver would be to first induce hepatocyte division by a partial hepatectomy and second, to perfuse the regenerating liver with a suspension of recombinant retroviral particles. For this purpose we have designed a surgical procedure illustrated in Fig. 2. The two large liver lobes were removed (two-third hepatectomy) and 24 to 48 hours later, the liver was temporarilly excluded from the systemic circulation by successively clamping the hepatic atery, the portal vein and the
supra-hepatic and infra-hepatic venae cavae. Infusion of the retroviral suspension was started through a canula inserted in the portal vein at a constant flow rate of 5 ml/min, for 10 minutes and the fluid was collected from the lower vena cava. After the perfusion, clamps were released and the regeneration was allowed to proceed until completion.

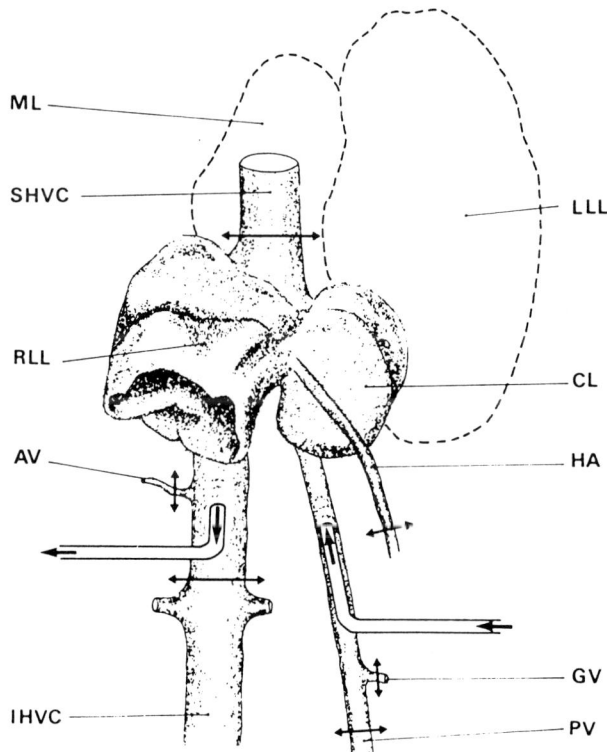

Fig. 2. Selective perfusion of remnant rat liver lobes after partial hepatectomy. The resected liver lobes appear as dotted lines. Double-headed arrows show the position of ligatures and clamping. The direction of the perfusion flow is indicated with arrows. LLL : left lateral lobe, ML median lobe, RLL: right liver lobe, CL : caudal lobe, AV : right adrenal vein, HA : hepatic artery, PV : portal vein, GV : gastroduodenal vein, IHVC : infrahepatic vena cava, SHVC : suprahepatic vena cava.

Under our conditions, liver regeneration in rats is complete after 7 days (Mito et al., 1979; Ponder et al., 1991; Woods et al., 1982). Perfused animals were sacrified 15 to 100 days after surgery and their liver was fixed and analyzed for expression of the transgene. X-Gal coloration revealing the presence of ß galactosidase activity could be directly performed on 5mm thick liver slices (Fig 3, panel B). Thiner (8μm) cryostat sections of the same liver were also incubated with X-Gal and a nuclear staining was observed (Fig 3 panel A). Beta-galactosidase activity only appeared in hepatocytes but never in macrophages, endothelial or non parenchymal epithelial cells. The positive cells were further identified as hepatocytes by immunohistochemical staining for albumin (Fig 3 panel C) or for a sinusoidal-specific membrane antigen (Fig 3 panel D).

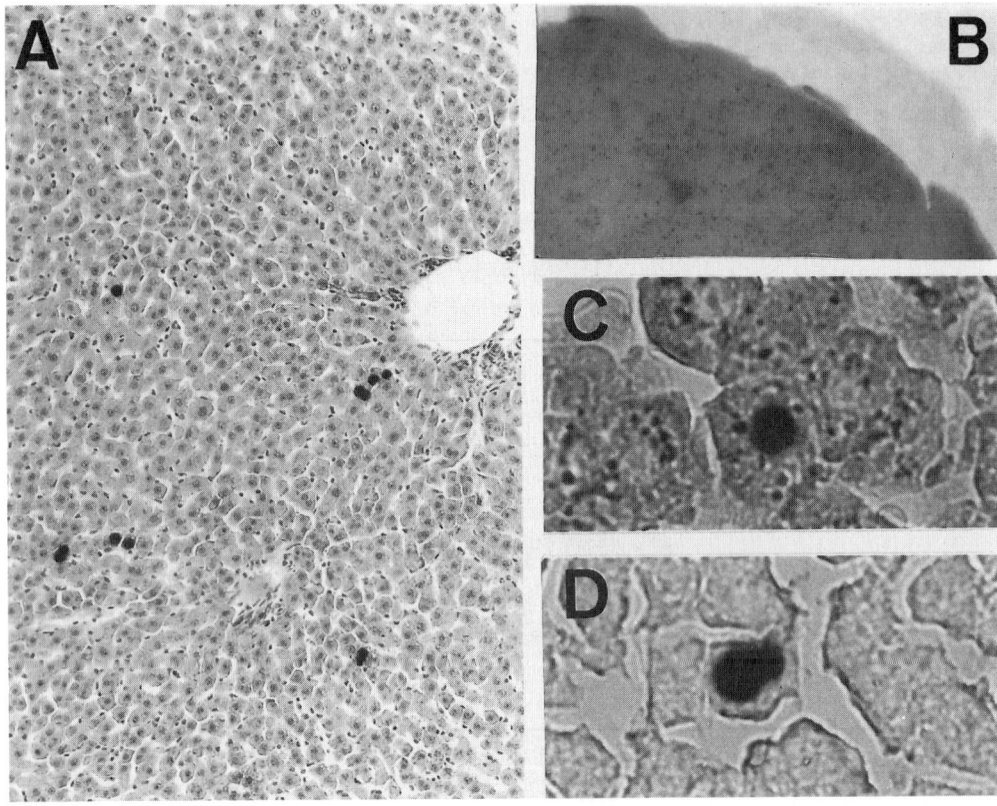

Fig. 3. Histochemical staining of livers from treated animals.
Panel B shows X-gal staining of 5 mm thick liver sections from rat number 9 examined with a binocular microscope. Panel A, C and D are representative cryostat sections stained with X-gal and counterstained respectively with hematoxylin-eosin (panel A, x60), a goat anti-serum directed against rat albumin (panel C, x500) and a monoclonal antibody directed against a sinusoïd membrane antigen specific of the hepatocyte (20) (panel D, x500).

Since we had used recombinant retroviruses preparation free of replication competent viruses, and since the liver was physically isolated from the rest of the organism during the asanguineous perfusion, we expected the gene transfer to be restricted to this organ. To check this point, we prepared DNA from liver, spleen, lung, kidney and brain of operated animals and looked for the presence of the recombinant provirus by polymerase chain reaction (PCR). The PCR assay could specifically detect one recombinant provirus in 10^4 cells and as shown in Fig. 4, the diagnostic 400 bp fragment was present in the liver DNA only. A sensitive virus mobilisation assay was used to detect the presence of replication competent virus in the tissues analysed by PCR. No virus was detected, even in the nlslacZ positive livers.

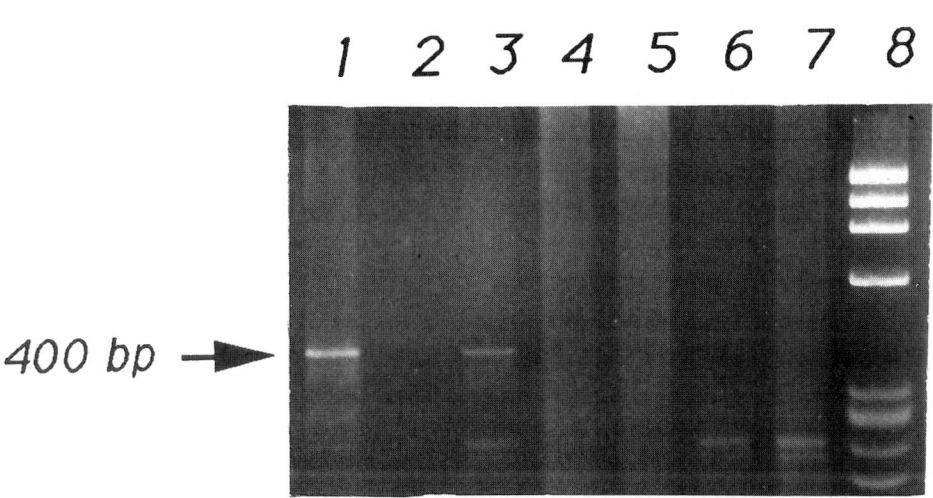

Fig. 4. PCR analysis of the MFG-NB provirus in the tissues of treated animals. PCR were performed using synthetic oligodeoxynucleotides primers and 1 µg of high molecular weight DNA. The reactions products were run on 3% agarose gels and revealed by ethidium bromide. DNA samples were prepared from NIH/3T3 cells containing one copy of integrated NB5 genome (lane 1), liver (lane 3), spleen (lane 4), lung (lane 5), brain (lane 6), kidney (lane 7) of rat 4. Lane 2 shows a control reaction performed in the absence of added DNA, and lane 8 molecular weight markers (phiX174 DNA digested with *Hae* III). After transfer to nylon membrane, the diagnostic 400 bp fragment shown by the arrow specifically hybridized with a ^{32}P labeled *lac* Z DNA probe (not shown).

Table 1 summarizes the data obtained with 10 animals. For each animal, the average number of blue nuclei per cm2 was counted on cryostat sections. Blue nuclei appeared in small groups of sister cells, with an average number of 1.7 nuclei per cluster. This is consistent with the notion that most hepatocytes

Animal	Interim period between hepatectomy and perfusion	ß-galactosidase positive nuclei per cm^2 §	Average number of nuclei per cluster *	Days between perfusion and sacrifice
1	48 hours	12.5 ± 1.5	1.19	15
2	"	21.3 ± 11	1.16	21
3	"	31.6 ± 10	1.25	21
4	24 hours	160 ± 85	1.32	21
5	"	260 ± 34	1.55	21
6	"	239 ± 86	2.07	43
7	"	210 ± 30	1.45	15
8	"	570 ± 150	1.78	15
9	"	> 1500	N.D.¶	15
10	"	297 ± 54	N.D.¶	100

Table 1. Number of *nlslac Z* positive cells in the livers of rats after a partial hepatectomy followed by a selective perfusion of the remnant lobes with the MFG-NB amphotropic retroviral vector. § Data are the mean numbers of nuclei expressing ß-galactosidase activity per cm^2 of liver section ± standard deviations. Positive cells were scored on different sections representing a total area of 10 to 30 cm^2. * Data are the ratios of the mean number of positive nuclei per cm^2 by the mean number of clusters per cm^2. ¶ : not determined.

participated in the regeneration process and divided once or twice on the average. Our data also indicates that gene transfer is more efficient when the perfusion is carried out 24 hours after hepatectomy. This time point corresponds to the peak of DNA synthesis after partial hepatectomy (Fabrikant, 1968) and we observed a direct relationship between the score of blue nuclei per cm2 and the amount of DNA replication at the time of perfusion.

We have estimated that 1 to 5% of the hepatocytes expressed the transgene. This represents 20 to 80×10^6 cells, a number that could be high enough to complement a deficiency. We are now trying to improve the proportion of genetically modified cells by optimizing the lag period between hepatectomy and perfusion, studying the beneficial effects of concentrating our viral preparation and adding hepatic specific growth factors to the perfusion medium.

The procedure that we describe here could possibly be adapted to human patients. We have been able to infect human hepatocytes in culture with our amphotropic retroviral vector and selective perfusion of liver lobes as well as partial hepatectomy are surgical procedures currently carried out in patients undergoing treatment for liver tumors. However, proposing a protocol for human gene therapy supposes previous demonstration of its capacity to cure a genetic disease in the available animal models. We are currently using the Gunn rat which lacks bilirubin glucuronosyl transferase, accumulates unconjugated bilirubin in its serum and develops jaundice, to test our ability to complement the genetic defect and to restore a normal phenotype using our liver perfusion procedure.

REFERENCES

Fabrikant, J. I. (1968). The kinetics of cellular proliferation in regenerating liver. J. Cell. Biol. *36*, 551-565.

Flowers, M. E. D., Stockschlader, M. A. R., Schuening, F. G., Niederwieser, D., Hackman, R., Miller, A. D. and Storb, R. (1990). Long-term transplantation of canine keratinocytes made resistant to G418 through retrovirus-mediated gene transfer. Proc. Nat. Acad. Sci. USA *87*, 2349-2353.

Higgins, G. M. and Anderson, R. M. (1931). Experimental pathology of the liver I. Restoration of the liver of the white rat following partial surgical removal. Arch. Pathol. *12*, 186-202.

Ledley, F. D., Darlington, G. J., Hahn, T. and Woo, S. L. C. (1987). Retroviral gene transfer into primary hepatocytes : implications for genetic therapy of liver-specific functions. Proc. Natl. Acad. Sci. USA *84*, 5335-5339.

Mito, M., Ebata, H., Kusano, M., Onishi, T., Saito, T. and Sakamoto, S. (1979). Morphology and function of isolated hepatocytes transplanted into rat spleen. Transplantation *28*, 499-.

Nabel, E. G., Plautz, G., Boyce, F. M., Stanley, J. C. and Nabel, G. J. (1989). Recombinant gene expression *in vivo* within endothelial cells of the arterial wall. Science *244*, 1342-1344.

Ponder, K. P., Gupta, S., Leland, F., Darlington, G., Finegold, M., DeMayo, J., Ledley, F. D., Chowdhury, J. R. and Woo, S. L. C. (1991). Mouse hepatocytes migrate tp liver parenchyma and function indefinitely after intrasplenic transplantation. Proc. Nat. Acad. Sci. USA *88*, 1217-1221.

Wilson, J. M., Birinyi, L. K., Salomon, R. N., Libby, P., Callow, A. D. and Mulligan, R. C. (1989). Implantation of vascular grafts lined with geneticaly modified endothelial cells. Science *244*. 1344-1346.

Wilson, J. M., Jefferson, D. M., Chowdhury, J. R., Novikoff, P. M., Johnqron, D. E. and Mulligan, R. (1988). Retrovirus-mediated transduction of adult hepatocytes. Proc. Natl. Acad. Sci. USA *85*, 3014-3018.

Woods, R. J., Fuller, B. J., Attenburrow, V. D., Nutt, L. H. and Hobbs, K. E. F. (1982). Functional assessment of hepatocytes after transplantation into rat spleen. Transplantion *33*, 123-.

RESUME : Le transfert stable de gènes dans des hépatocytes pourrait être utilisé soit pour compenser des déficits génétiques touchant la fonction hépatique soit pour délivrer des facteurs diffusibles dans le courant sanguin. Nous avons combiné chez le rat le transfert de gène médié par les rétrovirus avec un procédé chirurgical consistant à exclure temporairement le foie de la circulation et à l'infecter in-vivo. Une hépatectomie partielle a été pratiquée 24 à 48 heures avant la perfusion de virus afin d'induire une division hépatocytaire et faciliter ainsi l'intégration virale. Un rétrovirus recombinant dénué d'helper et codant pour une bêta-galactosidase à localisation nucléaire a été utilisé pour dénombrer les cellules exprimant le transgène. Jusqu'à 5% des hépatocytes expriment la bêta-galactosidase nucléaire au delà de trois mois suivant le transfert de gène. Tandis que la réimplantation in-vitro d'hépatocytes génétiquement modifiés s'est avérée jusqu'à présent infructueuse, notre approche constitue une alternative plausible.

Approaches to cell targeting by murine recombinant retroviruses

Maryse Etienne-Julan [1], Pierre Roux [1], Serge Carillo [1], Philippe Jeanteur [1, 2] and Marc Piechaczyk [1]*

[1] *Laboratoire de Biologie Moléculaire, UA CNRS 1191, Génétique Moléculaire, USTL, place E. Bataillon, 34095 Montpellier Cedex 05, France;* [2] *Laboratoire de Biochimie, Centre Paul Lamarque-Val d'Aurelle, 34094 Montpellier Cedex 05, France*

* Author for correspondence

Summary

    Cell targeting by murine retroviruses carrying recombinant genes will have numerous applications such as immortalization of under-represented cell types from complex cellular mixtures, improvement of infection of hematopoietic stem cells in the case of gene therapy through graft of autologous bone marrow and delivery of specific genes at any location and at any moment of the life-time of living animals. To this aim, we are currently developping techniques that allow binding of viral particles to specific cell membrane markers different from the natural viral receptors. The use of bi-specific molecular adaptors recognizing, on one side, the virus and, on the other side, the targeted cell has already proved successful. Our experiments have led to the notion that both the cell type and the membrane receptor mediating infection influence cell targeting efficiency. Genetic engineering of the envelope glycoprotein as an alternative approach is discussed.

    Recombinant retroviruses are considered the most efficient vectors for stable gene transfer into culture cells and living animals (Varmus, 1988), even though modified Adenovirus, parvoviruses and Herpes Simplex viruses have now emerged as new candidates for this purpose. The reasons for this are multiple and include the efficiencies of cell infection and integration of proviruses as well as the usual absence of detectable effects upon the viability and the physiology of infected cells. However, in its current state the recombinant retroviruses technology falls short of the efficiency required for human gene therapy. Among its main limitations, one can note : (i) the relatively low titers of viral suspensions despite the availability of numerous packaging cell lines and recent methods for increasing retroviruses production (Bestwick and Kabat, 1988), (ii) the difficulty of adequately regulating transcription of carried genes, even when using self-inactivating vectors (Yu et al., 1986), (iii) the random insertion of proviruses into infected cells DNA that can potentially lead to activation of oncogenes or inactivation of tumor suppressor genes and (iv) the broad cell type spectrum of infection of mouse retroviruses that prevents their concentration onto defined cells.

Definition and applications of cell targeting by recombinant retroviruses

It is commonly agreed that cell infection by retroviruses is initiated by the binding of the *env* gene-encoded envelope glycoprotein to specific receptors residing at the surface of host cells (For reviews see : Weiss et al., 1985; Goff and Lobel, 1987; Varmus, 1988). Based on this observation, cell targeting by recombinant retroviruses can be defined as cell infection through the interaction with membrane molecules differing from the natural viral receptor. From an experimental point of view, changing the cell receptor will have two non-mutually exclusive consequences. The first one is the possibility to concentrate recombinant retroviruses onto specific cell types either *in vitro* or *in vivo*. The second is the possibility of overcoming the species barrier in the case of murine ecotropic viruses, the infection spectrum of which is naturally restricted to murine cells. Both uses should have numerous and immediate applications *in vitro* and *in vivo* in fields as diverse as Oncology, Developmental Biology and Gene Therapy depending on the gene to be expressed and the mode of targeting (see Table 1). As a few examples, one can note the development of *in vitro* models of pathological situations by allowing immortalization of under-represented cell types from complex mixtures of cells as those in biopsies, the improvement of infection of hematopoietic stem cells in the case of gene therapy through autologous bone marrow graft, the study of oncogenes (or combinations of oncogenes) action in specific organs of adult animals....

Table 1 : Applications of cell targeting by recombinant retroviruses

	TARGETING METHOD	APPLICATIONS	P3 LABORATORY
IN VITRO	Bispecific adaptors	Immortalization of under-represented Cell types from complex mixtures (Development of in vitro models of Pathological situations)	Not required
IN VITRO	Gene Engineering of the Envelope Glycoprotein	Gene therapy involving autologous grafts	Required
IN VIVO	Gene Engineering of the Envelope Glycoprotein	Gene therapy (gene desorders, AIDS, cancer) Targeted carcinogenesis in living animals Developmental biology	Required

Strategies for cell targeting by recombinant retroviruses.

Only Mo-MuLV-derived (Moloney Murine Leukemia virus) recombinant retroviruses will be considered below since they constitute the most common vectors used for gene delivery into mammalian cells. However, most of the following remarks and conclusions also hold for avian retroviruses.

The envelope glycoprotein of Mo-MuLV is synthesized as a 90 KD precursor (*gp90*) which, after proteolytic maturation, gives rise to two proteins associated by a disulphide bound. The first one, *p15 (E)*, is a transmembrane protein necessary for the budding of viral particles outside the cell. The second one, *gp70*, is an external protein whose main role is to bind the viral receptor located on the surface of host cells. Differences in infection tropisms of the multiple murine retrovirus strains characterized so far having been correlated to sequence variations in the NH_2 moiety of *gp70*, this region of the molecule has been proposed to be responsible for, or at least instrumental in, the specific binding to the receptor (see Weiss et al., 1985 and Goff and Lobel, 1987). On these grounds, two approaches for cell targeting by recombinant retroviruses can be designed. The first one consists in the development of "molecular adaptors" able to recognize, on one side, the *env* glycoprotein (which is the main, if not the only, specific and accessible structure determinant on the surface of viral particles) and, on the other side, specific membrane markers of host cells. The second one consists in genetically modifying the *env* protein either by substituting

Table 2 : Cell targeting methods by recombinant retroviruses

TARGETING METHOD	RECOGNITION OF THE RECEPTOR	TROPISM	IN VIVO / IN VITRO USES
MOLECULAR ADAPTORS	*Agent recognizing the env protein:* Anti-gp70 antibody *Agents recognizing the receptor:* Antibodies Cytokines Hormones Hybrid protein A proteins	Viruses conserve their initial tropism The species barrier can be overcome	Unusuable in vivo or in vitro in the presence of complement
GENE ENGINEERING OF THE ENV PROTEIN	Substitution of hormones, cytokines or antibodies for the NH2 moiety of gp70	Loss of the initial tropism	In vitro and in vivo uses
	Insertion of adhesiotopes	Can conserve the initial tropism	

cytokines, hormones or antibodies for the NH_2 part of the molecule or by inserting short adhesiotopes conferring a new binding specificity. Clearly, each approach has its advantages and drawbacks. Although most of these features are listed in Table 2, we would like to emphasize two of them. Molecular adapters would certainly be interesting for safety concerns in the case of gene therapy since high amounts of murine ecotropic retroviruses could be prepared, stored and handled with minimal risks and rendered infectious for human cells at will. However such an approach appears inappropriate for *in vivo* targeted infection in mice for multiple reasons. The main one is that not all *env* glycoprotein will be complexed with adaptors, thus allowing viruses to conserve their initial tropism. In this case, engineering new specificities into the *gp70* envelope protein in place of the natural binding site might be appropriate.

Molecular adaptors-mediated infection of human cells

To test the possibility that cell infection by recombinant retroviruses could be mediated by membrane markers different from the natural viral receptor, we developed the following assay : naturally resistant human cells of various types were incubated in the presence of low amounts of murine ecotropic retroviruses (cell/virus ratio of 1 or less) in the presence or the absence of molecular adaptors that would allow specific binding to arbitrarily chosen membrane markers. To facilitate monitoring of cell infection, we used vectors expressing both the G418 drug resistance and the Polyoma virus middle T antigen (Jat et al., 1986). After infection, cells were cultured for at least 15 days in the presence of 1mg/ml G418. Resistant clones were then counted and tested for their ability to express Polyoma virus middle T antigen using an immunochemistry assay. The ratio of positive clones to the initial input of infectious viruses, as assayed onto murine NIH 3T3 cells, was considered as the infection yield. In some experiments, attachment of retroviruses onto target cells was monitored by immunofluorescence using monoclonal antibodies directed against the envelope glycoprotein (Chesebro and Wehrly, 1985). Our main results are presented in Table 3 and summarized below.

Since the *env* protein is glycosylated, we first tested the possibility that lectins would allow infection of human HeLa cells through the interaction with lipids- and proteins-conjugated carbohydrates. Although virus binding was shown by immunofluorescence, no G418-resistant clone was obtained in any experiment, thus showing that virus attachment to the cell surface is not sufficient to allow successfull infection. As a second step in our investigations, we developed adaptors specifically recognizing retroviruses on one side and cell membrane receptors on the other side. In all of our experiments, recognition of viruses was achieved with antibodies. For this purpose, the 273, 500 or 715 anti-gp70 monoclonal antibodies developed by Chesebro and co-workers were used since they are not inhibitory for cell infection (see Chesebro and Wehrly, 1985; kind gift from Dr Chesebro). Recognition of cell membrane receptors was however achieved with various types of molecules. Antibodies were first used. They allowed infection of human cells via MHC class I and class II antigens as well as via the Epidermal Growth Factor (EGF) receptor. Interestingly, infection yields varied significantly from one cell type to another in the case of

MHC class I-mediated infection. Moreover, integration and stable expression of retroviruses were not obtained in the of case the transferrin receptor although specific association of viral particles with hepatic and epithelial cells was detected by us and others (Gould et al., 1988), respectively. In all successful situations, antibodies were biotinylated and linked with streptavidin (For details see Roux et al., 1989). For unknown reasons no infection was obtained when *Staphylococcus aureus* protein A was used as an alternative coupling agent. Biotinylated insulin and biotinylated EGF were also used successfully for infecting human cells. Remarkably, infection yields were lower when EGF was used instead of anti-EGF receptor antibodies. However, no infection was detected when biotinylated asialo-fetuin was used to link viruses to the hepatic galatose receptor. Finally, an Apo A-1-protein A chimeric protein (Monaco et al., 1987 ; kind gift from Dr R. Cortese) failed to

RECEPTOR	BRIDGE	CELL LINE	VIRUS BINDING	RELATIVE EFFICIENCY
Membrane glycoprotein and glycolipids	Lectins :PWM, PNA, SBA, WGA UcA-F, Ricin B	HeLa	+	0
MHC class I	A/S/A	HeLa A431 Hep G2 EJ MCF 7		1 5 0.2 20 2.5
	A/P-A/A	HeLa		0
MHC class II	A/S/A	HeLa		5
EGF-receptor	A/S/A EGF/S/A	A431 A431		1 0.01
Galactose Receptor	Asialofetuin/S/A	Hep G2	+	0
Transferrin Receptor	A/S/A	Hep G2	+	0
Insulin Receptor	Insulin/S/A	HeLa	+	0.1

Table 3 : Cell targeting experiments using the molecular adaptor method

To compare cell targeting methods efficiencies, the following assay was developed (for details see Roux et al., 1989). 2×10^5 cells in a 35 mm diameter culture dish were washed with cold PBS and placed on ice for one hour in the presence of an excess of the agent binding the cell surface marker. After washing with cold PBS, cells were incubated in the presence of an excess of streptavidin or *Staphylococus aureus* protein A for one hour and wahsed again with PBS. 2×10^4 viruses (Jat et al., 1987), assayed on NIH 3T3 fibroblasts, coated with either 273, 500 or 715 anti-gp70 antibodies were then added. After one hour at 0°C, cells were transfered at 37°C and cultured 15 days in the presence of 1 mg/ml G-418. Resistant colonies were then counted and, if needed, expression of Polyoma virus middle T antigen was monitored using a specific immunofluorescence assay. **Abbreviations** : *PWN* : Pokweed mitogen, *PNA* : peanut agglutinin, *SBA* : Soybean agglutinin, *WGA* : Wheat germ agglutini, *A/S/A* : Biotinylated antibody/Streptavidin/Biotinylated antibody, *A/P-A/A* : Antibody/Protein A/Antibody, *EGF/S/A* : Biotinylated epidermal growth factor/Streptavidin/Biotinylated antibody, *Asialofetuin/S/A* : Biotinylated asialofetuin/Streptavidin/Biotinylated antibody, *Insulin/S/A* : Biotinylated insulin/Streptavidin/biotinylated antibody. HeLa cells infection *via* MHC class I antigens using bi-specific antibodies was used as reference for estimating relative infection efficiencies. It approximately corresponds to an infection yield of 1% in our assay (see text).

permit retroviral infection of human hepatic cells through the interaction with the high density lipoprotein receptor.

Discussion and perspectives

The above data demonstrate that cell targeting by recombinant retroviruses is possible since infection of human cells by murine ecotropic retroviruses was easily achieved using molecular adaptors. Moreover, it appears that at least two parameters may influence infection yields. The first one is the targeted cell type. This is illustrated by the fact that MHC class I antigens are not equally efficient in mediating infection of different human cell types. For example A431 cells are 100-fold more sensitive to infection than Hep G2 cells (Roux et al., 1989 ; see Table 3). The second one is the nature of the targeted cell membrane marker. Several lines of evidence support this notion since (i) bridging retroviruses and membrane glycolipids or glycoproteins with lectins do not allow infection, (ii) MHC class II antigens are 5-fold more efficient than MHC class I molecules in the case of HeLa cells even though they are 10 times less abundant (Roux et al., 1989) and (iii) Hep G2 cells cannot be infected via transferrin and galactose receptors although they can be infected via the natural receptor for amphotropic viruses or MHC class I antigen (see Table 3). Whether this is related to the turn-over or the intracellular fate of internalized receptors or to the lack of appropriate helper molecules is not known. This latter possibility is supported by the observation that human viruses such as HIV (Maddon et al., 1986) or EBV (Cantaloube et al., 1990), albeit efficiently internalized, are not able to actually infect mouse fibroblasts expressing the cognate receptors upon transfection. Finally, we suspect that the chemical composition of the link also influences infection efficiency since, on one hand, a molecular adaptor made up of a combination of antibodies was more efficient for infecting cells via the EGF receptor than the association of an antibody and a cytokine and, on the other hand, protein A, when used to associate antibodies, turned out to be inefficient in our infection assay.

The major limitation of the methods presented above is the relatively low yields of infection in our assay since, in the best situation, only 1% of input viruses turned out to infect cells and stably expressed the G418-resistance and Py MT genes. Various predictible factors can account for this : (i) we used a sequential addition protocol in which each component of the bridge, including viruses, was added onto cells kept on ice (see legend to Table 3), that is a condition where targeted receptors are neither internalized nor replaced at the cell surface, (ii) most viral particles from producer cell supernatants are void of genomic RNA and act as competitors for viable viruses and (iii) along the same line, *gp70* also acts as a competitor since it is relatively loosely attached to *p15(E)* and is consequently released by both viral particles and virus producer cells. Adding purified bi-specific adaptors to growing human cells cultured in the presence of murine ecotropic retroviruses should help overcoming the receptor cycling limitation and to improve infection yields.

Even when efficient the molecular adaptor method will remain restricted to *in vitro* infections since the anti-*gp70* antibody moiety of the bridge would certainly initiate a cellular immune response against viral particles *in vivo*. Gene engineering of the *env* glycoprotein, as discussed above, should probably reveal more appropriate for this purpose. However, it is already clear that structural modifications will have to be designed so as not to interfere with the complex biology of the *env* molecule (see Weiss et al., 1985) and to maintain the following properties : association to the endoplasmic reticulum, proteolytic maturation generating a functional *p15(E)*, *env* protein multimerization in the endoplasmic reticulum, migration to the cell membrane and budding of virions. This requires a thorough structure/function study of the envelope glycoprotein of Mo-MuLV which is currently under way in our laboratory.

Acknowledgments

This work was supported by grants from the Centre National pour la Recherche scientifique, the Institut National de la Santé et de la Recherche Scientifique, the Association pour la Recherche contre le Cancer, the Ligue National contre le Cancer, the Fondation pour la Recherche Médicale and the Association Française contre les Myopathies. M. E-J. is supported by a fellowship from the Association Française contre les Myopathies. We thank our colleagues of the Laboratoire de Biologie Moléculaire for valuable discussions and K. Grimsrud for careful reading of the manuscript. Experiments were performed in accordance with the safety guidelines of the French National Commitee for Biological Hazards.

References

Bestwick, R.K., Kozak, S.L. and Kabat, D. (1988) Overcoming interference to retroviral superinfection results in amplified expression and transmission of cloned genes. Proc. Natl. Acad. Sci. USA 85, 5404-5408.

Cantaloube, J-F., Piechaczyk, M., Calender, A., Lenoir, G., Minty, A., Carrière, D., Fischer, E. and Poncelet, P. (1990) Stable expression and function of EBV/C3d receptor following genomic transfection into mouse fibroblasts. Eur. J. Immunol. 20, 409-416

Chesebro, B. and Wehrly, K. (1985) Different murine cell lines manifest unique pattern of interference to superinfection by murine leukemia viruses. Virology 141, 119-129

Goff, S. P. and Lobel. L. I. (1987) Mutants of murine leukemia viruses and retroviral replication. Bioch. Biophys. Acta 907, 93-123

Goud, B., Legrain, P. and Buttin, G. (1988); Antibody-mediated binding of a murine ecotropic Moloney retroviral vector to human cells alloww internalization but not the establishement of the proviral state. Virology 163, 251-254

Jat, P.J., Cepko, C.J., Mulligan, R. and Sharp, P. A. (1986) Recombinant retroviruses encoding Simian Virus 40 Large T antigen and Polyoma Large and Middle T antigens. Molec. Cell. Biol. 6, 1204-1217

Maddon, P.J., Dalgleish, A.G., Dougal, J.S., Clapham, P.R., Weiss, R.A. and Axel, R. (1986) The T4 gene encodes the AIDS virus receptor and is expressed in the immune system and the brain. Cell 47, 333-348

Monaco, L., Bond, H., Howell, K. and Cortese R. (1987): A recombinant apoA-1-protein A hybrid reproduces the binding parameters of HDL to its receptors. EMBO J. 6, 3253-3260

Roux, P., Jeanteur, P, and Piechaczyk, M. (1989): A versatile and potentially general approach to the targeting of specific cell types by retroviruses. Proc. Natl. Acad. Sci. USA 86, 9079-9083

Varmus, H. (1988) Retroviruses. Science 240, 1427-1435

Weiss, R., Teich, N., Varmus, H. and Coffin, J. (Eds) (1985) in RNA Tumor Viruses, Vol 2 Cold Spring Harbor Laboratory, Cold Spring Harbor, NY.

Yu, S-H., van Rüden, T., KAntoff, P.W., Garber, C., Seiberg, M., Rüther, U., Anderson, F.W., Wagner, E. and Gilboa, E. (1986) Self-inactivating retroviral vectors designed for transfer of whole genes into mammalian cells. Proc. Natl. Acad. Sci. USA 83, 3194-3198.

Résumé

Le ciblage cellulaire par des rétrovirus murins portant des gènes recombinants pourrait avoir de nombreuses applications telles que l'immortalisation de cellules peu représentées dans des mélanges complexes comme les biopsies, l'amélioration de l'infection des cellules souches hématopoiétiques dans le cadre de la thérapie génique faisant intervenir la greffe de moelle osseuse autologue ou bien encore la transgénèse somatiques à n'importe quel stade de développement d'animaux vivants. Dans ce but, nous developpons des techniques qui permettent la liaison des rétrovirus murins à des marqueurs membranaires des cellules hôtes différents du récepteur naturel. L'utilisation d'adaptateurs moléculaires reconnaissant, d'un coté, le virus et, de l'autre, la cellule ciblée s'est déjà révélée efficace. Nos expériences ont montré qu'à la fois le type cellulaire ciblé et la nature du récepteur membranaire utilisé influencent l'efficacité d'infection.

The multidrug resistance (MDR1) gene as a selectable marker in gene therapy

Michael M. Gottesman* and Ira Pastan [1]

Laboratory of Cell Biology and [1] Laboratory of Molecular Biology, Building 37, Room 1B22, National Cancer Institute, National Institutes of Health, Bethesda, Md, 20892, USA

* Author for correspondence

ABSTRACT

We have used the multidrug resistance (MDR1) gene as a model selectable marker for gene therapy. The MDR1 cDNA encodes an energy dependent multidrug efflux pump which confers resistance to many different anti-cancer drugs such as doxorubicin, vinblastine and taxol. Resistance can be conferred on virtually all drug sensitive cell types *in vitro* using an MDR1 retroviral vector. This selectable marker can be used to co-transfer and amplify unselected genes by co-transfection of two vectors, transfection in the same vector, or the formation of a chimeric protein between the multidrug transporter and the unselected gene product. In the latter case, expression of both the MDR1 gene product and the unselected gene product is guaranteed. Transgenic mice in which the MDR1 gene is expressed in drug sensitive tissues such as bone marrow demonstrate that the MDR1 cDNA can confer drug resistance *in vivo*.

INTRODUCTION

The successful somatic therapy of human genetic diseases will require the stable insertion of DNA sequences into somatic cells. This type of therapy depends on the development of adequate vectors for safe high frequency introduction and expression of genes in recipient cells, and may well require a means of selecting cell populations which have received the genes of interest. Currently, there are no reliable ways of selecting *in vivo* for cells which have received donor genes. In this work, we will describe a selection system based on the multidrug resistance (MDR1) gene which works both *in vitro* and *in vivo* to select cell populations into which this gene has been introduced.

The phenomenon of multidrug resistance was first observed in the tumors of patients undergoing chemotherapy, but this phenomenon also occurs in cultured cells selected for resistance to anti-cancer drugs. In its broadest sense, multidrug resistance refers to simultaneous resistance to multiple, structurally unrelated drugs, when cells (or cancers) are selected for resistance to a single agent only. In its best understood form, multidrug resistance results from the expression of a 170,000 dalton surface glycoprotein, called P-glycoprotein, which acts as an energy-dependent efflux pump for many hydrophobic natural product chemotherapeutic agents (Gottesman & Pastan, 1988; Endicott & Ling, 1989; Kane et al., 1990). Drugs pumped out of resistant cells by this multidrug transporter include the commonly used anti-cancer agents doxorubicin, daunomycin, vinblastine, vincristine, etoposide (VP-16), teniposide (VM-26), and actinomycin D as well as colchicine, puromycin, gramicidin D, and taxol.

VECTORS CARRYING THE *MDR1* GENE CAN CONFER MULTIDRUG RESISTANCE ON DRUG SENSITIVE CELLS

Both human and mouse cDNAs which encode the multidrug transporter have been isolated (Gros et al., 1986; Ueda et al., 1987). When inserted into retroviral expression systems, these cDNAs confer the complete pattern of multidrug resistance on recipient cells (Pastan et al., 1988; Guild et al., 1988). The cDNA for the human gene encodes a protein of 1280 amino acids, which has two homologous halves. Each half consists of 6 transmembrane regions with associated extracellular and cytoplasmic loops, and a nucleotide binding site (Chen et al., 1986). Because of this overall structure, and the extensive sequence identity in the nucleotide binding regions with many other energy dependent transport systems, the multidrug transporter belongs to a superfamily of transporters known as the ABC (ATP-Binding Cassette) Family (Hyde et al., 1990) or the family of Traffic ATPases (Ames & Joshi, 1990).

Although the precise mechanism of action of the multidrug transporter is not known, studies of transport of drugs in vesicles isolated from multidrug resistant cells indicate that it uses the energy of ATP to pump hydrophobic drugs against a concentration gradient (Horio et al., 1988). Because of the known hydrophobicity of these drugs, and because of evidence suggesting that the transporter removes drugs directly from the plasma membrane (Raviv et al., 1990), we have proposed the model shown in cartoon form in Figure 1. In this model, the drugs are shown as amphipathic molecules with both hydrophobic and charged moieties which are able to diffuse across the plasma membrane in their uncharged form. The function of the multidrug transporter is to recognize these drugs in the context of the membrane and expel them from the cell.

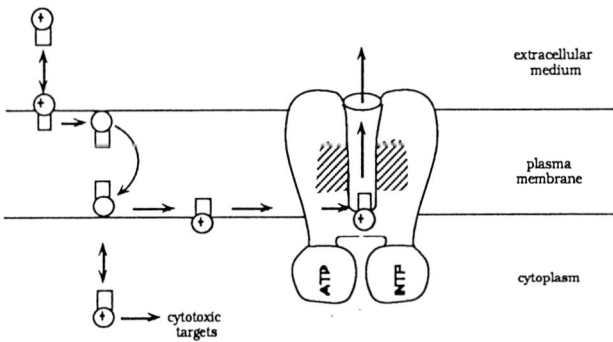

Fig. 1. Cartoon showing postulated mechanism of action of the multidrug transporter.

INTRODUCTION OF THE *MDR1* GENE INTO MOUSE BONE MARROW CELLS *IN VITRO* and *IN VIVO* IN TRANSGENIC ANIMALS

Studies on the multidrug transporter using antibodies specific for this transporter and specific cDNA probes have indicated that many rodent and human tissues do not express appreciable amounts of this transporter. Thus, tissues such as bone marrow, skin, and skeletal muscle do not normally express the transporter and are therefore suitable potential targets for gene therapy with the *MDR1* gene, whereas transporting epithelia and endothelia of the liver, kidney, intestine, brain and testis are already protected by expression of the multidrug transporter (Thiebaut et al., 1987; Thiebaut et al., 1989).

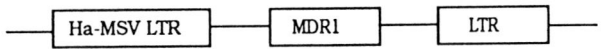

Fig. 2. pHaMDR1/A retroviral vector for expression of the *MDR1* cDNA.

To test the possibility of using the *MDR1* gene as a selectable marker in normal animal tissues, we infected mouse bone marrow *in vitro* with the *MDR1* cDNA cloned as the retroviral vector shown in Figure 2 (McLachlin et al., 1990). This vector uses a Harvey sarcoma virus LTR as a promoter, and was derived from a *ras*-expressing vector (Ellis et al., 1980). As shown in Table 1, bone marrow cells, detected as granulocyte and monocyte-colony forming units (GM-CFU) become resistant to both vinblastine and colchicine after infection with this vector (McLachlin et al., 1990). These infected cells could be detected as splenic foci, since 16-30% of such foci contained human *MDR1* sequences as revealed by Southern blotting (McLachlin et al., 1990). In these initial studies, no attempt was made to select for *MDR1*-expressing bone marrow cells *in vivo*, since we did not know what optimal selection conditions would be.

Table 1

Frequency of drug resistant GM-CFU
from mouse bone marrow infected with pHaMDR1/A

Drug Concentration (ng/ml)	Uninfected control*		pHaMDR1/A infected*	
	Colchicine	Vinblastine	Colchicine	Vinblastine
10	67	28	39	17
15	0	0	23	9
20	0	0	10	9
25	0	0	7	5
30	0	0	7	2

* Numbers are moderate to large GM-CFU per 10^5 cells. 78 GM-CFU were obtained without drug selection.

To demonstrate that the human *MDR1* gene could be used as a selectable marker for bone marrow cells *in vivo*, we constructed a transgenic mouse in which the human *MDR1* gene was expressed almost exclusively in bone marrow. The vector used for these studies consists of a truncated β-actin promoter from the chicken driving the human cDNA. Several mouse founder lines carrying this transgene were identified, and one line had a low copy number of the gene and expression of the *MDR1* cDNA in most bone marrow cells (Galski et al., 1989). Levels of *MDR1* RNA in bone marrow cells from the transgenic mice were comparable to those found in drug resistant human cancers, or in cultures of cells after initial infection with our retroviral vectors. Challenge of these mice with several different anti-cancer drugs such as daunomycin, vinblastine, and taxol revealed that their bone marrow was relatively resistant to the cytotoxic effects of these drugs (Galski et al., 1989; Mickisch et al., 1991). This resistance was demonstrated by a normal white blood count (WBC) after challenge with chemotherapeutic drugs, whereas non-MDR mice show a drop in peripheral WBC.

To establish that the multidrug resistant phenotype of the bone marrow of these transgenic mice was due to expression of the *MDR1* gene in bone marrow, we have transplanted bone marrow from the transgenic mice to drug sensitive recipient mice. These recipient mice are resistant to the same anti-cancer drugs as are the donor mice (unpublished data). This transplant system should now allow us to determine the conditions under which *MDR1*-expressing bone marrow can be selected in the presence of normal non-expressing bone marrow.

MDR1 GENE EXPRESSION IN SKELETAL MUSCLE

As noted above, skeletal muscle is another tissue which does not usually express appreciable amounts of the multidrug transporter, which therefore makes it a target for selections based on drug resistance imparted by this transporter. One advantage of using skeletal muscle is that as a recipient for gene transfer it is a differentiated tissue in which extensive cell division does not occur once it has matured. However, muscle can be stimulated to divide, and can therefore become a target for retroviral vectors, which might be stably expressed once the tissue has differentiated.

We have introduced the *MDR1* gene into cultured rat L6 myoblasts using the same retroviral vector shown in Figure 2. These myoblasts, transformed with the *MDR1* vector, express high levels of the multidrug transporter and can be transplanted into the soleus muscle of cyclosporin A immunosuppressed rats. These L6 myoblasts fuse to form myotubes after transplantation into rats. Expression of the multidrug transporter can be detected several weeks after transplantation in the rat L6 myotubes (Salminen et al., 1991).

Expression of the *MDR1* gene has also been obtained in skeletal muscle, brain, and lung of transgenic mice carrying a *MDR1* cDNA under control of a metallotheinein promoter (P. Marino, M.M. Gottesman, I. Pastan, unpublished data). *MDR1* RNA can be induced in this system with zinc or cadmium. After induction, female transgenic animals are resistant to the lethal effects of colchicine, whose primary lethal toxicity may be on muscle. Although it is not possible to attribute colchicine-resistance in this case to skeletal muscle expression of the human *MDR1* transgene, this system suggests that *MDR1* cDNA expression may be selectable in tissues other than bone marrow.

USE OF THE *MDR1* cDNA TO CO-TRANSFER OTHER NON-SELECTABLE GENES

Expression vectors carrying the *MDR1* cDNA can be used as selectable markers to introduce non-selectable genes into cultured cells (Kane et al., 1988). At high levels of resistance to drugs such as colchicine, such *MDR1* transfected cell lines frequently show amplified copies of the *MDR1* cDNA, and amplified copies of the co-transfected, unselected DNA sequences (Kane et al., 1988). Thus, the *MDR1* cDNA can be used to co-transfect and co-amplify other genes. To facilitate this process of co-transfection and co-amplification, we have constructed a vector which includes the *MDR1* cDNA as well as a unique cloning site downstream from an SV40 promoter in the same vector. Such a vector has been successfully used to introduce and amplify an interleukin-2 cDNA (Kane et al., 1989).

One potential problem with gene therapy by selection of co-transfected or co-infected genes is that the non-selected gene may not be expressed if it is under control of a different promoter. To circumvent this problem, we have constructed an *MDR1* cDNA vector in which the unselected marker gene is linked to the 3' end of the *MDR1* cDNA to form a hybrid gene, which encodes a chimeric protein in which the unselected gene is attached to the carboxyl-terminus of the multidrug transporter. In the example shown in Figure 3, adenosine deaminase is the unselected gene. A chimeric protein which confers both multidrug resistance and human adenosine deaminase activity is encoded by this vector (Germann et al., 1989). A retrovirus which encapsulates this chimeric gene can transform KNIH cells to multidrug resistance and tumors formed from these transformed cells continues to express a bi-functional *MDR1*-ADA chimera after growth in animals for several weeks (Germann et al., 1990).

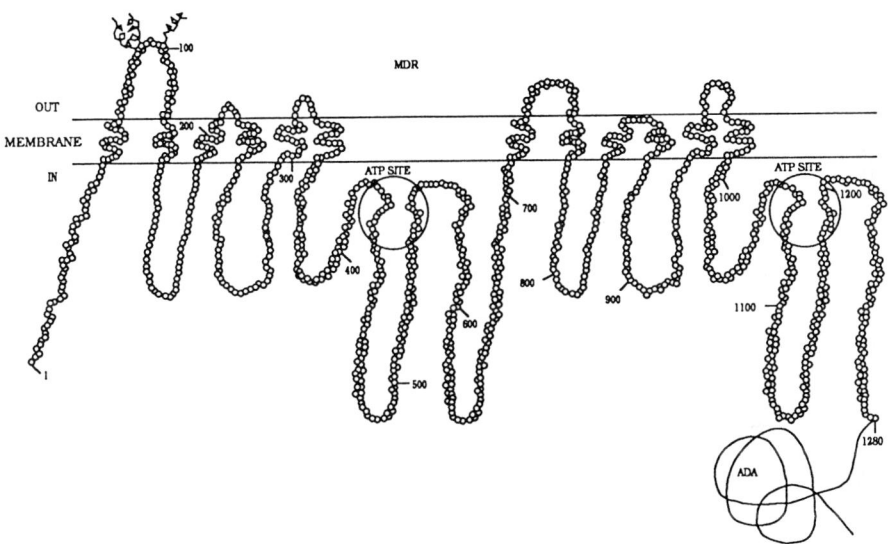

Fig. 3. Model of the chimeric protein comprising the multidrug transporter and adenosine deaminase.

CONCLUSIONS

The *MDR1* cDNA described in this work is a flexible selectable system for introduction of non-selectable genes into cultured cells and bone marrow cells of intact animals. Preliminary studies using transgenic mice expressing the human *MDR1* gene indicate that the multidrug resistance phenotype can be selected in intact animals. Since foreign genes often cease to function upon prolonged passage, the presence of a selectable drug resistance element such as MDR1 linked genetically or physically to the gene of interest combined with repeated selection may be necessary to preserve the functional expression of foreign genes.

REFERENCES

Ames, G.F.-L., and Joshi, A.K. (1990): Energy coupling in bacterial periplasmic permeases. *J. Bacteriol.* 172: 4133-4137.

Chen, C.-j., Chin, J.E., Ueda, K., Clark, D., Pastan, I., Gottesman, M.M., and Roninson, I. (1986): Internal duplication and homology with bacterial transport proteins in the *mdr1* (P-glycoprotein) gene from multidrug-resistant human cells. *Cell* 47: 381-389.

Ellis, R.W., DeFeo, D., Maryak, J.M., Young, H.A., Shih, T.Y., Chang, E.H., Lowy D.R., and Scolnick, E.M. (1980): Dual evolutionary origin for the rat genetic sequences of Harvey murine sarcoma virus. *J. Virology* 80: 408-420.

Endicott, J.A., and Ling, V. (1989): The biochemistry of P-glycoprotein-mediated multidrug resistance. *Annu. Rev. Biochem.* 58: 137-171.

Galski, H., Sullivan, M., Willingham, M. C., Chin, K.-V., Gottesman, M. M., Pastan, I., and Merlino, G. T.(1989): Expression of a human multidrug-resistance cDNA (*MDR1*) in the bone marrow of transgenic mice: resistance to daunomycin-induced leukopenia. *Mol. Cell. Biol.* 9: 4357-4363.

Germann, U. A., Gottesman, M. M., and Pastan, I. (1989): Expression of a multidrug resistance-adenosine deaminase fusion gene. *J. Biol. Chem.* 264: 7418-7424.

Germann, U. A., Chin, K-V., Pastan, I., and Gottesman, M. M. (1990): Retroviral transfer of a chimeric multidrug resistance-adenosine deaminase gene. *FASEB J.* 4: 1501-1507.

Gottesman, M. M. and Pastan, I. (1988): The multidrug-transporter, a double-edged sword. *J. Biol. Chem.* 263: 12163-12166.

Gros, P., Ben-Nen-Neriah, Y.B., Croup, J.M., and Housman, D.E. (1986): Isolation and expression of a complementary DNA that confers multidrug resistance. *Nature* 323: 728-731.

Guild, B.C., Mulligan, R.C., Gros, P., and Housman, D.E. (1988): Retroviral transfer of a murine cDNA for multidrug resistance confers pleiotropic drug resistance to cells without prior drug selection. *Proc. Natl. Acad. Sci. USA* 85: 1595-1599.

Horio, M., Gottesman, M. M., and Pastan, I. (1988): ATP-dependent transport of vinblastine in vesicles from human multidrug-resistant cells. *Proc. Natl. Acad. Sci. USA* 85: 3580-3584.

Hyde, S.C., Emsley, P., Hartshorn, M.J., Mimmack, M.M., Gileadi, U., Pearce, S.R., Gallagher, M.P., Gill, D.R., Hubbard, R.E., and Higgins, C.F. (1990): Structural model of ATP-binding proteins associated with cystic fibrosis, multidrug resistance and bacterial transport. *Nature* 346: 362-365.

Kane, S. E., Troon, B. R., Cal, J., Ueda, K., Pastan, I., and Gottesman, M. M. (1988): Use of a cloned multidrug-resistance gene for co-amplification and overproduction of MEP, a transformation-regulated secreted acid protease. *Mol. Cell. Biol.* 8: 3316-3321.

Kane, S. E., Reinhard, D. H., Fordis, C. M., Pastan, I., and Gottesman, M. M. (1989): A new vector using the human multidrug resistance gene as a selectable marker enables overexpression of foreign genes in eukaryotic cells. *Gene* 84: 439-446.

Kane, S. E., Pastan, I., and Gottesman, M. M. (1990): Genetic basis of multidrug resistance of tumor cells. Review. *J. Bioenerg. Biomembr.* 22: 593-618.

McLachlin, J. R., Eglitis, M. A., Ueda, K., Kantoff, P. W., Pastan, I. H., Anderson, W. R., and Gottesman, M. M. (1990): Expression of a human complementary DNA for the multidrug resistance gene in murine hematopoietic precursor cells with the use of retroviral gene transfer. *J. Natl. Cancer Inst.* 82: 1260-1263.

Mickisch, G., Merlino, G. T., Galski, H., Gottesman, M. M., and Pastan, I. (1991): Transgenic mice that express the human multidrug resistance gene in bone marrow enable a rapid identification of agents that reverse drug resistance. *Proc. Natl. Acad. Sci. USA* 88: 547-551.

Pastan, I., Gottesman, M. M., Ueda, K., Lovelace, E., Rutherford, A.V., and Willingham, M. C. (1988): A retrovirus carrying an *MDR1* cDNA confers multidrug resistance and polarized expression of P-glycoprotein in MDCK cells. *Proc. Natl. Acad. Sci. USA* 85: 4486-4490.

Raviv, Y., Pollard, H. B., Bruggemann, E. P., Pastan, I., and Gottesman, M. M. (1990): Photosensitized labeling of a functional multidrug transporter in living drug-resistant tumor cells. *J. Biol. Chem.* 265: 3975-3980.

Salminen, A., Elson, H. F., Mickley, L. A., Fojo, A. T., Gottesman, M. M. (in press): Implantation of recombinant rat myocytes into adult skeletal muscle: a potential gene therapy. *Human Gene Therapy*.

Thiebaut, F. Tsuruo, T., Hamada, H., Gottesman, M. M., Pastan, I., Willingham, M. C. (1987): Cellular localization of the multidrug resistance gene product P-glycoprotein in normal human tissues. *Proc. Natl. Acad. Sci. USA* 84: 7735-7738.

Thiebaut, F., Tsuruo, T., Hamada, H., Gottesman, M. M., Pastan, I., and Willingham, M. C. (1989): Immunohistochemical localization in normal tissues of different epitopes in the multidrug transport protein, P170: evidence for localization in brain capillaries and cross-reactivity of one antibody with a muscle protein. *J. Histochem. Cytochem.* 37: 159-164.

Ueda, K., Cardarelli, C., Gottesman, M. M., and Pastan, I. (1987): Expression of a full-length cDNA for the human "*MDR1*" (P-glycoprotein) gene confers multidrug resistance to colchicine, doxorubicin, and vinblastine. *Proc. Natl. Acad. Sci. USA* 84: 3004-3008.

Résumé

Le gène MDR1 qui est impliqué dans la résistance a de nombreux médicaments dont certains anticancereux a été utilisé comme marqueur de sélection en thérapie génique. La protéine codée par le cDNA correspondant au gène MDR1 est responsable du transport actif d'un certain nombre d'agents anti-néoplastiques tels que la doxorubicine, la vinblastine et le taxol. Cette résistance multiple peut être conférée *in vitro* à tous les types de cellules réceptrices sensibles en utilisant le vecteur rétroviral MDR1. Un gène non sélectionnable peut donc être transferé et amplifié soit par le cotransfert simultané des deux vecteurs, soit par la transfection d'un vecteur unique comportant les différentes informations, soit enfin par la production d'un protéine chimère entre le transporteur de la résistance multidrogue et la protéine codée par le gène associé. Dans ce dernier cas, l'expression à la fois des protéines codées par le gène MDR1 et par le gène non sélectionné est assurée. L'utilisation de souris transgéniques dans lesquelles le transfert du gène MDR1 entraîne l'expression de la multirésistance dans des tissus sensibles tels que la moëlle osseuse, a permis de démontrer que le transfert du cDNA de la MDR1 est capable de conférer la résistance multidrogue *in vivo*.

Homologous recombination and animal models

Recombinaison homologue et modèles animaux

Animal models of human genetic diseases

Jean-Louis Guénet

Unité de Génétique des Mammifères, Institut Pasteur, 25, rue du Docteur Roux, 75724 Paris Cedex 15, France

Abstract

Several mutations have been discovered in the mouse over the past fifty years. Some of these mutations, because of similarities with a human affection, can be used as models to help the scientists and the pediatricians in the understanding of the human disorders. This chapter is a synthetic overview of the value and limits of those animal models.

The concept of animal models is almost as old as experimental medicine itself since, in 1865, referring to the use of animals in biomedical research in his famous "Introduction à l'étude de la médecine expérimentale", Claude Bernard wrote " I think that without experiments on animals practical medicine can never acquire a scientific character".
When infectious diseases represented the bulk of human pathology many animals were experimentally infected to help pathologists understand the evolution of the pathological processes and, thanks to this approach, many vaccines and many bacteriolytic drugs have been discovered. These days infectious diseases, with the exceptions of AIDS and malaria, no longer represent a burden, in terms of mortality, for human beings and even in these latter two cases it is not an overstatement to consider that the lack of suitable animal models for experimental research represents a serious drawback for the progress towards eradication of these diseases.

Nowadays many pathological conditions in man have been recognized as being more or less the direct consequence of a defective genetic make up and in order to try and understand as precisely as possible the contribution of genetics to the pathogenesis of these diseases it is of great utility, where possible, to be capable of using animal models which mimic as precisely as possible the condition in humans.

The purpose of this paper is to describe how animal models of human genetic diseases are discovered or produced and what their advantages and limitations are.

Instead of making a general review of the existing mouse models we have prefered to select a few didactic examples. Those among the readers who wish to know more in this field can refer to a review written by several investigators at the Jackson laboratory (Leiter et al 1988).

WHERE DO THE ANIMAL MODELS COME FROM ?
Most of the animal models which have proved useful tool so far are laboratory mice because this mammal has several invaluable advantages in addition to its small size and very high prolificity. Many strains of the laboratory mouse are highly inbred and with them it is possible to graft cells or tissues from one animal to the next without taking the risk of immunological rejection. With mice it is possible to perform a series of *in vitro* manipulations on embryos at an early stage of development. One can make for example allophenic or tetraparental chimeras clumping a mutant genotype and a normal one in order to check for the occurence of eventual extracellular complementations. With mice it is also possible to make transgenic animals by injecting a cloned DNA sequence in ovo. It is also possible to make parabiontic animals grafting a normal adult individual on a mutant one. This for example has made it possible to demonstrate that diabetic (*db/db*) mice are unable to respond to a circulating satiety factor which they therefore produce in great excess and which cause the normal partner of the parabiontic construction to die of starvation.

The mouse has also some trivial advantages which are unique to the species. For example it is possible, in many instances, to identify the individuals with a defective genotype well before the onset of a particular abnormal feature using genetic markers closely linked to the mutated alleles and setting up particular crosses. Finally, the mouse species seems to be one of the rare species where it is possible to breed viable and fertile offspring from interspecific matings what allows formal geneticists to set up crosses where genetic polymorphisms of all kind segregate extensively.

Most of the known animal models of human genetic diseases were the consequence of spontaneous mutations which were accidentally discovered in those facilities where inbred strains are bred in large quantities. Inbred strains of laboratory mouse result from the uninterrupted systematic mating of brothers with their sisters for many generations making the detection of mutations particularly frequent. Many mouse mutations have also been produced after treatment of progenitors with mutagenic agents such as radiations or chemicals. With the recent discovery of some particularly powerful chemical mutagens it has even become possible to design experiments aimed at the detection of a specific kind of mutation and, as we shall see, models of thalassemias and of phenylketonuria have been produced almost "upon request" using such protocols in the mouse.

Apart from this common source of models the possibility of transfecting mammalian enbryonnic cells *in vitro* with different sorts of alien DNAs, sometimes genetically modified, represents another important source of models and it is predictable that, in the near future, many interesting models will be made available as a consequence of that kind of experiments.

Mouse models resulting from spontaneous or induced mutations

Mouse geneticists generally classify animal models of human diseases in two types:
- homologous, when the same gene product is defective (or absent) in both species and,
- analogous, when, on the contrary, the model is recognized on the basis of a similar pathology with no precise knowledge of its genetic determinism;

Many mutations producing dwarfism, obesity (with or without diabetes), hair loss or change in structure, various skeletal defects, eye defects, inner ear defects, anemia, abnormal neuromuscular behavior, immunological disorders with a more or less severe phenotype, abnormal metabolisms, etc...have been reported. These are listed, with a brief description and bibliography, in a chapter written by Dr Margaret Green in the book edited by Drs Mary Lyon and Antony Searle "Genetic Variants and Strains of the Laboratory Mouse - 2nd Edition; Oxford University Press 1989. Regular updating of this list is published in "Mouse Genome" (Oxford University Press) twice a year.

Many of these mutations have proved interesting models for the understanding of some developmental processes. A lot of information, for example, has been collected on the cerebellar organization from the studies which have been carried out on the mouse mutants staggerer: *sg*, reeler: *rl*, Purkinje cell degeneration: *pcd*, weaver: *wv*, nervous: *nr*, etc... however, none of the genes involved have been cloned yet and very little is known at the molecular level about these defects.

More interesting examples have been the defects in myelination encountered in the mutants quaking: *qk*, jimpy: *jp*, Trembler: *Tr*, twitcher: *twi*, shiverer: *shi* etc... because many of these defects have been investigated in detail at the molecular level. Jimpy, for example, is the result of a mutation at the X-linked locus coding for myelin proteolipid protein (PLP) and one considers this mouse disease to be homologous to the X-linked Pelizaeus-Merzbacher disease in man. Twitcher mice (*twi/twi*) exhibit progressive weakness and wasting resulting from degeneration of myelin sheaths in both the central and peripheral nervous systems. These abnormalities closely resemble those of human globoid cell leukodystrophy or Krabbe's disease. The shiverer mutation affects the myelination process in a completely different way (MBP) but the human homologue has not been reported so far.

Many neuromuscular diseases resulting from spontaneous mutations have been reported in the mouse and some of them have now also been identified as models of human defects. The recessive mutation myotonia: adr^{mto}, exhibits the classical myotonia similar to that described in man and *dy*, dystrophia muscularis, which is characterized by progressive weakness and paralysis, has been extensively studied by muscle physiologists as a model of neurogenic dystrophy.

The most popular mouse muscular mutant nowadays is certainly the X-linked muscular dystrophy *mdx*. This mutation arose spontaneously and was accidentally discovered several years ago because hemizygous males and homozygous females have elevated plasma levels of muscle creatine kinase and pyruvate kinase. However, no clinical symptoms appear until about 12 months of age when the affected mice develop mild incoordination. Homozygous *mdx/mdx* mice show dystrophic changes in muscle histopathology beginning at 3 weeks with repeated alternate episodes of muscle fiber necrosis and regeneration. The *mdx* locus has been recognized, at the molecular level, as homologous with the Duchenne (DMD) muscular dystrophy locus in man because mutant mice, like their human counterparts, do not synthesize the protein dystrophin.
Several other mouse mutations with predominantly neuromuscular effects are known in the mouse (muscle deficient, *mdf* and myodystrophy, *myd* for example) but, surprisingly, these have so far received little attention.

Three mutations, with a neuromuscular phenotype, have been identified in the mouse producing progressive ataxia. These are motoneuron degeneration: *mnd*, progressive motor neuronopathy: *pmn* and wobbler: *wr*.

mnd/mnd mice are characterized by hindlimb weakness and ataxia progressing to severe spastic paralysis of all limbs with death usually occuring by 9 to 14 months. Histological examination of the nervous system of affected animals shows degeneration of the motoneurons of the spinal cord and cranial nerves. Wobbler homozygotes: *wr/wr*, also develop progressive ataxia, but the syndrome is more severe (affected mice die by 2 or 3 months of age) and concerns mostly the anterior part of the body. Both mutations as well as the recently discovered mutation progressive motor neuronopathy *pmn* somewhat resembles amyotrophic lateral sclerosis and Werdnig-Hoffmann disease in man. So far these mutations are considered analogous models but, as we shall see, with the rapid progress of gene mapping in the mouse and the concomitant discovery of chromosomal homologies some may shortly turn out to be homologous models.

In the mouse many mutations affect to various degrees bone and/or cartilage and animals exhibiting conditions of osteopetrosis, chondrodysplasia, and limb deformities (sometimes with polydactyly, syndactyly, or hypodactyly) as well as animals with degenerative joint diseases are available as models. There are, for example, four genetically distinct osteopetrotic mutants in the mouse; grey-lethal: *gl*, microphthalmia: *mi*, osteopetrosis: *op* and osteosclerotic: *oc* which, to some extent, mimic human osteopetrosis (Albers-Schönberg syndrome or "marble bone disease"). With these models transplantation of bone marrow from normal sibs to affected animals, which, as we already mentionned, can be easily performed in mice since these animals are entirely histocompatible, have been shown to cure completely the disease in *gl/gl* and *mi/mi* mice but not in *op/op* indicating different etiology. The treatment of children with congenital osteopetrosis by bone marrow transplantation has greatly benefited from experiments on mice.

Many mouse models of osteochondrodysplasia (achondroplasia: *cn*, brachymorphic: *bm*) are also available in the mouse which may prove useful for the study of this heterogeneous group of disorders in man.

Gene mutations affecting the immune system of mice are also very common. Many of these mutations represent interesting "ready made deficiencies" and affected animals have been extensively used as universal acceptors for all kind of transplantations including xenografts. They have also contributed to our understanding of the complex relationships between the various components of the immune system. There is little doubt that several of these mutant genes have potential human homologues but to date, with the exception of the X linked immunodeficiency: *xid*, which is analogous with Wiskott-Aldrich syndrome, none of these homologies has been established with certainty. On another hand no deficiency in the enzymes Adenosine deaminase (*Ada*) or Nucleotide phoshorylase (*Np*) have ever been reported in the mouse. This can be considered surprising given the relative frequency of the homologous mutations in the human.

In addition to the mutations described above, there are many situations in the mouse where autoimmune diseases have been found to result from a clear cut genetic determinism. Some mouse inbred strains for example (MRL, NZB, BXSB, etc...) are known to represent analogous models of human syndromes. Here however little is known concerning the genetic determinism of the condition because of its relative complexity.

Several mouse models of metabolic disorders identified in the humans are now available. Together with V. Bode (Bode et al. 1988) we found the first mouse model of

Phenylketonuria (P.K.U.) by checking with the same diagnostic test used in man, the Guthrie test, the offspring of E.N.U. treated males. The mutant which we reported (hph-1) is deficient in a cofactor instead of phenylalanine hydroxylase itself but several other mutations have been induced with a similar protocol, in William Dove's laboratory in Madison, representing almost perfect models of the human disease, with various alterations of the phenylalanine hydroxylase (Pah) gene. It is interesting to note that several deleterious alleles at the same Pah locus, independently discovered by these investigators, can result in syndromes with various degree of severity.

Because they are relatively easy to detect, mouse models of red blood cell dyscrasias (hemoglobinopathies, spectrin-deficient anemias, microcytic and macrocytic anemias) are relatively numerous even if many of them have been recognized only recently. Many mutations at both the Hba and Hbb loci have been induced either by radiations or by chemical mutagenesis. Mice homozygous for these mutations generally die *in utero* but, in the heterozygotes, the absence of one α or one β form results in α or β thalassemias.

Some mutations resulting in an abnormal globin β chain are viable in the homozygous state and this produces either in hypochromic microcytic anemia (Hbb^{d3}) or polycytemia (Hbb^{d4}). The affected mice are good models for stem cell transfer experiments and may also be good recipients of their own marrow cells transfected with normal globin genes. The hemoglobinopathy, Hbb^{a4} which results from a single amino acid alteration (from Tyr to Cys at position 145) in the major adult mouse β-globin is a homolog of hemoglobin Rainier in man. Spectrin-deficient anemias are known in the mouse and the mutations spherocytosis: sph, hemolytic anemia: sph^{ha}, and jaundiced: ja, are examples.

Defects in iron metabolism are known in mice with four different mutations that cause microcytic anemia: sex-linked anemia: sla, microcytic anemia: mk, flexed tail: ft and hemoglobin deficit: hbd.

Mice with macrocytic anemias are extremely common and occur repeatedly. They are represented by the numerous alleles at the dominant spotting locus: W, the numerous alleles at the Steel: Sl locus and the recessive mutation Hertwig anemia, an. In W/W homozygotes the defect results from a stem cell defect while in steel (Sl/Sl) mutants mice have an environmental defect that decreases the number of erythroid cells. The defect in an/an mice is not yet completely understood but may be the consequence of an unequal distribution of chromosomes during successive divisions. It may be in fact a general cell disease which is more obvious in the erythroid lineage because the cells are dividing more rapidly. Finally hypotranferrinemia (hpx: Bernstein 1987) is a mutation which closely resembles human atransferrinemia and the recently discovered ferrochelatase deficiency (fcd: our laboratory) mimics the human protoporphyria

Mouse models resulting from transgenesis

Transgenic animals result from the *in vitro* addition of an alien genetic information to the mouse genome. This can be achieved either by mechanical injection of a cloned gene, eventually genetically engineered, into one of the two pronuclei or by transfection of embryonnal stem cells (E.S. cells) grown *in vitro* then reinjected into the blastocel of a developing embryo. Many transgenic strains have been produced which are potentially interesting models and it is predictable that many other strains will be produced in the future as new genes will be cloned. Due to limitation in space we must limit ourself to the presentation of some examples but several reviews are now available.

Some transgenic strains result in pathological conditions because they overexpress a gene which is normally precisely regulated. This is the case for example for the strains where the transgene is constructed from the coding sequence of a cellular oncogene linked *in vitro* to a ubiquitous promoter. Many mouse strains of that kind develop neoplasias with a very high frequency. When the promotor is tissue specific then the cancer occurs in specific tissue. In other instances the transgene codes for a chimeric, abnormal or mutant protein producing deleterious effects. For example a transgenic mouse line has been successfully produced by Ryan et al. (1990) inserting the human α and β^s globin genes immediately downstream of the erythroïd-specific DNase I super hypersensitive sites normally located 50 kb upstream of the human β-globin gene. When erythrocytes from these mice were deoxygenated, greater than 90 percent of the cells displayed the same characteristic sickled shapes as erythrocytes from humans with sickle cell disease, and compared with controls the mice also had decreased hematocrits, lower hemoglobin concentrations, splenomegaly and anemia symptoms which are associated with human sickle cell disease. Hopefully, new drugs and therapies can be designed and tested in these animals and therefore provide new strategies for treating this debilitating disease.

Making transgenic mice with a chimeric DNA stretch resulting from the *in vitro* adjunction of the first 5' exon of the *bcr* gene to the 3' exons of the c-Abelson oncogene Heisterkamp et al. (1990) have produced a model of the acute human leukemia resulting from the 9q34-22q11 reciprocal translocation (Philadelphia chromosome). In so doing they have unraveled the causal relationship between the presence of the Philadelphia chromosome and the development of the acute leukemia but the model they have produced is not very useful for the study of the evolution of human leukemia because the mice die at very early age.

Mice are genetically resistant to experimental infections with HIV, the retrovirus responsible for AIDS in human beings, or HBV, the virus responsible for the B type hepatitis. This acquired, or natural, resistance to the infection is a consequence of the absence of the viral receptor at the cell surface. Transgenic mice resulting from the integration of a complete or nearly complete viral genome have permitted the analysis and study of the liver specific activity of the viral genomes. Although some transgenic mice have a very active transcription and produce many viral copies these are not capable of infecting other cells due to the lack of cell receptor. When the gene coding for HBV cell receptor will be cloned it may then become possible to develop a mouse model susceptible to HBV infection. This is may also be applicable to HIV. Finally several models of human pathological conditions have been produced by crossing independant transgenic strains carrying different transgenes the pathological condition resulting either from the mere addition of the elementary effects or from an deleterious interaction.

THE MOUSE AS A MODEL FOR MORBID CYTOGENETICS

The mouse has long been a poor model for cytogenetics. All mouse chromosomes are acrocentric or telocentric, with virtually no cytologically visible short arm and little difference in length. This situation has dramatically changed with the discovery of selective staining techniques and nowadays each chromosome can be readily identified by its characteristic Q, G, or R banding pattern.

A large number of reciprocal translocations and inversions have been produced in the mouse and many of these chromosomal rearrangements can be used experimentally. X-autosome reciprocal translocations for example have played (and continue to play) an important role in our understanding of the X chromosome inactivation process. Robertsonian translocations are numerous, they exist in several combinations, involving all chromosomes but the Y. They have been used to determine the frequency of chromosome nondisjunction or chromosome loss and the effect of various agents on chromosome behavior during meiosis. They also provide a model system for producing specific autosomal trisomies and monosomies. The most common approach is to mate a normal mouse to a partner doubly heterozygous for two different Robertsonian translocations with one chromosome arm in common. This technique has been extensively used by Gropp and his coworkers, in the '80s, to produce all kind of individual trisomies. Trisomy for chromosome 16 has received particular attention as a possible mouse model for Down's syndrome because mouse chromosome 16 carries several of the genes that have been assigned to the segment of human chromosome 21 and, as showed by Epstein (1986) mice with trisomy 16 indeed share clinical features with patients affected with Down syndrome. Unfortunately every mouse autosome has homologues on more than one human chromosome and it is clear that no mouse trisomy will provide a true homologous model for any human trisomy. However, it is possible that some partial trisomies for mouse chromosomes would yield suitable models. For example, trisomy for the distal part of mouse 11 might provide a model for trisomy of human 17

Cattanach and coworkers have used a large variety of chromosomal rearrangements in the mouse to elucidate the question of chromosome imprinting. Nowadays a map of imprinted chromosomal segments is available in the mouse.

MOUSE MODELS OF HUMAN DISEASE AND CHROMOSOME HOMOLOGIES

The mouse genetic map represents a total haploid length of about 1600 centimorgans, spanning over 19 autosomes, a X and a Y chromosome with around 1600 gene loci now mapped on it. In man the density of markers is almost the same order of magnitude. About 600 of these mapped genes can be considered as homologous to one another because they are known to code for similar products, to have the same function or because they have been assigned to a particular locus, in both species, using the same "molecular" probe and thus have the same DNA sequence. When two or more genes of that kind are found to be linked on the same chromosome arm this results in the materialization of a conserved segment.

To date approximately half of the mouse map (800cM) is made of such segments where both synteny and gene order have been conserved since the divergence of lineages leading to either mouse or man. Such maps (Lyon and Kirby, 1991, Nadeau and colleagues, 1991) are invaluable tools when human geneticists wish to list candidate models for a particular human disease and vice versa.

Mouse chromosome 1 for example is made up of two large conserved segments, one with homology to human 2q, and the other to human 1q. The latter segment spans 35 cM, contains 20 genes with known mapped homologues and the linear arrangement of 16 of these genes does seem to have been largely conserved as reported by Seldin and colleagues (Seldin et al 1989). Human chromosomes 17 and 20 are syntenic with mouse chromosomes 11 and 2 respectively. Human 17 is probably entirely integrated into mouse chromosome 11 but, being a metacentric chromosome in man, one must expect some reshuffling in the gene order as suggested by Buchberg et al (1989).

An application of these homology maps is in mapping a gene in one species when its position is already known in the other. We have recently discovered, for example, the mouse homologue of human alcaptonuria (the first inborn error of metabolism as reported by Sir A. Garrod). This mutation has not yet been assigned to a mouse chromosome but this should not be a problem given the strategies available nowadays. When the chromosomal location of alcaptonuria will be known then it may be possible to define a candidate region for the human locus by checking the map of already known homologies. This will be of great value for human geneticists because alcaptonuria is a relatively uncommon disease thus making its localization difficult. The mouse muation *dt*: dystonia musculorum which maps to mouse chromosome 1 is another example.

Histologically the nervous system of affected homozygous shows degenerative changes and progressive loss of nerve fibers in the central and peripheral branches of the sensory ganglion cells of the spinal and cranial nerves and in longer surviving animals there is evidence of lower motor neuron involvement. Together with C. Sotelo (Sotelo & Guénet 1988) we have claimed that this mutation may represent a mouse model for some ataxic syndrome in man. Since the gene responsible for Friedreich's ataxia has been localized on human 9q (which is not homologous with mouse 1) we predict that another gene producing ataxia in man may be located somewhere on 2q.

Another recently discovered mouse mutation, *fcd*, a homologous model for the human syndrome of ferrochelatase deficiency, represents the opposite situation. Because of its similarities with the human syndrome it was predicted to map to the telomeric region of mouse chromosome 18, in a region syntenic with human chromosome 18q, and this prediction turned out to be true.

With the increasing knowledge of the mouse genetic map there will be further interesting examples in the future of the application that can be made of knowledge of man-mouse chromosome homologies. The mouse-man homology map may even become particularly important tool when the diseases with a multigenic determinism will be elucidated in the mouse. In this respect the NOD strain of mouse, which develops spontaneously an insulin dependent diabetes homologous to type I diabetes of man is a good example. It is reasonable to think that many of the genes involved in this pathologic condition will be mapped in the near future then human geneticists could use mouse parameters to try and detect homologous human regions. The same situation can be transposed to autoimmune diseases, and to the determinism of many infectious or parasitic diseases such as tuberculosis, leishmaniosis, sensitivity to *Salmonella* infection etc...

THE LIMITATIONS OF THE MOUSE AS A MODEL FOR HUMAN DISEASES
As more genetic models are identified in mice, more differences are being found between some of the mouse mutants and human diseases. The severity of the human dystrophic syndrome, with its ruthless consequences for the affected boys, contrast for example with the relative weakness of the mouse syndrome and this discrepancy in itself raises several puzzling questions to the biologists: how can a *mdx/mdx* mouse cope without dystrophin? Is there elsewhere in the mouse genome a gene which is able to compensate for the lack of dystrophin? In short what makes a *mdx/mdx* mouse different from a boy affected by the Duchenne muscular dystrophy.

According to Erickson (1989) this may be the consequence of three possible mechanisms: (1) Variation in biochemical pathways between mouse and man, (2) Variation in developmental pathways between mice and man or (3) Absolute time versus physiological time and rates of pathological processes.

To examplify point 1 Erickson notes that the Lesch-Nyhan syndrome, which is a severe human disease, has no equivalent in the HPRT negative mouse, and according to this author this may result from the fact that mice but not humans can convert uric acid to allantoin by oxidation with urate oxidase, and are protected from potentially toxic metabolites of uric acid. Thus, it may be necessary to eliminate both urate oxidase <u>and</u> HPRT activity to create an animal model of Lesch-Nyhan disease. Erickson also note that a mouse being much smaller than a human this may influence some developmental processes and he gives the example of bone remodeling. Humans deficient in carbonic anhydrase (CA)II suffer from osteopetrosis, renal tubular acidosis, intracranial calcifications, and mental retardation. Mice deficient in (CA)II on the contrary never develop osteopetrosis. This may be a consequence of the fact that rodents only remodel bone at the surfaces of their smaller bones and not internally, as larger mammals do. Finally to give some credit to his third hypothesis (absolute time versus physiological time and rates of pathological processes) Erickson emphasizes that physiological processes tend to occur faster in small animals than in larger ones. For example, mouse heart rates are 10 times those of man. Thus, it is usually assumed that pathological processes occur at similar rates as defined by life span, however, several examples suggest that some pathological processes are more closely related to absolute time. The C3H inbred strain of mice has low levels of liver β-glucuronidase comparable to deficiencies that are symptomatic in many human lysosomal storage diseases. However, stored material doesn't accumulate significantly until the mice are about a year old. Thus, this rate of accumulation seems comparable to rates in the human disorders in which patients are normal at birth but typically develop symptoms in the second half of the first year of life. A time-dependent rate of onset of symptoms may explain the mild phenotype of *mdx/mdx* mice.

In addition to Erickson's hypothesis it is also possible that the mouse models are different from humans simply because the mouse has specific peculiarities that are not yet understood. Transgenic rats that express the human class I major histocompatibility allele HLA-B27 and human- $β_2$microglobulin faithfully reproduce the human features of the B27-associated human diseases (spondyloarthropathies) while mice with the same transgenes did not.

CONCLUSIONS

In this review we have discussed the value of some selected mutations of the mouse with the view that knowledge acquired from an analysis of the disease in mice might be applicable to an understanding of the homologous conditions in man and to the development of effective therapies. The technologies so developed will probably influence the diagnosis and treatment of human disorders in the future.

REFERENCES

Bernstein, S.E. (1987): Hereditary hypotransferrinemia with hemosiderosis, a murine disorder resembling human atransferrinemia. *J. Lab. Clin. Med.* 110, 690-705.

Buchberg, A.M. Brownell, E. Shiguilazu, N. Jenkins, N.A. and Copeland, N.G. (1989): A comprehensive genetic map of murine chromosome 11 reveals extensive linkage conservation between mouse and human. *Genetics* 122, 153-161.

Erickson, R.P. (1989): Why isn't a mouse more like a man? *Trends in Genetics* 5, 1-3.

Epstein, C. (1986): The Consequences of Chromosome Imbalance: Principles, Mechanisms and Models Cambridge university Press.

Greaves, D.R. Fraser, P. Vidal, M.A. Hedges, M.J. Ropers, D. Luzzatto, L. & Grosveld, F. (1990): A transgenic mouse model of sickle cell disorder. *Nature* 343, 183-185.

Gropp, A. & Winking, H. (1981): Robertsonian Translocations: Cytology, Meiosis, Segregation Patterns and Biological Consequences of Heterozygosity. In *Biology of the House Mouse*, ed R.J. Berry, pp141-171. London: Academic Press.

Hammer, R. E. Maika, S.D. Richardson, J.A. Tang, J.P. & Taurog, J. (1990): Spontaneous Inflammatory Disease in Transgenic Rats Expressing HLA-B27 and Human β_2m: An Animal Model of HLA-B27-Associated Human Disorders. *Cell* 63, 1099-1112.

Heisterkamp, N. Jenster, G. ten Hoeve, J. Zovich, D. Pattengale, P.K. & Groffen, J.(1990): Acute leukemia in *bcr/abl* transgenic mice. *Nature* 344, 251-253.

Leiter, E. H. Beamer, W.G. Schultz, L.D. Barker, J. E. & Lane, P.W. (1987): Mouse models of Genetic Diseases in *Medical and Experimental Mammalian Genetics: A perspective.* ed V.A. Mc Kusick, T.H. Roderick, J. Mori, & N.T. Paul, pp. 221-257. Alan R. Liss, New York.

Lyon, M.F. & Kirby, M.C. (1991): Mouse chromosome atlas. *Mouse Genome* 89(1), 37-59.

Nadeau, J.H. (1989) Maps of linkage and synteny homologies between mouse and man. *Trends in Genetics* 5, 82-86.

Ryan, T.H. Townes, T. M. Reilly, M.P. Asakura, T. Palmiter, R.D. Brinster, R.L. & Behringer, R.R. (1990): Human Sickle Hemoglobin in Transgenic Mice. *Science* 247, 566-567.

Searle, A.G. Peters, J. Lyon, M.F. Hall, J.G. Evans, E.P. Edwards, J.H. & Buckle, V.J. (1989): Chromosome maps of man and mouse IV. *Ann. Hum. Genet.* 53, 89-140.

Seldin, M.F. Kingsmore, S.F. & Moseley, W.S. (1989): Analyses of gene linkage relationships in the mouse using an interspecific cross: comparative mapping of genes localized to human chromosome 1. *Cytogenet. Cell Genet.* 51, 1077.

Sotelo, C. & Guénet, J.-L. (1988): Pathologic changes in the CNS of Dystonia musculorum mutant mouse: an animal model for human spinocerebellar ataxia. Neuroscience 12,

---

Résumé

De nombreuses mutations de la souris on été isolées au cours des cinquante dernières années. Certaines reproduisent des affections héréditaires connues chez l'homme et peuvent donc servir de modèles pour les chercheurs ou les pédiatres qui étudient ces affections. Ce chapitre présente une revue synthétique des principaux modèles en soulignant leurs avantages et leurs limites.

Homologous recombination and gene targeting on ES cells*

Mario R. Capecchi

Howard Hughes Medical Institute, Eccles Institute of Human Genetics, Bldg. 533, Room 5440, University of Utah, Salt Lake City, UT 84112, USA

* Transcription made by Odile Cohen-Haguenauer

Introduction

In terms of contribution to the field of gene therapy we can look at gene targeting in two ways. The first one, which is immediate, is the ability to create mouse models for human genetic diseases and thereby have a vehicle in order not only to study the pathology of the disease but also to study different therapeutic protocols including gene therapy.

Principles

The protocols essentially consist in preparing an exogenous piece of genomic DNA, to which a modification can be added; that piece of DNA is then introduced into cells, searches the entire genome, binds the cognate sequence; and then subsequent homologous recombination brings that intentional modification in the chromosomal cognate. Inversely you could design this piece of DNA with the aim of repairing a deleterious mutation in the chromosome; towards this end, you could introduce a functional gene and then again by exchange of genetic information, it would correct that modification or mutation and result in a functional gene.

The general procedure used to generate germline chimeras consists of the following steps: you start out with embryo derived stem cells, and you introduce the targeting vector by some method, i.e. microinjection or electroporation; a very small proportion of those cells will actually undergo the targeting event; you thus have to design some means of getting to that specific clone either by screening and sib selection or by enriching through selection. Once you have isolated a pure population, you introduce those cells back in the pre-implantation embryo; you can reimplant that embryo back into a pregnant mouse and if you have appropriate code colour alleles, you can recognize a chimeric mouse. By doing appropriate crossing, you can recognize whether you actually have a germline transmission. The markers coat colour alleles that are most commonly used are agouti in the ES genome and black 6 in the recipient (blastocyst). The efficiency of the process can be very high since in some experiments in which about 7 chimeric animals were generated, all of them were greater than 90% derived from the ES cell genome; all of them were males and turned out to be germline. Germline transmission can be simply assessed by backcrossing to a black 6 mother and showing that the pups are agouti since the marker is coming from the ES cells ; the sperm produced by the chimeric male was thus generated from the ES cell line.

Parameters affecting the targeting frequency.

Insertion vectors and replacement vectors. Two main types of vectors can be used; either insertion vectors or replacement vectors. They contain the same sequence but are topologically different since one carries a double stand break within an homology and the other is colinear with the endogenous sequence; the difference is in the recombination process: in one case the recombination event takes place across a double strand break resulting in the insertion of the whole piece of DNA into the endogenous locus and duplication; whereas in the case of replacement vectors, particular sequences can be looped out; endogenous sequences are being replaced by exogenous ones. Either type of vector can be utilized with equal efficiency. The choice between insertion or replacement vectors only depends on the type of allele which is desired.

Extent of the homology. Some important parameters are the extent of homology between the endogenous sequence and the target; we have observed an exponential dependence for about 10 Kb and then it starts to slope off.

Size limitation. What we have been able to determine recently is that there is a wide latitude in what can be done, for example the amount of non homologous DNA can be increased without affecting the targeting frequency. This might in theory allow to generate any size deletion, any size insertion and even to correct large deletions in the genome by supplying appropriate homologous sequences on either side. This essentially means that perhaps any allele could either be created or corrected in a particular cell type.

Selection for homologous recombination events. But still, the targeting frequency is not very efficient in the sense that most of the time non-targeting events do take place. There is a subsequent need to identify the targeted cell clone. This can be achieved either by using very sensitive screening techniques like PCR or by enrichment techniques like positive-negative selection (PNS). PNS consists of introducing a positive selectable gene to mark for DNA integration whatever site in the whole genome is involved; and a negative selectable gene to essentially kill random events and thereby enrich for the targeting ones.

Homologous recombination in somatic cells. As with respect to gene therapy, the question is: "Do all somatic cells have equal targeting efficiencies?" Most of our work has been done with ES cells; however we have actually examined for example 6 independent somatic cell lines where the targeting frequency measurements were comparable; although in some cases reports of some cell lines, for example P 19, with a lower targeting frequency; but in this case it is allele specific and comparisons between certain alleles have led us to find sometimes much lower targeting frequencies. If other alleles or other genes are tried then comparable frequencies are observed. We thus conclude that it is locus specific as opposed to the concept of some cell lines having or not having the machinery in order to carry out the recombination events.

It appears that what we are taking advantage of is essentially a machinery which is very important to all cell types and that is DNA repair. We would assume that these machineries are ubiquitous to all cell lines.

Models

I will now describe essentially three different mutations that have been generated by gene targeting. We are actually interested in two sets of genes, which are directed mostly towards the analysis of development.

1. The Int gene family

One corresponds to genes involved in localized developmental decisions through cell-cell interaction. For that purpose we chose the *Int* family which was initially identified as a family of proto-oncogenes.

Varmus and co-workers showed that following infection mouse-strains with the mouse mammary tumor virus (MMTV), mammary tumors were generated at high frequency as a result of ectopic insertion of the provirus next to a particular gene; and these are called integration site 1, 2, 3, 4 and 5.

What is interesting about this set of genes is that all of them look like growth factors except for *Int-3* which looks like a growth factor receptor. None of these genes are either involved in the genesis of mammary tissues or actually expressed in mammary tissues. Whereas ectopic expression leads to mammary tumors. What is common about these genes, is that most of them are expressed exclusively during embryogenesis; this is very true of *Int-2* which is a member of the fibroblast growth factor family (FGF). In adult *Int-1* is only expressed during formation of the sperm. We thus felt that these were good candidates for being involved in induction processes and in cell-cell interactions. We thus started to knock out several of these genesgenes among what turns out to be a large family.

In order to find out what the normal function of these genes is, we simply created null alleles and observed the resulting phenotype.

Int-1

Int-1 turns out to have a homolog in drosophila which is *wingless*; a segment polarity gene which is required for the formation of the anterior/posterior compartment in each parasegment. *Int-1* expression pattern is observed in the neural tube just prior to closure, the cells at the very tip expressing *int-1* and then following closure it continues to be expressed to up to about 14 1/2 days of gestation.

ES cell line with a targeting event in that gene were selected to produce chimeras. Heterozygotes were then interbreeded and happened to be perfectly normal. The homozygotes showed severe ataxia as a result of macroscopic lesions in the cerebellum and midbrain. Around 17 1/2 days of gestation, just prior to birth, the whole region of the brain which should give rise to the cerebellum is missing. Amazingly, this mouse actually responds to light, touch, smell; the only striking feature is its incapability to coordinate its front and hind legs therefore giving rise to severe ataxia.

Int-2

The other gene we have analyzed in this family is *int-2* which is a member of the fibroblast growth factor family, without any known drosophila homolog. There is evidence that *int-2* may be involved in induction processes. In particular, it is expressed in cells which are going to give rise to the inner ear; ectopic transplantation of those cells results in generation of a new organ. In order to define the function of *int-2*, we again created null alleles. *Int-2* is very complicated in terms of expression pattern compared to *int-1;* it is expressed in many different sites during embryogenesis but exclusively during embryogenesis; what is in common to all these cell sites is that they are involved either in induction or in cell migration processes.

What we were interested to do was not only to create a null allele by placing the neo gene in the first coding protein exon (1 b) but also to target in the reporter *lacZ* gene which forms a fusion *int-2* protein in the process of being targeted; therefore all the cis elements that normally drive the *int-2* gene are now controlling *lac Z*. The neo gene is also added with its own promotor-enhancer in order to do positive selection. The *int-2-lac Z* reporter gene very accurately reflects the expected expression pattern of *int-2* and I should point out that even having the neo gene only a few Kbs away is not affecting this expression. This approach is important not only to follow the expression pattern in the heterozygote but more importantly, in the homozygote it results in a gene disruption; the cells which are responsible for the phenotype will be blue thus allowing the analysis of the phenotype at the cellular level. We are still in the process of analyzing the associated phenotype. The heterozygote is normal but the homozygote is very abnormal with a very complicated phenotype.

2. Hox-1.5

The final experiments I will present deal with *Hox-1.5* gene which belongs to a set of genes in mouse and man that correspond to the *drosophila UBX and antennapedia* complex. Gene order has been maintained throughout evolutions of both invertebrates and vertebrates; furthermore not only has the order been maintained but also there is an order to function correlation.

These genes are all transcription factors. In drosophila if you simply go down the 5' end to the 3' end of the complex, the first genes have a phenotypic effect in the expression pattern of the posterior end of the drosophila; down the sequence they have more and more anterior expression and phenotypic effects with respect to mutation. The same correlate with respect to expression holds in mouse and man.

We are interested not only in defining what a particular gene is doing, for instance here *Hox-1.5*, but also what this whole network is devoted to; and that means how it is actually involved in setting up the anterior-posterior boundaries and positioning of organs during embryogenesis; we are also interested in finding out how these different genes interact: 1°- who is talking to who? 2°- Is there a hierarchy with respect to these genes? This is obviously a long range project since this complex contains 38 genes.

Phenotype of newborn with targeted disruption of the Hox-1.5 gene

We have generated three independent germline chimeras with targeted disruption of the *hox-1.5* gene and bred them to black 6 mice. All the pups are agouti and half of those contain the mutant allele. Again, the heterozygote is perfectly normal, the homozygotes are born; there is no fatality during embryogenesis but they live approximately 6 to 12 hours, and they appear to die from pulmonary or cardiac dysfunction since they become purple, breath with difficulty and finally die.

Morphology and organs abnormalities. The first thing that is evident in looking at these mice is their altered shape. They have a very short neck and a whole region of the head has been shortened. One thing that became evident is that in the mutant there is no thymus. They also turn out to lack parathyroid glands and have reduced thyroid tissue. The other evident abnormalities consist of numerous cardiac and arterial defects like persistence of ductus arteriosis, atriums enlargement, size-reduction of the aorta also much thinner walled, stenosis of the arterial valve, missing of some large arterias and enlargement of all major veins.

Skeleton. The other thing we were interested in is to examine the skeleton because we have foreshortening of the whole region between the head and the neck. There is no deficiency in vertebrae but the whole region is constricted; the head shape is very different and that is mainly due to the jaws, the maxible and mandible being shorter and thicker relative to the wild type. The mutant also has other crano-facial abnormalities.

Bloated abdomen. They also have a bloated abdomen, and this was puzzling because all the defects first seemed region specific. When the mutant breathes the esophagus is not constricted, the upper glottis is not pulled back as they should be and the soft palate cannot swing over because it is missing. All these things indicate that the air passages are dysfunctional and this could either be due to muscular or neurological disorder or both. The muscles are also distorted and disorganized in this region as well. So when the mouse tries to breathe, instead of pumping air into the lungs, it pumps it into the stomach which builds up pressure and perforates, leading to the bloated phenotype.

What is in common is that most of the impaired stuctures are being derived from the pharyngeal arches. *Hox-1.5* disruption could thus distort the formation of tissues from these particular regions. A hypothesis that we favour is that the neural crest rather than the pharyngeal arches would be involved. One hypothesis that we are following is that this gene is involved in imprinting information to the migrating neural crest either in terms of the migration pattern themselves or in affecting the formation of these tissues through the interaction with tissues in the appropriate pharyngeal arches

Analogies with human DiGeorge syndrome

The other thing that should be underlined is that humans with DiGeorge syndrome are athymic, aparathyroid, have reduced thyroid tissue, bear craniofacial abnormalities and they show both heart and arterial defects. The coincidence of this phenotype with the mouse phenotype is remarkable. As I should point out there are important differences and as Guenet just mentioned, DiGeorge syndrome is autosomal dominant. It has also been associated with deletions that occur in chromosome 22, although a very small fraction of all the DiGeorge syndrome patients actually show any karyotypic abnormalities. *Hox-1.5* does not map to this chromosome in man. However, there is still a possibility that more than one gene is involved in DiGeorge syndrome.

Irrespective of whether it turns out that *Hox-1.5* mutations give rise to DiGeorge syndrome, what the similarity in phenotype tells us is that we are at least in the same developmental pathways, and in this respect the mouse model will be very useful in terms of studying DiGeorge syndrome itself.

REFERENCES

Introduction
Capecchi MR. Altering the genome by homologous recombination. Science 244: 1288-1292, 1989.

Int-1
Thomas K.R. and Capecchi M. Targeted disruption of the murin *int-1* proto-oncogene resulting in severe abnormalities in midbrain and cellular development. Nature, 346: 847-850, 1990.

Int-2
Mansour SL, Thomas KR and Capecchi MR. Disruption of the proto-oncogene int-2 in mouse embryo-derived stem cells: a general strategy for targeting mutations to non-selectable genes. Nature 336: 348-352, 1988.

Hox-1.5
Chisaka O and Capecchi M. Regionnally restricted developmental defects resulting from targeted disruption of the mouse homeobox gene *hox-1.5*. Nature, 350: 473-479, 1991.

RESUME : Le ciblage génique peut contribuer au domaine de la thérapie génique selon deux axes. Le premier, est représenté par la capacité à générer des modèles murins de maladies génétiques humaines et disposer ainsi d'un moyen d'étudier non seulement la physiopathologie de la maladie mais aussi des protocoles thérapeutiques. Les principes généraux de la recombinaison homologue et les paramètres affectant la fréquence du ciblage génique sont rappelés. L'interruption génique ciblée des gènes Int1, Int2 et Hox-1.5, sur des cellules souches embryonnaires (ES) de souris a pu être transmise à la lignée germinale. Le phénotype des souriceaux homozygotes pour l'interruption du gène Int1 est décrite, ainsi que celui de ceux homozygotes pour la mutation du gène Hox-1.5. L'analogie de ce dernier avec le phénotype des patients atteints du syndrome de DiGeorge est soulignée.

A substitution mutation in the *c-abl* gene introduced into the murine germ line by targeted gene disruption in embryonic stem cells

Pamela L. Schwartzberg [1], Elizabeth J. Robertson [2] and Stephen P. Goff [1]

Departments of Biochemistry and Molecular Biophysics [1] and Genetics and Development [2], Columbia University College of Physicians and Surgeons, New York, NY 10032, USA

Summary

We have introduced a substitution mutation into the c-abl locus of murine embryonic stem (ES) cells by homologous recombination between exogenously added DNA and the endogenous gene. We used a promoterless neomycin resistance gene embedded in c-abl genomic sequences derived from the 3' portion of the gene to enrich for homologous recombination events. ES cells carrying a single disrupted allele were used to generate chimeric mice. We have shown that the c-abl mutation is transmitted in the germ line of male chimeras. Mice bearing such engineered mutations should be critically important in increasing our understanding of gene function and in developing models of human genetic disorders.

Introduction

The introduction of mutations into the germline of an organism is one of the most powerful genetic methods for determining the functions of a specific gene product (for example, see Botstein and Fink, 1988). Recent advances in the detection of rare homologous recombination events have facilitated the modification of defined chromosomal loci in mammalian cell lines. The use of these techniques in combination with cultured pluripotent embryonic stem (ES) cells now allows the transfer of defined genetically modified copies of normal cellular genes to the mouse germ line (Capecchi, 1989; Rossant and Joyner, 1989).

We are interested in the function of v-abl, the oncogene carried by the Abelson murine leukemia virus (A-MuLV). A-MuLV causes the rapid induction of lymphosarcomas in susceptible mice and can transform both fibroblasts and lymphocytes in culture (Abelson and Rabstein, 1970a, 1970b; for review see Rosenberg and Witte, 1988). The v-abl gene encodes a tyrosine-specific protein kinase and is an altered version of a normal mouse gene, the proto-oncogene c-abl (Goff et al., 1980; Wang et al., 1984). While much is known about the oncogenic potential of both v-abl and c-abl, little is known about the function of the normal gene in development or in the life of the adult organism. The generation of defined mutations in c-abl in the mammalian germ line could provide critical insights into the function of the gene product.

Embryonic stem cells (ES cells) provide a powerful experimental system for manipulating the genome of mice. These cells are pluripotent cells derived from preimplantation mouse embryos (Evans and Kaufman, 1981; Martin, 1981) which can be propagated in culture and subsequently reintroduced into mouse blastocysts by microinjection to form chimeric mice. Such chimeras, if constructed using euploid ES cells, have been shown to have high rates of transmission of the embryonic stem cell component in the germ line (Bradley et al., 1984). Thus it is now possible to introduce mutations into the germline using ES cell clones that have been pre-selected as carrying mutations at specific loci. We have used homologous recombination to introduce a substitution mutation into the c-abl locus of mouse embryonic stem cells. The mutation affects the large C-terminal portion of the c-abl protein, leaving the tyrosine kinase function intact. The resulting ES cell clones have been used, in combination with embryos derived from a variety of genetic backgrounds, to generate chimeric mice and transmit that mutation through the germline into progeny. This work constituted the first example of the introduction of a mutation into the mouse germline at a non-selectable locus modified by molecularly cloned DNA. This technology has enormous potential for elucidating the function of gene products for which the physiological role is poorly understood.

Experimental strategy for disruption of the c-abl locus

To select for the rare homologous recombination of DNA with the endogenous c-abl locus, we designed DNA constructs in which a promoterless neomycin resistance gene (neo^r) is embedded in c-abl genomic sequence; the DNA would confer resistance to the drug G418 only after certain recombination events. Expression of the neo gene in the construct could be activated either when a nonhomologous integration event places the sequence next to an arbitrary cellular promoter, or, alternatively, when homologous recombination inserts the DNA into the c-abl locus and places the gene under control of the c-abl promoter. Since activation by cellular promoters occurs in only about 1/100 of random integration events, selecting for G418 resistance should enrich for homologous recombination events approximately 100-fold (Jasin and Berg, 1988; Sedivy and Sharp, 1989). A requirement of the procedure is that the c-abl locus be expressed in the target cell line; we have shown by Northern blots that the CCE ES cell line used in this study does indeed express the two normal c-abl mRNAs.

We chose to introduce mutations affecting only the carboxy-terminal third of the c-abl protein, downstream from the tyrosine kinase domain. Since c-abl is expressed ubiquitously, we were concerned that introduction of a null mutation would have severe deleterious effects on the development of the mouse, or might even be lethal, at a very early stage. Mutations limited to this region might not represent null mutations and might generate a less severe phenotype. Deletions affecting the C-terminus of v-abl have shown that this domain is not needed for tyrosine kinase activity or for the transformation of fibroblasts, but is important for transformation of lymphocytes (Goff et al., 1981; Watanabe and Witte, 1983; Prywes et al., 1983). The tissue specificity of the effects of these mutations in A-MuLV suggested that we might obtain informative tissue-specific phenotypes from similar mutations in c-abl.

Construction of v-abl-neo fusions: tests of model gene fusions

To ensure that the planned promoterless neo constructs would indeed confer resistance to the drug G418 when homologous recombination occurred, we first inserted the neo gene into A-MuLV and tested the constructs for biological activity. We generated v-abl-neo constructs which would express the neo gene sequences in either of two ways (Fig 1).

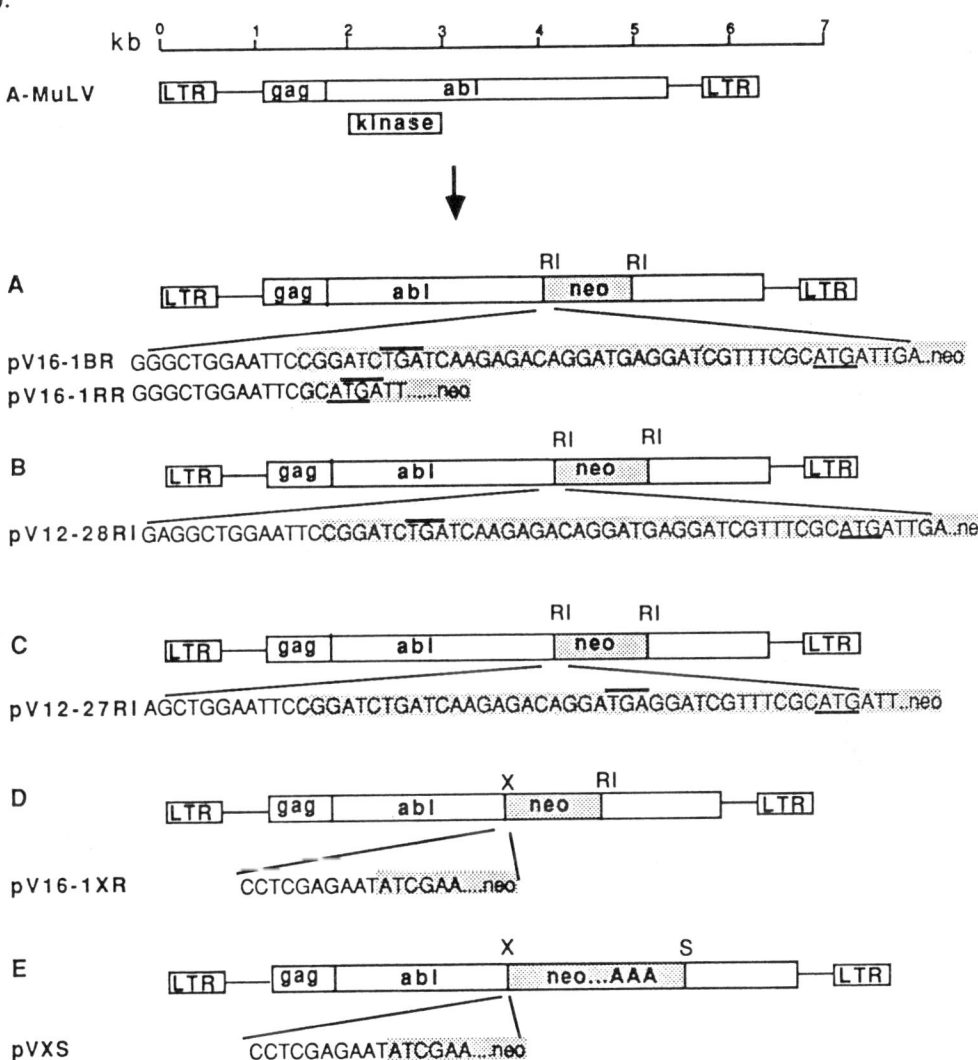

Fig. 1. Structures of v-abl-neo constructs and nucleotide sequences at the abl-neo boundaries. Top line: structure of the wild type A-MuLV genome; the position of the tyrosine-specific protein kinase domain is indicated by the box. Lines A-E: structure of v-abl-neo genomes. The neo sequences are shaded, and restriction sites flanking the neo sequences are indicated. The sequences at the abl-neo boundary for each of the constructs are shown in the expanded region underneath. In lines A-C, the translational restart constructs, the introduced terminator codons are overlined and the AUG initiator codons for neo expression are underlined. From Schwartzberg et al., 1990.

In some constructs, one or more stop codons were placed in the v-abl sequence, immediately followed by the AUG of the neo coding region. Expression of the neo gene in these constructs depends on translational restart by ribosomes terminating in v-abl and restarting at the inserted AUG (Peabody and Berg, 1986; Kozak, 1987). In two other constructs, the neo sequences were simply introduced in frame into the c-abl sequence, so as to encode a large fusion protein. Since these constructs introduced alterations in the v-abl coding region downstream of the tyrosine kinase domain, we expected them simultaneously to transform fibroblasts and confer G418 resistance.

The v-abl-neo constructs were introduced into NIH/3T3 fibroblasts along with DNA of the helper virus Moloney murine leukemia virus (M-MuLV). Virus was allowed to spread through the culture for three days, and the cells were plated to assay either for focus formation or for G418 resistance. All constructs were able to produce both foci and G418-resistant colonies. However, only some of the transformed foci from the translational restart constructs were able to grow in G418; and the majority of the colonies initially selected for drug resistance were not morphologically transformed. This result suggests that the two markers were not simultaneously expressed at high efficiency. Examination of the viral DNA from the recipient cells revealed that the integrated proviruses were generally rearranged. In contrast, the constructs encoding v-abl-neo protein fusions were able to express both markers stably. Thus, foci of morphologically transformed cells derived from the protein fusion viruses grew in G418. Furthermore, most colonies selected in G418 appeared morphologically transformed, and the viral DNA integrated in these cells was unrearranged as judged by from Southern analysis of the proviral DNA. We therefore concluded that the fusion virus was indeed able to express both functions and was stably transmitted through rounds of viral replication.

The v-abl-neo constructs are expressed at high levels from the potent transcriptional promoter contained in the retroviral long terminal repeat (LTR). To ensure that this high level of transcription was not required for the expression of drug resistance, we made an additional construct in which the fusion was placed downstream of the relatively weak promoter of the Herpes simplex virus thymidine kinase gene. Transformation of cells with this construct demonstrated that even weak transcription was sufficient to provide drug resistance.

Homologous recombination of c-abl-neo fusions into the endogenous c-abl gene of ES cells

The region of v-abl containing the neo fusion was excised from the A-MuLV genome of plasmid pVX16-1R and used to replace the corresponding region of the c-abl gene in a cloned 7.5-kb Xba I fragment of the c-abl genomic sequence (Fig. 2). Since this fragment lacks any functional transcriptional promoter, expression of the neo^r gene depends on the juxtaposition of a promoter at the 5' end of the DNA either by chance or by homologous recombination into the c-abl gene sequences. When this construct was introduced into fibroblasts, at least 75-fold fewer G418^r colonies per µg were obtained than with the construct containing the viral promoter. The plasmid containing the c-abl-neo fusion was digested with XbaI, the DNAs were introduced into CCE ES cells by electroporation, and the cells were plated into medium containing G418. Drug-resistant colonies were isolated, and DNA preparations from these cell lines was examined for rearrangements by Southern blotting.

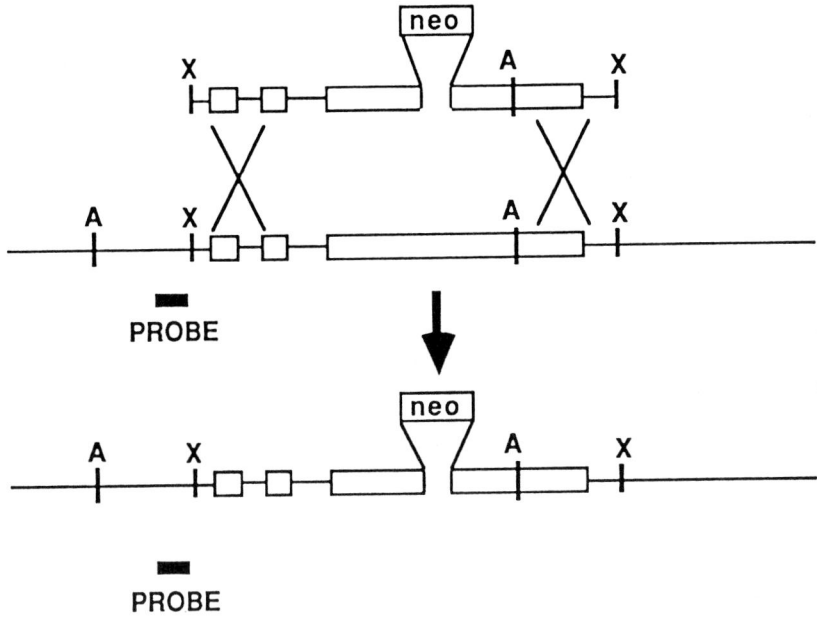

Fig. 2. Scheme for the replacement of the normal c-abl gene with a c-abl-neo fusion by homologous recombination. A linear DNA containing the neo gene embedded in c-abl sequences, but devoid of signals for transcription and translation, is introduced by electroporation. A double crossover in the flanking c-abl sequences replaces the normal gene with the fusion and activates expression of the neo gene. After digestion with ApaL1 and XbaI, hybridization with the flanking probe EX detects DNA fragments of novel sizes from the mutant allele, as well as fragments of the normal size from the unaltered allele.

Genomic DNAs from G418^r clones were digested with ApaLI, separated by electrophoresis, transferred to nitrocellulose, and hybridized with a labelled probe (EX) homologous to a region of c-abl outside the introduced DNA fragment. Integration of the neo sequences by homologous recombination should convert one copy of the 6.5-kb ApaLI wild-type fragment detected by this probe to a novel 7.1-kb fragment. Examination of DNAs from many clones revealed the presence of such an alteration in several cases. In 4 separate experiments, we identified a total of 7 independent (single copy) homologous integration events out of 239 colonies screened, giving a frequency of 1 in 34 G418^r clones. In these seven cases, reprobing the blots with a probe containing neo sequences showed hybridization only to the 7.1-kb rearranged band.

Examination of the genomic DNA from five of the clones by digestion with several other restriction enzymes demonstrated that, in 4 of the 5, the alteration of restriction pattern was as expected for a simple substitution of the c-abl region by the added DNA. In one case, however, integration was accompanied by a rearrangement at the 3' end of the recombination region. We also obtained 9 clones that contained multiple, probably tandem, copies of the added DNA integrated at the c-abl locus. Perhaps a low level of expression of drug resistance produced from the fusion construct enriched for the recovery of clones containing multiple, tandem inserts. If we include these clones, the proportion of the drug-resistant clones that underwent recombination at the c-abl locus was 1 in 15. Although these clones contained mutations at the c-abl locus, the complex structure of the inserted DNA dictated against further use of these lines.

Generation of Chimeric Mice

The overall procedure for the introduction of a mutation into the germ line is summarized in fig. 3. The CCE cell line used for these experiments was originally derived from a single XY blastocyst of the 129/Sv//Ev strain (Robertson et al., 1986), and the cells are therefore homozygous at the black (B) and agouti (A) loci. Additionally, the strain is homozygous for the GPI-1c allele, encoding a rare electrophoretic variant of the glucose phosphate isomerase enzyme. This line was chosen because it has been shown reproducibly to colonize the germ line of male chimeras with high efficiency (Robertson et al., 1986). For the generation of chimeras, host blastocysts were obtained from CD-1, MF1, and C57Bl/6 mouse strains. The CD-1 and MF1 outbred strains are both albino (homozygous for the c allele), whereas the C57Bl/6 inbred strain is black, nonagouti (BB aa). Thus, chimeric mice could be scored by the presence of pigmented coat hair in the CD-1 and MF1 genetic background, and by the presence of agouti hair in the C57Bl/6 background.

Cells of one clone (2b1) were introduced into blastocysts and the resulting hybrid embryos were transferred to the uterine horns of pseudopregnant hosts. The overall frequency of formation of chimeric animals was approximately equal in all backgrounds (32-52% of live-born examined). Interestingly, the degree of ES cell colonization to the coat was markedly influenced by the genetic background of the host blastocyst. We consistently found that the ES cells contributed very extensively in combination with C57Bl/6 blastocysts. In the CD-1 background coat pigmentation was less pronounced. This poor contribution in CD-1 mice could not be attributed to the use of outbred albino recipients; injections of 2b1 cells into blastocysts of MF1 mice, another outbred albino strain, yielded better chimeras, intermediate between the CD-1 and C57Bl/6 chimeras. We conclude that the genetic background provided by the CD-1 outbred strain does not favor the incorporation of 129 derived ES cells.

Germline transmission of the c-abl-neo allele

To screen for germ line transmission, phenotypically male chimeras were caged with tester females. The CD-1-based chimeras were mated to albino females (CD-1) while the C57Bl/6-based animals were mated to nonagouti (genotype (C57Bl/6 X DBA/2) F_1) females. From both series of test matings, the litters were inspected for progeny carrying ES cell-derived agouti pigmentation. GPI isozyme analysis of peripheral blood samples was used to verify that the agouti progeny were derived from the CCE cells.

Of the first 9 male C57Bl/6-based chimeric mice that were proven to be fertile, we obtained 3 which produced agouti progeny. These three chimeras have to date sired a total of 10 agouti offspring in a total of 9 litters. Southern analysis of DNA from the first 3 agouti progeny of the chimeric male designated "J" demonstrated that one of them carries the c-abl mutation originally present in the 2b1 cell line . Similarly, analysis of the DNA of 2 agouti progeny of male "C" showed germline transmission to one of these animals. Thus, we successfully introduced the original mutant allele into the mouse germline.

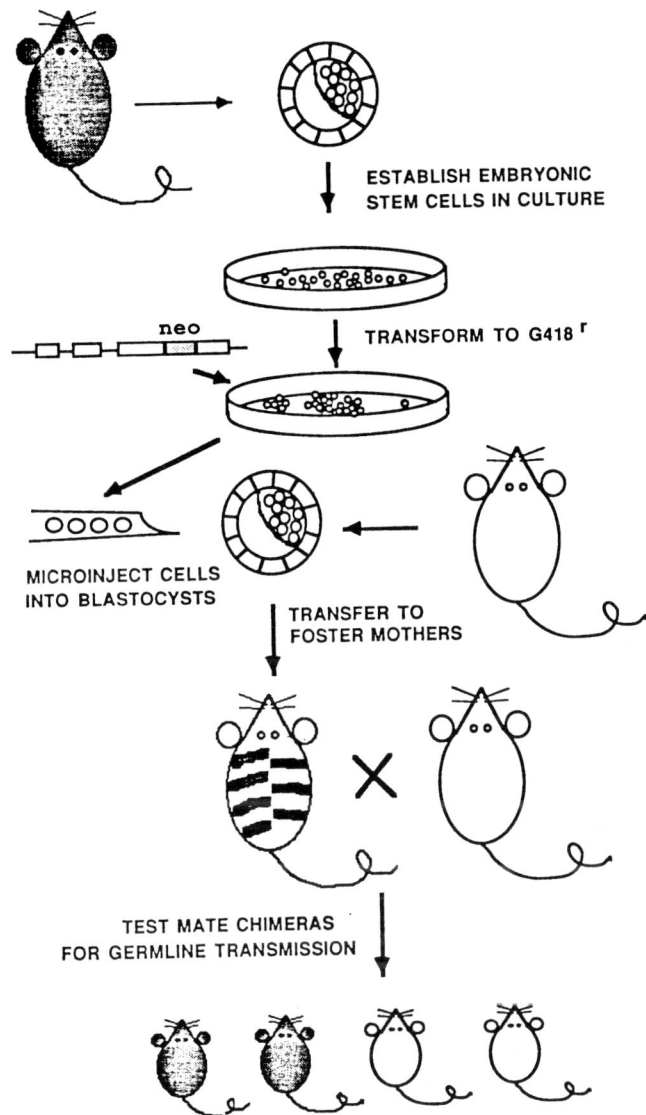

Fig. 3. Flowchart for the introduction of a mutation into the mouse germ line. At top, ES cells are established from a day 3.5 blastocyst. Cell lines are isolated after transformation with a DNA fragment containing an altered version of the target gene, and representative lines are screened for clones that have taken up the DNA by homologous recombination into the endogenous gene. 12-15 cells from these clones are injected into blastocysts, and the blastocysts are transferred to foster mothers to generate chimeric offspring (striped). Chimeric males are mated to tester females to generate animals carrying the mutant gene in the germ line.

Discussion

The use of promoterless selectable markers as a means of selecting for rare homologous recombinants has been described by several investigators to target mutations to defined regions of the genome of tissue culture cells (Jasin and Berg, 1988; Sedivy and Sharp, 1989). Our work adds to a small but growing list of genes that have been disrupted and shows that this method can be used for introducing mutations at defined chromosomal loci with acceptable frequencies. In the case of c-abl, we found that 1 in 34 drug-resistant clones had undergone a homologous recombination event. If we assume an approximately 100-fold enrichment using this technique, the ratio of unselected homologous to nonhomologous integration events is approximately 1/3400, comparable to frequencies observed at other chromosomal loci. Similar or better rates have been obtained by other investigators using similar approaches with promoterless selectable markers (Jasin and Berg, 1988; Sedivy and Sharp, 1989; J. Charron; L. Jeannotte, Columbia University). The different efficiencies of homologous recombination at different target loci could depend on the level of expression of the target gene, but other factors may be important (Smithies et al., 1985; Mansour et al., 1988).

When we used the mutant ES cell clones to generate chimeric mice, we found a significant difference in the degree of contribution of the embryonic stem cells introduced into recipient blastocysts of different mouse strains. In particular, when CCE cells and clones derived from them were introduced into blastocysts derived from C57Bl/6 mice, many chimeras were obtained which showed a greater than 95% contribution to the coat by the ES cells, with very fine and evenly distributed patterns of mosaicism. In contrast, chimeras generated in the CD-1 background had much lower levels of contribution to their coat hairs. The differences among strains in the relative efficiency of ES cell contribution to somatic tissues is also reflected in efficiency of contribution to the germ line.

These experiments constituted the first demonstration that a mutation can be introduced into an endogenous nonselectable gene in ES cells by homologous recombination and that the mutation can be transmitted through the germline of the resultant chimeric mice. The results suggest that it will be possible to generate mutations in mice at any locus defined by a cloned DNA sequence. Using these techniques, we have introduced a mutation which abolishes the carboxy terminal portion of the c-abl protein. Mice heterozygous for the mutation show no growth or developmental defects, demonstrating that this allele does not act in a dominant fashion. Analysis of homozygous abl-/abl- mice should ultimately reveal much about the function of the normal gene.

This report is a summary of published work (Schwartzberg et al., 1989, 1990).

References

Abelson, H. T., and Rabstein, L. S. (1970a). Influence of prednisolone on Moloney leukemogenic virus in BALB/c mice. Cancer Res. 30, 2208-2212.
Abelson, H. T., and Rabstein, L. S. (1970b). Lymphosarcoma: Virus-induced thymic-independent disease in mice. Cancer Res. 30, 2213-2222.
Botstein, D., and Fink, G.R. (1988). Yeast: an experimental organism for modern biology. Science 240, 1439-1443.
Bradley, A., Evans, M., Kaufman, M. H., and Robertson, E. (1984). Formation of germline

chimeras from embryo-derived teratocarcinoma cell lines. Nature 309, 255-256.
Capecchi, M. (1989b). The new mouse genetics: altering the genome by gene targeting. Trends. Genet. 5, 70-76.
Evans, M. J., and Kaufman, M. J. (1981). Establishment in culture of pluripotent cells from mouse embryos. Nature 292, 154-156.
Goff, S. P., Gilboa, E., Witte, O. N., and Baltimore, D. (1980). Structure of the Abelson murine leukemia virus genome and the homologous cellular gene: Studies with cloned viral DNA. Cell 22, 777-785.
Goff, S. P., Witte, O. N., Gilboa, E., Rosenberg, N., and Baltimore, D. (1981). Genome structure of Abelson murine leukemia virus variants: proviruses in fibroblasts and lymphoid cells. J. Virol. 38, 460-468.
Jasin, M., and Berg, P. (1988). Homologous integration in mammalian cells without target gene selection. Genes Dev. 2, 1353-1363.
Kozak, M. (1987). Effects of intercistronic length on the efficiency of reinitiation by eukaryotic ribosomes. Mol. Cell Biol. 7, 3438-3445.
Mansour, S. L., Thomas, K. R., and Capecchi, M. R. (1988). Disruption of the proto-oncogene int-2 in mouse embryo-derived stem cells: a general strategy for targeting mutations to non-selectable genes. Nature 336, 348-352.
Martin, G. (1981). Isolation of a pluripotent cell line from early mouse embryos cultured in medium conditioned by teratocarcinoma stem cells. Proc. Natl. Acad. Sci. USA 78, 7634-7638.
Peabody, D. S., and Berg, P. (1986). Termination-reinitiation occurs in the translation of mammalian cell mRNAs. Mol. Cell Biol. 6, 2695-2703.
Prywes, R., Foulkes, J. G., Rosenberg, N., and Baltimore, D. (1983). Sequences of the A-MuLV protein required for fibroblast and lymphoid cell transformation. Cell 34, 569-579.
Robertson, E.J., Bradley, A., Kuehn, M., and Evans, M. (1986). Germ-line transmission of genes introduced into cultured pluripotent cells by retroviral vectors. Nature 323, 445-447.
Rosenberg, N., and Witte, O.N. (1988). The viral and cellular forms of the Abelson (abl) oncogene. in Advances in virus research. (Academic Press, Inc., San Diego) v. 35, pp. 39-81.
Rossant, J., and Joyner, A. L. (1989). Toward a molecular genetic analysis of mammalian development. *Trends in Genetics, in press.*
Schwartzberg, P., Goff, S.P., and Robertson, E.J. (1989) Germ-line transmission of a c-abl mutation produced by targeted gene disruption in ES cells. Science 246, 799-803.
Schwartzberg, P., Robertson, E.J., and Goff, S.P. (1990) Targeted gene disruption of the endogenous c-abl locus by homologous recombination with DNA encoding a selectable fusion protein. Proc. Natl. Acad. Sci. USA 87, 3210-3214.
Sedivy, J.M., and Sharp, P.A. (1989). Positive genetic selection for gene disruption in mammalian cells by homologous recombination. Proc. Natl. Acad. Sci. USA 86, 227-231.
Smithies, O., Gregg, R. G., Boggs, S. S., Koralewski, M. A., and Kucherlapati, R. S. (1985). Insertion of DNA sequences into the human chromosomal β-globin locus by homologous recombination. Nature 317, 230-234.
Wang, J. Y. J., Ledley, F., Goff, S., Lee, R., Groner, Y., and Baltimore, D. (1984). The mouse c-abl locus: Molecular cloning and characterization. Cell 36, 349-356.
Watanabe, S. M., and Witte, O. N. (1983). Site-directed deletions of Abelson murine leukemia virus define 3' sequences essential for transformation and lethality. J. Virol. 45, 1028-1036.

RESUME : Nous avons introduit par remplacement génique une mutation dans le locus c-abl de cellules souches embryonnaires murines (ES) par recombinaison homologue entre un ADN exogène ajouté et le gène endogène. Nous avons utilisé un gène de résistance à la Néomycine dépourvu de promoteur inclus dans des séquences génomiques de c-abl dérivées de l'extrémité 3' du gène afin d'enrichir pour les évènements de recombinaison homologue. Les cellules ES portant un seul allèle interrompu ont été utilisées pour produire des souris chimères. Nous avons pu démontrer la transmission de la mutation c-abl dans la lignée germinale de chimères de sexe masculin. Les souris porteuses de mutations établies intentionnellement auront une importance décisive pour faire progresser notre compréhension de la fonction d'un gène et développer des modèles animaux de maladies génétiques humaines.

Transgenic mouse models for bone and vascular diseases and gene transfer into hematopoietic cells*

Erwin F. Wagner

Research Institute for Molecular Pathology (IMP), Dr Bohr-Gasse 7, A1030 Vienna, Austria
* *Transcription made by Odile Cohen-Haguenauer*

I would like to present today three short synopses of our research efforts. First, from a more developmental point of view and with the theme of growth control and oncogenesis, to elaborate on the role of particular oncogenes on mesenchymal cell development; I will then show what we have done with endothelial cells, trying to understand the specific role of a particular oncogene in that cell compartment and how this oncogene is involved in disrupting blood vessel formation. Finally, I would like to consider some aspect of gene therapy; I will thus show you how we are attempting to cure a known mouse mutant, the *W* mutant, at least as far as the hematopoietic compartment is concerned.

c-fos expression and mesenchymal cell development.

The mesenchymal lineage has a stem cell. The mesenchymal lineage, like muscle and hematopoietic tissues, also has a stem cell; this lineage comprises 5 different cell types; muscle cells, adipocytes, chondroblasts, osteoblasts and fibroblasts. There is very good evidence that there is a common precursor cell, but very little is known about the growth factors which are responsible for the differentiation of a pluripotent progenitor into one of these differentiated cells. I would like to present some clues that one particular set of transcription factors interacts in a very specific way with the chondrocytic and the osteoblastic lineage, i.e. some molecular data which suggest how we can explain its effects.

c-fos gene transfer to the mouse germ line. c-fos is a common transcription factor which is expressed in almost every cell type upon stimulation with growth factors and thought to be involved in cellular regulation and growth. *fos*-transgenic mice show a quite remarkable phenotype. We will just concentrate on a single construct, H2-c-*fos* LTR which yields stable expression in the animal. The resulting phenotype is very specific and it is always observed in osteogenic cells. We have worked for 2 or 3 years describing this phenotype and we know exactly at what time the transgene is expressed, and how the phenotype develops. *fos* expression affects every single bone, from the long bones, to the vertebra, the skull, the pelvis etc... The animals breed but they are severely affected.

Specific involvement of the osteogenic compartment. What we learned from this set of experiments is that this transcription factor, in spite of being expressed in many different tissues, specifically affects the mesenchymal, osteogenic compartment. We know from many experiments that only osteoblasts do proliferate in these lesions. Expression occurs after birth in 2 to 3 weeks and the phenotype develops later according to the general hypothesis on multistep oncogenesis. We have no idea in this particular case of what the secondary events are; but the penetrance of the phenotype is 100% since every single mouse has an identical phenotype.

c-fos gene transfer into ES cells. Many cell lines have been established from these lesions to identify the possible target cells, but I would like to concentrate on a different set of experiments using the same vectors in a different system, i.e. ES cells. We thus wanted to express the transcription factor during development and see if we could still obtain a specific effect in the embryo where many cells have to divide very rapidly; in that case, we were not dealing with loss of function in the ES cells, but with gain of function. Cells carrying c-*fos* were expressing the corresponding protein 5 to 10 times more than normal embryonic stem cell. We then selected 5 to 10 clones, assessed the pattern of expression in the cultured cells, introduced them back into blastocysts and then looked at the phenotype that we obtained. To our surprise, we got chimeras which were completely normal. In situ hybridizations starting from day 8 to birth showed that the gene is expressed in almost all lineages. Therefore, it is no turned-off; the abnormal phenotype developed from 3 and 4 weeks up to 10 weeks depending on the clones we used. The phenotype that we obtained in a mouse with low chimerism happened to be a very specific one; again, with several clones, the penetrance almost reached 100% whatever the level of expression of the transcription factor was.

The target cell is a chondrogenic cell. We have done a very careful analysis on the target cells which are effective, depicted here as cartilage cells to rule out at what time these lesions occur. In one particular clone they occur around 2 to 3 weeks along the spine, in the long bones. Some sort of chondrocytic focus developed together with highly proliferating lesions which then evolved in full chondrosarcomas. Histological and in situ hybridization analyses on tumor tissues verified that the target cell is indeed a chondrogenic cell. We have taken these lesions at different times during development to establish cell lines and shown that they prove to be chondrogenic cells expressing type 2 collagen as a specific marker. When these cells were reintroduced into a mouse, the same chondrogenic tumors phenotype developed again. More importantly, we could observe chondrogenic cells together with osteoblastic cells. Our hypothesis is that we have indeed immortalized a precursor cell in this lineage.

c-jun and c-fos interaction and timing of the expression. We have a possible molecular clue to what is happening: c-*jun* is expressed only in highly proliferating chondrocytes during development and when the ES cell differenciates into a chondrogenic cell c-*fos* basically settles this cell in a state where it continues to divide. As a summary, neither *fos* nor *jun* has any effect on either differentiation or growth parameters of undifferentiated ES cells. Chimeric mice seem like pre-conditioned since 100% develop these chondrogenic cartilage tumors implying a specific effect on chondrogenic cells; this goes along with a 5 to 10 fold upregulation of c-*jun* in all these cells. The transgenic mice develop osteogenic tumors as we have documented in many publications; thereby affecting a related mesenchymal target cell. This is important to understand since we think that the timing of expression is responsible for the differential activity we see in these particular cell types; and may account for the different phenotypes.

Through these experiments we have learnt that despite assuming that *fos* is very important in every cell type, it has a very restricted target cell specificity when it is analysed either in chimeric mice or in transgenic mice. We have tried to identify genes downstream but we have nothing to report on.

Middle T oncogene expression and vascular tumors

I will move to my second part which again is related to oncogenesis and to endothelial cells. Many transgenic studies have underlined that converting a normal cell into a cancer cell requires multiple steps. What our studies tend to address is: 1°-

what is the target cell; 2°-what might be the target genes; 3°-can we come up with a concept which could explain multistep oncogenesis; 4°-and finally what strategy can we derive from this concept in order to prevent the disease from developing.

Polyoma middle T antigen also interacts with other proteins, e.g. c-*src*, thereby stimulating c-*src* tyrosine kinase activity. We thus are modulating somehow tyrosine kinase activities.

Middle-T specificity to endothelial cells. When middle-T is transferred into ES-cells and the cells introduced into blastocysts, the resulting phenotype is very clear and reproducible with hemangiomas developing into the yolk sac. Cell lines have been derived and they have been identified as endothelial cell lines by lots of markers; they also grow very rapidly. Identical cell lines can be derived by direct infection with middle T, of primary endothelial cells from brain and other sources. Therefore, this oncogene appears to exert a very specific effect on endothelial cells.

Hemangiomas and high fibrinolytic activities. When these endothelioma (End) cell lines are put back into an animal, they again induce rapid formation of hemangiomas within 12 to 18 hours by recruiting non proliferating host endothelial cells into the lesion. 99% of the cells lining the hemangioma are host-derived. How can we get a molecular understanding of that phenotype? A section through one of these tumors shows very nicely rounded cavernas hemangiomas. We next were seeking an *in vitro* system, outside the animal where we could analyze that particular phenotype. We used an *in vitro* fibrin gel system in the presence of plasminogen; the resulting morphology was almost identical (this was done with the help of Roberto Montesano). Experts in the field know that such a structure can only be formed in the presence of a very high fibrinolytic activity and we actually were able to detect such a very high proteolytic activity.

In vitro phenotypic reversion with proteases inhibitors. One target gene as we think is urokinase plasminogen activator (u-PA). The latter is upregulated very specifically in these endothelioma cell lines and the antagonist to urokinase, the plasminogen activator inhibitor is completely downregulated. We were able to demonstrate that there was a causal relationship with what we observed since the presence of protease inhibitors could completely revert the abnormal morphogenetic behaviour of these cells to normal cells *in vitro*; they were able to form tube structures like primary endothelial cells. We did very similar experiments *in vivo* the data of which are not so clear and need statistical analysis. We nevertheless think that also *in vivo,* when these cells are added in the presence of protease inhibitors, a reduction in hemangiomas formation is observed. We finally have to prove this by direct gene transfer of urokinase or plasminogen activator inhibitor.

Proteolytic activity imbalance could account for the observed phenotype. Here is a summary of what we think is happening: due to the high proteolytic activity, the cells migrate very rapidly through tissues and are incorporated into blood vessels; the membrane binds urokinase, sets off a cascade which degrades the extra-cellular matrix via plasmin leading to the rupture of the blood vessel; the whole recruitment comes into play through unknown mechanisms and is responsible for host-derived lesions. In this particular set of experiments, the endothelial cells are the prime target, though we observe expression of the transgene in other cell types. The genes that are activated are urokinase plus urokinase-receptor. Candidates which could mediate this upregulation such as *ets1* all proved to be negative. The molecular basis for this oncogenesis might thus be the proteolytic activity. Imbalance of these proteases is likely to be responsible for that phenotype.

Hematopoiesis

The third part will be devoted to some experiments dealing with the hematopoietic system.

Hemopoiesis from in vitro differentiated embryonic stem cells

ES cells differentation into hemopoietic primitive progenitors. I first would like to describe how we can possibly induce the differentiation of an embryonic stem cell into a hematopoietic stem cell. The system is very simple: ES cells are explanted into semi-solid medium and conditioned to favour hematopoietic differentiation and to form embryoid bodies; this can be done very efficiently since 80-90% of all cells plated in methylcellulose develop redness within these embryoid bodies over a period of 6 to 26 days; these embryoid bodies can be harvested and stained in order to perform cytological analysis and determine the nature of the cells. These structures may alternatively be disrupted and the cells replated into a colony assay to look for specific progenitor cells. Primitive erythrocytes, megacaryocytes, macrophages, eosinophils and mast cells, all lineages develop in that system.

Prospects for further developments of this system. These cells can be explanted, cultured and permanent cell lines can be established. Oncogenes can be introduced in these ES cells and subsequent effects on hematopoietic differentiation can be studied. At present no hematopoietic reconstitution of an irradiated host can be obtained from these cells. We think that the hematopoietic development which we are observing in that system most likely reflects early yolk sac hematopoiesis. If you transplant yolk sac or these cells which appear to be equivalent to yolk sac hematopoietic cells, back into an irradiated recipient, signals for e.g. homing receptors, which would tell them to go into the spleen and form CFUs, might lack.

Rescue of the mouse W/W mutant phenotype

W/W mutant phenotype. The last result which will be presented is an attempt to rescue a known mutant-phenotype in the mouse, i.e. the W/W phenotype by gene transfer with c-*kit* a sort of gene therapy experiment. W affects three lineages, pigmentation, fertility, hematopoiesis; all these stem cell lineages have something in common which is that they are migratory cells. There are severities of W alleles available and the most severe W allele in the homozygote state is not viable. The target cells in terms of hematopoietic cells are either primitive stem cells or mast cells and the CFUs compartment.

Retroviral mediated c-kit gene transfer. What is needed in order to cure that disease is an efficient gene transfer system but it turned out not to be so simple. We also wanted to express c-*kit* in ES cells and investigate: 1°- what kind of stem cells are affected; 2°- what is the basis for *kit* differential activity on these three lineages; 3°- and to rescue W mutants with a gene transfer system. Vectors were tested towards this end and this was quite frustrating because vectors that worked very well in other systems with other genes did not work with *kit*. The only vector which worked was a vector where the mouse c-*kit* is expressed from the LTR and also carries a selectable marker. This vector was tested on fibroblasts, growth factor dependent hematopoietic cells and obviously in the mutant W system.

Infection of growth factor dependent hematopoietic cells. IL 3 dependent hematopoietic cells infected with the retroviral construct nicely respond to the ligand MGF. Growth factor dependent cell lines can thus be easily established. Established primary W/Wv or W/W mutant cells, proliferate in the presence of the stem cell factor. The W/Wv mast cells infected with the LTR-*kit* virus nicely repond to MGF in a proliferation assay, whereas with the control parental construct cells do not respond.

Infection of fetal liver cell. When fetal liver cells from W/W animals are being infected, they grow in the presence of the ligand and you can see that these cells are cured with respect to their growth defect and to mast cell proliferation.

CFUs. As for the CFUs compartment we have performed experiments which are preliminary. CFUs can partly be rescued with W/Wv cells since in one animal distinct spleen colonies are observed and the vector seems to be present. No long term rescue experiments have yet been done and fetal rescue experiments are on their way.

In summary, we can efficiently express this receptor with an LTR-*kit* virus in fibroblasts, in established myeloid cell lines and in addition, we are on the way of rescueing the W phenotype with respect to the mast cell deficiency, *in vitro* and *in vivo*.

REFERENCES

c-fos expression and mesenchymal cell development.
Wang Z-Q, Grigoriadis AE, Möhle-Steinlein U and Wagner EF. A novel target cell for c-fos induced oncogenesis: development of chondrogenic tumours in embryonic stem cell chimeras. EMBO J. 10, 1991 (in press).

Middle T oncogene expression and vascular tumors
Williams RL, Courtneidge SA and Wagner EF. Embryonic lethalities and endothelial tumors in chimeric mice expressing polyoma virus middle T oncogene. Cell 52: 121-131, 1988.

Williams RL, Risau W, Zerwes H-G, Drexler H, Aguzzi A and Wagner EF. Endothelioma cells expressing the polyoma middle T oncogene induce hemangiomas by host cell recruitment. Cell 57: 1053-1063, 1989.

Montesano R, Pepper MS, Möhle-Steinlein U, Risau W, Wagner EF and Orci L. Increased proteolytic activity is responsible for the aberrant morphogenetic behaviour of endothelial cells expressing the middle T oncogene. Cell 62: 435-445, 1990.

Hematopoiesis
Burkert U, von Rüden T and Wagner EF. Early fetal hematopoietic development from in vitro differentiated embryonic stem cells. The New Biol 3, July 1991, in press.

Alexander WS, Lyman SD and Wagner EF. Expression of functional c-kit receptors rescues the genetic defect of W mutant mast cells. EMBO J., submitted.

RESUME : Avec la biologie du développement pour toile de fond et le thème du contrôle de la prolifération cellulaire et de l'oncogénèse, trois grands axes de recherche sont décrits. Le premier tente de préciser le rôle de certains oncogènes sur le développement des cellules mésenchymateuses ; dans ce but, le phénotype de cellules transgéniques pour l'oncogène c-fos, et de souris chimères après transfert génique de l'oncogène c-fos dans des cellules souches embryonnaires, a été étudié. Bien que le transgène soit exprimé de façon ubiquitaire, le phénotype observé se limite au compartiment ostéogénique, avec des tumeurs ostéogènes chez la souris transgénique et des tumeurs chondrogéniques chez la souris chimère. De même, le transfert d'un second oncogène, l'antigène moyen T du virus polyome dans les cellules ES, est responsable du développement d'hémangiomes dans le sac vitellin. Il semble que le phénotype observé puisse être relié à de hautes activités protéolytiques ; en effet, une réversion phénotypique est obtenue in-vitro lorsque des inhibiteurs de protéase sont ajoutés. D'autre part, l'induction d'une différenciation des cellules ES vers des progéniteurs hématopoïétiques avec obtention d'une hématopoïèse essentiellement érythroide mais aussi mégacaryocytaire et myéloide est rapportée. Enfin, un rétrovirus contenant l'oncogène c-kit et un marqueur de sélection a été construit afin de normaliser sur le plan hématologique le phénotype de la souris mutante W/W. Après infection par ce virus d'une part d'une lignée cellulaire de cellules hématopoïétiques dépendant de facteurs de croissance, et d'autre part de cellules mastocytaires dérivées de la souris W/W, une réponse au MGF est obtenue. Il en va de même pour les cellules du foie foetal des animaux W/W ; quant aux données concernant le compartiment des CFUs, elles sont en cours d'évaluation.

Vaccines

Vaccins

Avirulent bacteria expressing heterologous genes : implications for vaccines

David O'Callaghan, Alain Charbit, Jean-Marie Clément, Pierre Martineau, Susie Muir, Sévec Szmelcman, Claude Leclerc (*) and Maurice Hofnung

Unité de Programmation Moléculaire et Toxicologie Génétique, CNRS URA 1444 and (*) Biologie des Régulations Immunitaires, Institut Pasteur, 25, rue du Docteur Roux, 75015 Paris, France
* Author for correspondence

Summary

Foreign genes can be expressed in avirulent bacteria which persist in mammalian hosts. One possible development is multivalent live bacterial vaccines. Three main components can be distinguished in such vaccines: the bacterial vehicle strain, the critical immunogen, and the expression system for the immunogen. This paper illustrates the potential of, and some of the questions raised by this type of vaccine. We describe two systems which allow the expression of peptide sequences as engineered fusions to bacterial envelope proteins.

There are striking homologies between certain bacterial and mammalian proteins which are suggestive of possible horizontal gene transfer (see for example Hofnung, 1987; Hyde et al., 1990). Techniques are also available to transfer genes from bacterial protoplasts to mammalian cells (Schaffner, 1980). To our knowledge, there is however no case where a direct transfer from bacteria to mammalian cells has been demonstrated. Such a demonstration would offer new possibilities for human gene transfer. Since our expertise on the pathways for bacterial invasion (Finlay & Falkow, 1989) and on specific interactions between bacteria and mammalian cells (Finlay, 1990) is rapidly increasing, this may even allow the targeting of foreign genes to particular cell lines *in vitro*, and possibly *in vivo*.

A number of bacteria are able to persist in mammalian hosts as beneficial symbionts or without pathogenic effects (Davis et al. (Eds),1990). When such bacteria are programmed to express foreign genes, this may affect their interactions with their host. In particular, especially well studied bacteria such as *E.coli* or *S.typhimurium*, can now be genetically modified so as to be (i) non-pathogenic (ii) still capable of invading and persisting, (iii) programmed to express foreign polypeptides.

One potential advantage of using bacteria instead of viruses to carry or express foreign genes is that bacteria can be controlled with a number of antibiotics. The problems of unwanted dissemination or adverse effects on immunosupressed subjects are thus less critical with live bacteria. On the other hand, bacteria are complex association of many antigens and one has to be careful of potential side effects.

The foreign polypeptides expressed in the recombinant bacteria may be hormones or mediators playing a direct role on the host. They may also represent or synthesize critical antigens from pathogens. In the latter case, the recombinant bacteria are likely to trigger an immune response towards the pathogens as well as towards themselves. This is the basis for live recombinant bacterial multivalent vaccines (for a recent symposium see Schödel and Hofnung (Eds), 1990).

1 - LIVE RECOMBINANT BACTERIAL VACCINES

Three main components can be distinguished in live bacterial vaccine: the vehicle strain, the critical antigen (or immunogen), and the expression system for the antigen.

Bacterial vehicles based upon many different bacterial species are being developed. The most studied is *Salmonella* which we will discuss below. Another interesting possibility is BCG, which has already been used extensively in the man (Jacobs et al., 1987). Among other possibilities, we could mention *Shigella flexneri* (Sansonetti & Arondel, 1989; Verma & Lindberg, 1991), *Vibrio cholerae* (Taylor et al., 1988), *Bordetella pertussis* (Roberts et al., 1989), and *Yersinia enterocolitica* (Sory et al., 1990; O'Gaora et al., 1990).

The number of protective antigens defined as candidates for inclusion in a recombinant vaccine is growing rapidly. Each component of a pathogen playing a critical role in pathogenicity is likely to be such an antigen. Antigens are being analyzed in terms of their basic antigenic determinants, in particular B- and T-cell epitopes (review in Dougan et al., 1991).

2 - BACTERIAL VEHICLES

Bacterial vehicles used to deliver the foreign antigens to the immune system may be either non-pathogenic bacteria or attenuated strains derived from erstwhile pathogen (Schödel and Hofnung (Eds), 1990). This may allow protection, at the same time, against this pathogen. To express foreign antigens, a minimum of genetic knowledge of the strain is necessary. Extensive work has already been performed with attenuated *Salmonella* strains (see 3 below).

When administrated orally to mice, *Salmonella typhimurium* attaches to, invades and proliferates in the gut-associated lymphoid tissue (GALT). Delivery of an immunogen to the GALT is able to elicit a generalized mucosal secretory immune response, affecting other mucosal surfaces such as in the lungs and the mouth (Chatfield et al., 1989 and references therein). A number of mutations which attenuate *Salmonella* have been described. In the most interesting cases, these mutations do not impair the ability of the strains to home to the GALT. From the GALT, virulent strains of *S.typhimurium* invade draining mesenteric lymph nodes and so to the other organs of the reticuloendothelial system (RES), such as the liver and spleen, where they are resistant to killing by phagocytic cells (Collins, 1972). It seems that persistence is a necessary, but not a sufficient, condition for efficient immunization (O'Callaghan et al., 1988b, and references therein).

A vehicle strain should retain its virulence properties such that it is still capable of invasion and of persisting in the RES. It should, however, be attenuated enough to be harmless. Such a compromise is difficult to attain. Attenuation may be obtained by mutations resulting in limited growth in the host. These mutation may result in sensitivity to a compound present in the host (Germanier & Furer, 1971) or to requirement for a growth factor which is not provided by the host (Stocker, 1988; O'Callaghan et al., 1988b). In this second case, *in vivo*, growth is limited by this factor. One must be sure that, under no circumstances, such as special diet, will the host provide the factor, otherwise the virulent phenotype of the bacteria may be restored. Another approach consists of using mutations affecting directly growth such as thermosensitive mutations (Fahey and Cooper 1970a,b). There are two potential problems. First, such mutations are generally point mutations and may revert at a significant rate. Second, there may be parts of the body with lower temperature (extremities) where virulence would be expressed (Hormaeche et al., 1981). Recently, mutations affecting the regulation of the expression of certain genes by cyclic AMP, have been shown to result in attenuation, possibly through the turning off of genes involved in virulence (Curtiss & Kelly, 1987). The direct selection for *S.typhimurium* mutants unable to survive in macrophages, has also provided a collection of avirulent strains affected in a series of different genetic loci (Fields et al., 1986).

3 - EXPRESSION VECTORS FOR FOREIGN ANTIGENS

The simplest situation is when the foreign antigen is a protein. However, genes involved in the synthesis of a non-protein antigen can also be transferred and expressed in a vehicle strain. Both types of antigen are discussed below.

Non-protein antigens
A plasmid encoding the genes responsible for the synthesis of form I antigen from *S.sonnei* was transferred to and expressed in *S.typhi* Ty21a. This antigen has altruonic acid as a component of its O-specific side chain. Protection against virulent *Shigella* challenge was induced in human volunteers immunised orally with this strain (Black et al., 1987).

E.coli K1 polysaccharide was expressed at the surface of a *S.typhimurium aroA* vaccine strain. Mice vaccinated with the recombinants were protected against challenge with virulent *S.typhimurium*. However, even delivery by a live *Salmonella* was not sufficient to enhance the poor immunogenicity of the K1 polysaccharide (O'Callaghan et al., 1988a).

Protein antigens
When the expression signals are compatible between the donor and the recipient strain, foreign protein antigens can be expressed from their original genes. In other cases, the elements needed for expression of the foreign gene may have to be modified. In general, cloning the

foreign gene under the control of an appropriate promoter leads to expression, although the level of expression may not be optimal.

A number of foreign proteins have been expressed in attenuated *Salmonella*. Humoral and mucosal responses were induced against *E.coli* heat labile toxin B subunit (LT-B) and the serum antibodies neutralised LT *in vitro* (Maskell et al., 1987). Mice immunised orally with an *aroA Salmonella* expressing the C-fragment of tetanus toxin developed antitoxin antibodies and were protected against challenge with purified toxin (Fairweather et al., 1990). Attenuated *Salmonella* can also generate protective cellular immune responses to heterologous antigens. When mice were immunised with a strain expressing the nucleoprotein from Influenza A virus, they developed a strong humoral response, and a specific T-cell proliferative response and a $CD4^+$ class II restricted cytotoxic lymphocyte response (CTL) (Tite et al., 1990). Immunisation of mice with a strain expressing the *Plasmodium berghei* circumsporozoite protein (CS protein) induced $CD8^+$, class I restricted CTLs (Aggarwal et al., 1990).

Expression of the complete foreign protein may result in difficulties: the foreign protein may be toxic to the vehicle, or produced in a non-immunogenic form. The foreign protein may also be harmful to the host. One example of such toxicity to the host is found in certain serotypes of the M protein of streptococci, which contain tissue cross-reactive epitopes (Beachey and Dale, 1988). It is possible to avoid toxicity to the host by expressing mutant forms of the foreign antigen; thus, if this antigen is a toxin, a non-reverting form of a toxoid would be a potential solution.

One solution to these difficulties is to express only the relevant epitopes in the form of peptides. This should be feasible at least when the epitopes correspond to continuous sequences. This approach would also have the advantage of allowing easier construction of strains expressing a (large) number of different epitopes, a situation favorable for multivalent vaccines.

One difficulty is that foreign peptides expressed in either *E.coli* or in *Salmonella* are usually unstable. Foreign peptides can often be stabilised by expressing them as genetic fusions to "recipient" proteins normally expressed in these bacteria (review in Hofnung and Charbit, 1991). By using various recipient proteins, one may be able to vary the presentation of an epitope to the immune system and hopefully to find favorable situations for obtaining a protective response. There are probably many factors which are important for the immunogenicity of a peptide genetically fused to a protein (review in Hofnung and Charbit, 1991). The site for insertion of the peptide, its localization with respect to the immunodominant epitopes of the protein, and the location of the protein within the vehicle strain are likely to play a role. Some of these factors may affect the mode of processing of the protein by the immune system.

4 - "PERMISSIVE SITES AND ENGINEERED PROTEIN FUSION"

When a foreign peptide is inserted within a protein by genetic means, it is likely to lead to an unstable or to a toxic hybrid protein. The folding and/or the routing of the initial protein may be perturbed.

We have developed a genetic procedure which allows us to search for "permissive" sites within a protein (Hofnung et al., 1988). These sites accept insertion of a foreign sequence without deleterious effects on protein stability, activity or localization. Interestingly, this procedure can be used without prior knowledge of the organization of the protein. Depending on the protein used as "recipient" for the insertion, the hybrid protein generated may have very different properties.

We have used two proteins from the gram-negative bacterium *E.coli*-K12: LamB, an outer membrane protein, and MalE, a periplasmic protein. With both proteins foreign epitopes could be expressed and the intact bacteria could be used as live immunogens without any adjuvant to obtain an immune response against the inserted epitopes (O'Callaghan et al., 1990 and references). The influence of the exact cellular location of the foreign epitope is currently under study. Preliminary results indicate that the cellular position plays an important role in determining the intensity and the quality (isotypes) of the antibody response (Leclerc et al., submitted).

a/ LamB

Eleven permissive sites have been identified in the LamB protein (Charbit et al., 1991). Insertion at three sites lead to the cell surface exposure of the foreign epitope (residues 153, 253, 374), while at three other sites, the epitope is exposed on the periplasmic side of the membrane (sites 183, 219, 352). It is thus possible to study the influence of the position of the foreign epitope on the immune response (Leclerc et al., submitted).

We have shown that a broad variety of foreign sequences in terms of length and sequence could be expressed at the surface of *E.coli* by insertion at site 153 of LamB. The hybrid proteins essentially retain their biological activities with inserts up to about 60 residues (Charbit et al., 1988).

The immunogenicity of several viral epitopes, genetically coupled to LamB, was explored (Hofnung, 1988; Leclerc et al., 1989; O'Callaghan et al., 1990; Charbit et al., 1990; Leclerc et al., submitted). Recombinant *E.coli* expressing the hybrid proteins, as well as purified hybrid proteins were immunogenic and induced high titre antibody responses against the inserted epitopes and against the corresponding viruses (poliovirus, Hepatitis B virus). Using hybrids, the amount of peptide required to induce an antibody response was 100 fold less than that used with synthetic peptides chemically conjugated to a protein carrier.

These experiments revealed that several parameters influence the humoral response to the inserted epitope : the route of administration, the preparation of the immunogen, and the location on the carrier protein. By the i.v. route, anti-epitope antibody responses are induced with live, heat killed or sonicated recombinant bacteria. By the s.c. route, anti-epitope antibody responses are induced only when soluble proteins are used as immunogens (semi-purified protein solubilized in detergent).

LamB hybrid proteins constructed in *E.coli* can be expressed at high levels in attenuated strains of *Salmonella*. Preliminary immunization experiments with recombinant *Salmonella* indicated that they could be efficient for the induction of anti-foreign epitope antibodies (O'Callaghan et al., 1990). However, optimal conditions for achieving stable and adequate levels of expression by the *Salmonella* within immunized animals must be found.

b/ MalE

MalE is a periplasmic binding protein involved in the transport of maltose and maltodextrins in *E.coli*. This protein is synthesized in the cytoplasm and exported to the periplasm. It binds maltose and maltodextrins with high affinity. It can be purified by a simple and efficient procedure which involves binding onto an amylose column and elution in mild conditions with maltose (Martineau et al., 1990 and references). Recently, the structure of MalE has been solved at high resolution (Spurlino et al., 1991).

"Permissive" sites in this protein (Hofnung et al., 1988) have been determined. We have analysed in detail insertions in two such sites of MalE, one after residue 133 and the other after residue 303 of the protein. These sites can accommodate peptide insertions up to 80 amino acids without major deleterious effects upon protein expression, localization and function. At site 133 all the hydrophilic insertions retain a Mal+ phenotype and the ability to bind cross-linked amylose column. In addition, at this site, it was possible to insert and express in the periplasmic space a peptide as hydrophobic as the signal sequence of the MalE protein. The versatility of the system allowed us to insert, in the continuity of MalE, a large variety of peptides of immunological interest (Martineau et al., 1991).

The immunogenicity of two epitopes inserted at two sites of MalE was extensively analysed. The first one is a neutralizing epitope from poliovirus type 1 and the second a dominant B epitope from the pre-S(2) region of hepatitis B virus. The immunologic activities of the hybrid proteins were analysed not only with purified protein but also with live bacteria expressing the hybrids in the periplasm. These studies showed that immunization with either bacteria or purified protein could induce high titers of antibodies not only against the peptide but also against the native viral proteins. In addition, the antibodies against the VP1 peptide were able to neutralize polio virus *in vitro* (Leclerc et al., 1990).

MalE-PreS(2) hybrids were transferred to *aroA Salmonella*. The proteins were expressed stably at high level, and immunised mice developed a specific anti peptide antibody response (O'Callaghan et al 1990). One of the advantages of the MalE system is that the peptide is inserted within the continuity of a protein with known structure. Such insertions, in comparison with classical coupling of peptide either chemically or by C-terminal fusions, limit the mobility of the inserted peptide. We are currently investigating the effects of this constraint, using either an approach with polyclonal and monoclonal antibodies directed against the peptide, either by 3-D modeling of the peptide structure by molecular dynamic and energy minimization technics, or by solving the structure of hybrids by X ray analysis (Rodseth et al., 1990). It was shown that depending on the insertion site and on the peptide, antigenicity was greatly affected. For example, the poliovirus epitope C3 was more antigenic in site 133 than in site 303, presumably because its structure is closer to the structure in the native viral particles.

Such studies should help to correlate the antigenicity and the immunogenicity with the 3-D structure of a peptide. By controlling the structure and context of a peptide, it may be possible to induce a response directed specifically against the native protein of a pathogen. It should be also possible to use such constructions to measure the antibodies directed against the native conformation of a peptide.

5 - EXTRAPOLATION TO THE FUTURE FOR LIVE BACTERIAL VACCINES

We are still in an early phase in the identification and epitopic analysis of relevant immunogens and in the design and development of new vehicle strains and of new expression vectors (Schödel and Hofnung (Eds), 1990; Dougan et al. (Ed.), 1991).

We may expect that for any given pathogen there will be a number of critical "target" antigens and that, in turn, these will be reducible to simple antigenic determinants, of which B and T epitopes are presently the most readily definable. It will then be an important step to evaluate the best combination of determinants to ensure effective protection to a population of genetically heterogeneous individuals in different environments. The mode of presentation will certainly play an essential role for immunization with these determinants. The immediate molecular environment of the epitope, its localization within the bacterial vehicle, delivery of the vehicle to the relevant part of the body and persistence of the immunogen will be relevant factors. They are likely to influence processing of the hybrid proteins and the determination of the components of the immune system which are triggered.

We have first examples of vehicle strains and expression vectors. It is important to explore further these systems and to develop others. Indeed, depending on the pathogen and on the antigenic determinant, the optimal presentation system may be different. Many other factors such as economics, conservation, transportability and convenience may play a role in the choice of a delivery system. One important aspect to consider also is the fact that protection against an increasingly large number of pathogens is desirable. It is quite likely that the same presentation systems may not be adequate for multiple administrations with different epitopes. For example, presentation within vaccinia virus, which is one of the promising approaches with live viral vaccines, seems to become less effective following prior immunization against vaccinia (Rooney et al., 1988). Thus, even with the view that multivalent vaccines will be able to protect against several pathogens, it appears desirable to have different presentation systems available to avoid this type of interference.

We can expect, in the coming years, to see a continuing extension in our capacity to present epitopes so as to devise better vaccines and to create vaccines against pathogens for which none exists to day.

6 - ACKNOWLEDGEMENTS

Work in the laboratory of the authors benefits from Grants from the World Health Organization ("Transdisease Vaccinology Program") the "Fondation pour la Recherche Médicale", the "Ligue Nationale Française Contre le Cancer" and the "Association pour la Recherche sur le Cancer" and the North Atlantic Treaty Organization. David O'Callaghan was supported by a Wellcome Trust Travelling Fellowship and Susie Muir by a CNRS-NIH fellowship.

7 - REFERENCES

Aggarwal, A., Kumar, S., Jaffe, R., Hone, D., Gross, M., and Sadoff, J. (1990): Oral *Salmonella*: malaria circumsporozoite recombinants induce specific CD8+ cytotoxic T cells. *J. Exp. Med. 172*: 1083-1090.

Beachey, E.H., and Dale, J.B. (1988): Multivalent Synthetic vaccines against group-A Streptococci. In *Vaccines 88*, eds Ginsberg H., Brown F., Lerner R.A. and Chanock R.M., pp. 95-98. USA: Cold Spring Harbor Laboratory.

Black, R.E., Levine, M.M., Clements, M.L. et al. (1987): Prevention of shigellosis by a *Salmonella typhi-Shigella sonnei* bivalent vaccine. *J. Infect. Dis. 155*, 1260-1265.

Charbit, A., Molla, A., Saurin, W., and Hofnung, M. (1988): Versatility of a vector to express foreign polypeptides at the surface of Gram⁻ bacteria. *Gene 70* :181-189.

Charbit, A., Molla, A., Ronco, J., Clément, J.-M., Favier, V., Bahraoui, E.M., Montagnier, L., Le Guern, A., and Hofnung, M. (1990): Immunogenicity and antigenicity of conserved peptides from the envelope of HIV1 expressed at the surface of recombinant bacteria. *AIDS 4*: 545-551.

Charbit, A., Ronco, J., Michel, V., Werts, C., and Hofnung, M. (1991): Permissive sites and the topology of an outer-membrane protein with a reporter epitope. *J. Bacteriol. 173*: 262-275.

Chatfield, S.N., Strugnell, R.A., and Dougan, G. (1989): Live Salmonella as and carriers of foreign antigenic determinants. *Vaccine 7*: 495-498.

Collins, F.M., (1972): Salmonellosis in orally infected specific pathogen free C57B1 mice. *Infect. Immun. 5*: 191-198.

Curtiss III, R., and Kelly, S. (1987): *Salmonella typhimurium* deletion mutants lacking adenylate cyclase and cyclic AMP receptor protein are virulent and immunogenic. *Infect. Immun. 55*: 3035-3043.

Davis, B.D., Dulbecco, R., Eisen, H.N., and Ginsberg, H.S. (eds.)(1990): *Microbiology. Fourth edition*. J. B. Lippincott Company, Philadelphia.

Dougan, G., Hofnung, M., Lanzavecchia, and Leclerc, C. (eds.) (1991): *Immune response to proteins with recombinant epitopes, perspectives for vaccines* (Conférence Philippe Laudat, Nov. 11-15, 1990, Bischenberg-Obernay, France), INSERM Paris. In press.

Fahey, K.J., and Cooper, G.N. (1970a): Oral immunization against experimental Salmonellosis. I. Development of temperature-sensitive mutant vaccines. *Infect. Immun. 1*: 263-270.

Fahey, K.J., and Cooper, G.N. (1970b): Oral immunization against experimental Salmonellosis. II. Characteristics of the immune response to temperature-sensitive mutants given by oral and parental routes. *Infect. Immun. 2*: 183-191.

Fairweather, N.F., Chatfield, S.N., Makoff, A.J., Strugnell, R.A., Bester, J., Maskell, D.J., and Dougan, G. (1990): Oral vaccination of mice against tetanus by use of a live attenuated *Salmonella* carrier. *Infect. Immun. 58*: 1323-1326.

Fields, P.I., Swanson, R.V., Haidaris, C.G., and Heffron, F. (1986): Mutants of *S.typhimurium* that cannot survive within the macrophage are avirulent. *Proc. Nat. Acad. Sci. USA 83*: 5189-5193.

Finlay, B.B. and Falkow, S. (1989): Common themes in microbial pathogenicity. *Microbiol. Rev. 53*: 210-230.

Finlay, B.B. (1990): Cell adhesion and invasion mechanisms in microbial

pathogenesis. *Current Opinion in Cell Biology* 2: 815-820.
Germanier, R., and Furer, E. (1971): Immunity in experimental salmonellosis. II. Basis of the avirulence and protective capacity of *galE* mutants of *Salmonella typhimurium*. *Infect. Immun.* 4: 663-673.
Hofnung, M. (1987): Protéines: un module énergétique, qui se branche et s'éclate. *La Recherche 18*: 1106-1108.
Hofnung, M. (1988): Engineered protein fusions and live recombinant bacterial vaccines. In *Proceedings of the 8th International Biotechnology Symposium*. II. eds Durand, G., Bobichon, L., Florent, J. pp. 713-724. Paris: Société Française de Microbiologie.
Hofnung, M., Bedouelle, H., Boulain, J.C., Clement, J.M., Charbit, A., Duplay, P., Gehring, K., Martineau, P., Saurin, W. and Szmelcman, S. (1988): Genetic approaches in the study and the use of proteins : random point mutations and random linker insertions. *Bull. Inst. Pasteur 86*: 95-101.
Hofnung, M., and Charbit, A. (1991): Expression of antigens as recombinant proteins. In *Structure of antigens* vol.1. ed. M.H.V. Van Regenmortel. The Telford Press, N.J. USA. In press.
Hormaeche, C.E., Pettifor, R.A., and Broock, J. (1981): The fate of temperature-sensitive Salmonella mutants in vivo in natural resistant and susceptible mice. *Immunology 42*: 569-576.
Hyde, S.C., Emsley, P., Hartshorn, M.J., Mimmack, M.M., Gileady, U., Pearce, S.R., Gallagher, M.P., Gill, D.R., Hubbard, R.E., and Higgins, C.F. (1990): Structural model of ATP-binding proteins associated with cystic fibrosis, multidrug resistance and bacterial transport. *Nature 346*: 362-365.
Jacobs, W.R., Tuckman, M., and Bloom, B.R. (1987): Introduction of foreign DNA into mycobacteria using a shuttle plasmid. *Nature 327*: 532-535.
Leclerc, C., Charbit, A., Molla, A., and Hofnung, M. (1989): Antibody response to a foreign epitope expressed at the surface of recombinant bacteria: importance of the route of immunization. *Vaccines 7*: 242-248.
Leclerc, C., Martineau, P., Van Der Werf, S., Deriaud, E., Duplay, P., and Hofnung, M. (1990): Induction of virus neutralizing antibodies by bacteria expressing the C3 poliovirus epitope in the periplasm. *J. Immunol.* 144: 3174-3182.
Martineau, P., Saurin, W., and Hofnung, M. (1990): Progresses in the identification of interaction sites on the periplasmic maltose binding protein from *E. coli*. *Biochimie 72*: 397-402.
Martineau, P., Charbit, A., Leclerc, C., Werts, C., O'Callaghan, D., and Hofnung, M. (1991): A genetic system to elicit and monitor anti-peptide antibodies without peptide synthesis, *Bio/Technology 9*:170-172.
Maskell, D., Sweeney, K.J., O'Callaghan, D., Hormaeche, C.E., Liew, F.Y., and Dougan, G. (1987): *Salmonella typhimurium aroA* mutants as carriers of the Escherichia coli heat-labile enterotoxin B subunit to the murine secretory and systemic immune systems. *Micro. Pathogen.* 2: 211-221.
O'Callaghan, D., Maskell, D., Beesley, J.E., Lifely, M.R., Robert, I., Boulnois G., and Dougan, G. (1988a): Characterization and *in vivo* behaviour of a *Salmonella typhimurium aroA* strain expressing *Escherichia coli* K1 polysaccharide. *FEMS Microbiol. Letters 52*: 269-274.

O'Callaghan, D., Maskell, D., Liew, F.Y., Easmon, C.S.F., and Dougan, G. (1988b): Characterization of Aromatic and Purine dependant *Salmonella typhimurium*: attenuation, persistence and ability to induce protective immunity in Balb/c mice. *Inf. Imm.* 56: 419-423.

O'Callaghan, D., Charbit A., Martineau P., Leclerc C., Van Der Werf S., Nauciel, C., and Hofnung, M. (1990): Immunogenicity of foreign peptide epitopes expressed in bacterial envelope proteins. *Res. Microbiol.* 141: 963-969.

O'Gaora, P., Roberts, M., Bowe, F., Hormaeche, C., Demarco de Hormaeche, R., Cafferkey M., Tite, J., and Dougan, G. (1990): *Yersinia enterolitica* aroA mutants as carriers of the B subunit of the *Escherichia coli* heat-labile enterotoxin to the murine immune system. *Microbial Pathogenesis* 9: 105-116.

Roberts, M., Maskell, D., Novotny, P., and Dougan, G. (1989): Construction and characterisation *in vivo* of *Bordetella pertussis* aroA mutants. *Infect. Immun.* 58: 732-739.

Rodseth, L.E., Martineau, P., Duplay, P., Hofnung, M., and Quiocho, F.A. (1990): Crystallization of Genetically engineered active maltose-binding proteins, including an immunogenic viral epitope insertion. *J. Mol. Biol.* 213: 607-611.

Rooney, J. F., Wohlenberg, C., Cremer, K.J., Moss, B., and Abner, L.N. (1988): Immunization with a vaccinia virus recombinant expressing simplex virus type 1 glycoprotein D: long term protection and effect of revaccination. *J. Virol.* 62: 1530-1534.

Sansonetti, P.J., and Arondel, J. (1989): Construction and evaluation of a double mutant of *Shigella flexneri* as a candidate for oral vaccination against shigellosis. *Vaccine* 7: 443-450.

Schaffner, W. (1980): Direct transfer of cloned genes from bacteria to mammalian cells. *Proc. Natl. Acad. Sci. USA* 77: 2163-2167.

Schödel, F., and Hofnung, M. (Eds) (1990): *Oral immunization using recombinant bacteria* (International Symposium, Münich June 6-7 1990). *Res. Microbiol.* 141 n° 7-8.

Sory, M.-P., Hermand, P., Vaerman, J.-P., and Cornelis, G.R. (1990): Oral immunization of Mice with a live recombinant *Yersinia enterolitica* O:9 strain that produces the cholera toxin B subunit. *Infect. Immun.* 58. 2420-2428.

Spurlino, J.C., Lu, G.-Y., and Quiocho, F.A. (1991): The 2.3 Å resolution structure of the maltose- or maltodextrin-binding protein, a high affinity receptor for bacterial active transport and chemotaxis. *J. Biol. Chem.* In press.

Stocker, B.A.D. (1988): Auxotrophic *Salmonella typhi* as live vaccine. *Vaccine* 6: 141-145.

Taylor, R., Shaw, C., Peterson, K., Spears, P., and Mekalanos, J. (1988): Safe, live *vibrio cholerae* vaccines ? *Vaccine* 6: 151-154.

Tite, J.P., Gao, X.-M., Hughes-Jenkins, C.M., Lipscombe, M., O'Callaghan, D., Dougan, G., and Liew, F.Y. (1990): Anti-viral immunity induced by recombinant nucleoprotein of Influenza A virus. III. Delivery of recombinant nucleoprotein to the immune system using attenuated *Salmonella typhimurium* as a live carrier. *Immunology* 70: 540-546.

Verma, N.K., and Lindberg, A.A. (1991): Construction of aromatic dependent *Shigella flexneri* 2a live vaccine candidate strains: deletion mutations in the *aroA* and the *aroD* genes. *Vaccine* 9: 6-9.

Résumé

Des bactéries avirulentes capables de persister dans un mammifère peuvent être programmées pour exprimer des gènes étrangers. Un des développements possibles est l'élaboration de vaccins bactériens vivants multivalents. De tels vaccins comprennent trois composants principaux : la souche bactérienne véhicule, les immunogènes critiques, et le système d'expression pour les immunogènes. Cet article illustre certaines des possibilités ouvertes et des questions posées par ce type de vaccin. Il met l'accent sur deux systèmes d'expression par fusion à des protéines d'enveloppe bactérienne.

Recombinant E1A-defective adenoviruses expressing pseudorabies and Epstein-Barr virus glycoproteins induce immunological responses as live vaccines in rabbits and mice

Thierry Ragot [1]*, Marc Eloit [2] and Michel Perricaudet [1]

[1] Laboratoire de Génétique des Virus Oncogènes, Institut Gustave Roussy, Pavillon de recherche 2, Niveau 3C2, 39, rue Camille Desmoulins, 94805 Villejuif, France; [2] Laboratoire d'Epidémiologie et de Physiopathologie des Maladies Animales à Virus, INRA, Ecole Nationale Vétérinaire d'Alfort, 94704 Maisons-Alfort, France

* Author for correspondence

Different E1A-defective recombinant adenoviruses harboring membrane glycoprotein genes from two herpesviruses were engineered. They were found to highly express correctly glycosylated pseudorabies virus gp50 or gI and Epstein-Barr virus gp340/220 (membraneous or secreted form) in various infected cell lines. Inoculation of those recombinants elicited specific and persistent neutralizing antibodies in rabbits and mice. Moreover, protection against pseudorabies virus was obtained for some animals. In view of these results, improvement with regard to convenience of construction and efficiency of expression are discussed. Considerations are also given to the development of recombinant adenoviruses as live vaccines for veterinary or medical purposes and for experimental immunology.

INTRODUCTION

Human Adenovirus type 5 (Ad5) has been well characterized with regard to molecular biology and structure (for a review see Berkner, 1988). Furthermore, Ad vaccine have already been shown to be safe, with Ad effecting an asymptomatic intestinal infection protecting against Ad respiratory disease. Thus, adenoviral vaccine vectors have been constructed that express various foreign immunogenic glycoproteins including hepatitis B virus surface antigen (HBsAg) (Davis et al., 1985; Ballay et al., 1985; Morin et al., 1987; Levrero et al., 1988), herpes simplex virus gB (Johnson et al., 1988), measles virus hemagglutinin and fusion protein (Alkhatib and Briedis, 1988; Alkhatib et al., 1990), vesicular stomatitis virus glycoprotein (Schneider et al.,1989), human immunodeficiency virus type 1 gp120 (Dewar et al, 1989; Chanda et al., 1990) and rabies virus glycoprotein (Prevec, 1990). We present in this paper results dealing with recombinant human Ad expressing immunogenic glycoproteins from two herpes viruses involve in animal and human diseases.

One of them, pseudorabies virus (PRV), is the causative agent of a major disease in pigs. Furthermore, it represents a good model for animal vaccinations because easy and fast challenge could be made in all mammals except primates. Among the different glycoproteins of PRV, gp50 was chosen because it was demonstrated to be a major immunogen of the virus (Eloit et al., 1988; Marchioli et al., 1987; Wathen et al., 1985). GI, a glycoprotein which is often to be found deleted in recent PRV vaccine strains enable to allow one to differentiate infected pigs from vaccinated ones, is thought to be of minor importance in immunogenicity. We wanted to investigate this point by vaccinating mice with a recombinant Ad expressing gI.

The Epstein-Barr virus (EBV) is etiologically associated with endemic Burkitt's lymphoma and undifferentiated nasopharyngal carcinoma (NPC). The virus causes infectious mononucleosis and has been implicated in lymphomas arising in immunosuppressed patients and AIDS sufferers. The major envelope glycoproteins gp340/220, are both encoded by the same viral gene and are expressed on the outer surface of virions and infected cells. They are capable of eliciting neutralizing antibodies to EBV (Thorley-Lawson et al., 1980). As an alternative to the subunit vaccine based on purified gp340, which has been sucessfully used to protect cottontop tamarins against EBV-induced lymphoma (Epstein et al., 1985; Morgan et al., 1988b, 1989), we wanted to develop a live vaccine based on recombinant human Ad, expressing the EBV envelope glycoproteins gp340/220.

RESULTS AND DISCUSSION

Construction of the recombinant adenoviruses.
Methodology is described in Figure 1.

Expression of herpesvirus glycoproteins in infected cell lines.
Whatever the cell type, exogenous proteins expressed after infection of the different recombinant Ad appeared physically identical to the authentic products synthesized by PRV and EBV. Posttranslational modifications occured correctly (e.g. cleavage of signal peptide after translocation and glycosylation). Western blotting analysis of the recombinant PRV gp50 showed two bands with variations in Mr depending on the host cell. The lower band seems to be a non-glycosylated precursor of the mature glycoprotein (Petrovskis et al., 1986). Similarly, recombinant PRV gI expressed in 293, Hela (human), Vero (monkey), ST (swine), MDCK (dog) or BHK21 (hamster) cell lines showed different electrophoretic mobilities correlating with variations in the glycosylation patterns among mammalian cells. This emphasized the advantage of a viral vector to obtain correct species-specific posttranslational protein modifications. The EBV-derived membrane proteins produced after cell infection with Ad-gp340 and Ad-gp220 were found to be correctly processed. In the same way, efficient transportation and localization of the glycoproteins to the cell surface were also verified by membrane immunofluorescence. Secreted forms of gp340/220 could be detected by immunoprecipitation from infected cell culture media when recombinants Ad-gp340D and Ad-gp220D were used. Moreover, during the course of the infection, the secreted glycoproteins accumulated in the cell medium and could easily be purified. On the other hand, analysis of the corresponding cell extracts only showed glycosylation precursors of truncated gp340/220. This suggests the

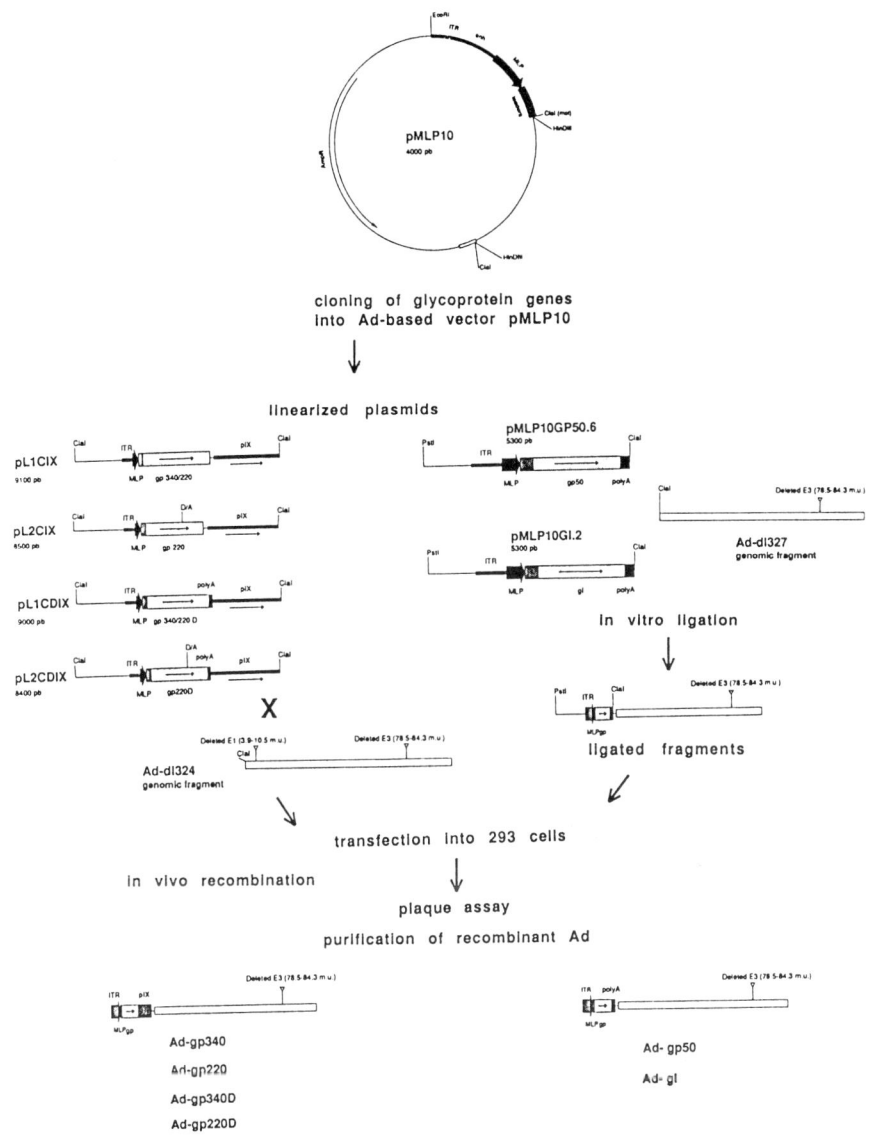

Fig. : Construction of recombinant adenovirus Ad-gp50, Ad-gI and Ad-gp340/220.
The glycoprotein genes were cloned into the eukaryotic expression vector pMLP10. This plasmid contains the extreme left end of the Ad5 genome (i.e. ITR: inverted terminal repeat, encapsidation sequence and E1A region enhancer) with the major late promoter (MLP) of Ad2 joined to its tripartite leader sequence (Ballay et al., 1985). The plasmids pMLP10GP50.6 and pMLP10GI.2 contain the PRV gp50 or gI genes followed by the polyadenylation signal from simian virus 40 early genes (Eloit et al., 1990). The plasmids pL1CIX, pL2CIX, pL1CDIX and pL2CDIX (Ragot et al., 1991) contain expression casssettes composed respectively of the coding region for EBV gp340/220, or the sequence of a cDNA clone corresponding to the

spliced mRNA coding region for gp220, or those constructs deleted for the region corresponding to the membrane anchor and cytoplasmic domains of the proteins (Tosoni-Pittoni et al., 1989). Recombinant Ad were obtained either by in vitro ligations (Ad-gp50, Ad-gI) or in vivo recombinations (Ad-gp340, Ad-gp220, Ad-gp340D, Ad-gp220D). Ligated DNA fragments or mixture of the viral genome fragment and linearized plasmid were respectively transfected into 293 cells (complementing E1 functions). Viruses from plaques isolated 10 days later were amplified.

Boxes: viral sequences (white: viral genome, light grey: glycoprotein genes, dark grey: Ad sequences, black: SV40 sequences); arrowed black box : MLP promoter; thin line: bacterial sequences. D/A: donnor and acceptor splice sites. 1 m.u. = 360 bp.

presence of a highly efficient posttranslational processing system secreting these peptide sequences as has previously been noticed by Whang et al. (1987).

Although high levels of glycoprotein expression could be detected in some infected cell lines, efficiencies of expression varied between them. Subsequent experiments were done to quantify more precisely the level and the temporal pattern of glycoprotein expression into 293 (complementing for the E1 functions), HeLa and Vero cell lines after infection with recombinant Ad. Results obtained with Ad-gp50 were summarized in Table 1. Although the kinetics of gp50 expression were faster in 293 cells, progressive accumulation of gp50 in HeLa cells led to levels of expression which were higher than in 293 cells. Comparable results were obtained for gp340/220 and have also been reported for the same kind of recombinant Ad expressing HBsAg or human a1-antitrypsin, both secreted proteins (Ballay et al., 1987; Gilardi et al., 1990). This observation can be probably explained by the rapid and extensive cytopathic effect seen in 293 cells , whereas in some other cell lines, an accumulation of recombinant products could compensate for the lack of E1A transactivation. Taken together, these results show that, in some cell lines other than 293, high levels of expression can be induced by E1A-defective recombinant Ad.

Table 1 : Cumulative amounts of gp50 in infected cells at different time post-infection.
(a): multiplicity of infection. (b): quantification by ELISA in μg of gp50/10^6 infected cells. Same quantities of infected cell extracts were used to coat microplate wells and the presence of gp50 was revealed by using the 10X16 monoclonal antibody (Eloit et al., 1988). The ELISA titer of cell extracts was considered to be the reciprocal of last dilution giving a signal higher than that of the negative control (Ad-dl327-infected cell extract). Conversion of ELISA titers to gp50 concentrations was made by using a cell extract with a known concentration of gp50 as a reference. ND : not done.

Days	293			HeLa			Vero		
	1(a)	10	100	1	10	100	1	10	100
1	ND	29(b)	15	ND	ND	ND	ND	ND	ND
2		15		ND	ND	ND	ND	ND	ND
3		ND		1,5	3	8	<1.5	<1.5	6
4		18		1,5	5	13	<1.5	<1.5	2
6		18		3	9	20	<1.5	<1.5	3
8		18		<1.5	5	40	<1.5	<1.5	2
13				<1.5	8	40	<1.5	<1.5	4

Antibody response in rabbits and mice inoculated with the recombinant Ad.
Antibody responses against gp50 and gp340/220 were monitored in rabbits and mice after injections of Ad-gp50 or in rabbits with recombinant Ad expressing different forms of gp340/220, from different routes. Immunization schemes are summarized in Table 2 and Table 3 respectively. After inoculation of a single dose of recombinant Ad-gp50 (Table 2), specific antibodies were detectable two weeks later in almost all but one rabbit (F). After a second injection, a boost effect was detected in the rabbits and they showed a strong antibody response one week later. Analysis of the serum of rabbit F with a Western blot proved that the detected antibodies were directed against gp50. Strong antibody responses were also detected in all groups of mice except in group 1 (probably due to the short interval between the inoculation and blood sampling).
Rabbits vaccinated with Ad-gp340 and Ad-gp220 (expressing membraneous glycoproteins) had a similar anamnestic response (Table 3). High levels of antibody that could recognize gp340/220 expressing cells by IF and gp340/220 proteins by immunoprecipitation and in Western blots were obtained. Relatively high titers were maintained 40 weeks after the last inoculation. There is no quantitative difference between gp340 and gp220 in their capacity to induce specific antibodies.
The anti-gp340/220 titers are much lower for the rabbits inoculated with recombinant Ad-gp340D (expressing secreted glycoproteins) and we have not observed a long term response. The difference found in the anti-gp340/220 titers between membraneous and secreted forms of gp340/220 might be explained by the processing of the antigen which probably involves T cell recognition of Ad-infected blood cells in the former case and soluble antigen pathway in the latter. No anti-gp340/220 response to the recombinant Ad-gp220 (expressing secreted protein) was observed even after repetitive injections in 14 rabbits. The truncated gp220 is either less stable *in vivo* or it is more likely that the conformation adopted by this recombinant protein where both the anchor domain and the domain unique to gp340 have been removed is poorly immunogenic in rabbits. The anti-gp340/220 positive sera from immunized rabbits were all strongly EBV neutralizing. These results correlated with the fact that secreted gp220 and protein with amino acid deletions from the C-terminus have been found to bind similarly to EBV B-lymphocyte receptor CR2 (Tanner et al., 1988). More precise deletions are necessary within the N-terminal end of gp340/220 to map the CR2 binding domain. Nevertheless, this work constitutes a preliminary stage towards delineating gp340/220 epitopes involved in the immune response in terms of antibody binding to gp340 and virus neutralization.

Protection of rabbits and mice from PRV challenge.
Rabbits and mice were challenged with 30 LD_{50} of virulent PRV (strain Kojnok). The results obtained are shown in the last column of Table 2. All the controls inoculated with Ad-dl327 died 3 to 5 days after the challenge. Of eight rabbits vaccinated with Ad-gp50, only three survived and they all exibited high levels of anti-gp50 antibodies. Similar results were obtained in mice, where surviving animals originated from groups 3 and 4, in which high levels of anti-gp50 antibodies were detected before challenge.
These results can be explained either by the animal models or by the method used for PRV challenge. It is known that rabbits frequently

give poorly reproducible results when used for the control of inactivated PRV vaccines. This is probably related to the high sensitivity to PRV of rabbits, which can be killed by a single p.f.u. of virus. Marchioli et al. (1987) reported that a recombinant vaccinia virus expressing the gp50 gene efficiently protected mice from a PRV injection. Nevertheless, the conditions of challenge which were used seem to be less severe than ours, because only 80% of the control mice died. To protect all mice against the same challenge conditions as ours, Ishii et al. (1988) would have needed to inject mice twice with 5 µg of purified gp50 emulsified in complete Freund's adjuvant. With two doses of only 1 µg, protection of mice was comparable to that described here for group 3. Thus under the conditions used, protection against PRV challenge could only be obtained in rabbits and mice that exhibited high titres of anti-gp50 antibodies.

Table 2 : Antibody response and protection from challenge in rabbits and mice vaccinated with Ad-gp50.
New Zealand white rabbits and BALB/c mice were inoculated by different routes (i.v.: intravenous, i.m.: intramuscular, i.n.: intranasal, i.p.: intraperitoneal) with recombinant Ad or Ad-dl327 as negative control (respectively 10^9 p.f.u. for rabbits and $10^{7.5}$ p.f.u. for mice per dose) and revaccinated as indicated. (a): interval between the last inoculation of Ad and the date of challenge. (b): anti-gp50 antibody titers on the day of challenge (sera from mice were pooled before testing) detected by ELISA (Eloit et al., 1989). Serum titers were expressed as the reciprocal of last dilution giving an absorbance reading greater than 0.15. (c): neutralization assay. Serum titers were expressed as the reciprocal of the dilution required to neutralize 50% of the input virus titrated on Vero cells (Eloit et al., 1990). (d): viral challenge involved intramuscular injection of 10^4 or 10^2 p.f.u. of PRV (titrated on PK15 cells) respectively into rabbits and mice. (e): rabbit D was not challenged with PRV, its blood was sampled 5 weeks after injection. NA: not appropriate.

Animal	Virus	Route	Number of injections (interval in weeks)	Weeks (a)	Antibodies ELISA (b)	Neutralizing (c)	Death (d)
Rabbit A	Ad-gp50	iv	2(3)	2	1024	128	Yes
Rabbit B	Ad-gp50	iv	2(3)	2	1024	64	Yes
Rabbit C	Ad-gp50	iv	2(3)	2	1024	256	No
Rabbit D	Ad-gp50	iv	1	NA(e)	128	16	NA
Rabbit E	Ad-gp50	im	2(3)	2	512	32	Yes
Rabbit F	Ad-gp50	im	2(3)	2	256	256	Yes
Rabbit G	Ad-gp50	in	2(3)	2	1024	128	Yes
Rabbit H	Ad-gp50	in	2(3)	2	1024	128	No
Rabbit I	Ad-dl327	iv	2(3)	2	<4	<4	Yes
Rabbit J	Ad-dl327	iv	2(3)	2	<4	<4	Yes
Rabbit 1	Ad-gp50	iv	2(11)	3	128	64	Yes
Rabbit 2	Ad-gp50	im	2(11)	3	256	32	No
Rabbit 3	Ad-gp50	in	2(11)	3	64	4	Yes
Rabbit 4	Ad-dl327	iv	2(11)	3	<4	<4	Yes
Mice group 1	Ad-gp50	ip	1	1	<2	<4	10/10
Mice group 2	Ad-gp50	ip	2(1)	1	64	<4	10/10
Mice group 3	Ad-gp50	ip	2(1)	3	256	8	7/10
Mice group 4	Ad-gp50	ip	3(1,2)	1	1024	16	9/10
Mice group 5	Ad-gp50	ip	3(1,2)	2	1024	16	9/10
Mice group 6	Ad-dl327	ip	3(1,2)	1	<2	<4	10/10

Table 3 : Antibody response in rabbits inoculated with Ad-gp340/gp220/gp340D/gp220D.
New Zealand white rabbits were inoculated by different routes with 10^{10} p.f.u. of recombinant Ad or Ad-dl324 as negative control and were revaccinated at weeks 5 and 10. (a): anti-gp340 antibody titers detected by immunofluorescence from fixed 293 cells previously transfected with a plasmid expressing gp340/220 (Tosoni-Pittoni et al., 1989). The serum titers were expressed as the reciprocal of the last positive dilution detected. (b): the neutralization assay is based on an abortive transformation of lymphoid cells with EBV. -: negative result, S: animal sacrificed or dead. ND: not done.

Virus type	Animal	Routes	Antibodies titers (a) (weeks after the first injection)					EBV neutralization (b)
			0	4	7	25	40	
Ad-gp340	30	iv	-	16	256	512	S	+++
	31	iv	-	512	1024	256	256	
	32	iv	-	128	256	256	S	
	33	iv	-	-	-	128	S	
	34	iv	-	512	1024	S		
	35	iv	-	512	2048	256	S	
	36	im	-	1024	1024	256	256	
	38	im	-	1024	2048	S		
	68	in	-	32	512	S		
Ad-gp220	40	iv	-	1024	1024	128	256	+++/++
	41	iv	-	2048	1024	64	64	
	42	iv	-	2048	1024	128	S	
	43	iv	-	256	128	-	S	
	44	iv	-	2048	512	256	64	
	45	iv	-	512	256	256	128	
	46	iv	-	1024	512	16	S	
	47	iv	-	1024	1024	256	S	
	48	im	-	512	256	128	S	
	49	im	-	1024	512	256	4	
Ad-gp340D	54	iv	-	128	16	-	S	++
	55	iv	-	256	-	-	S	
	56	iv	-	512	-	-	S	
	57	iv	-	64	-	-	S	
	58	iv	-	8	16	-	S	
	59	iv	-	64	8	-	S	
	60	im	-	256	8	-	S	
	61	im	-	64	32	8	S	
Ad-gp220D	65-67	iv	-	-	-	ND	S	ND
Ad dl324	80	iv	-	-	-	S		-

GENERAL DISCUSSION AND PERSPECTIVES

Improvement of foreign gene expression from recombinant Ad in infected cells.
We have demonstrated high levels of expression of foreign genes in various cell lines infected with the recombinant adenoviruses. In particular, the secreted form of EBV gp340/220 could be easily purified from a defined serum-free medium. This could provide a good source of antigen for a subunit vaccine without the risk of EBV DNA contamination. In our constructions, the foreign coding regions were placed under the control of the strong major late promoter of Ad2, followed by most of its tripartite leader sequence into E1 region. Indeed, mRNAs containing the tripartite leader have been shown to be translated in late infected cells at least 20-fold more efficiently than mRNAs containing only the first leader (Thummell et al., 1983;

Davis et al., 1985). Recent descriptions of recombinant adenoviruses engineered for in vivo expression of foreign genes used a cloning site in the E3 region without deletion of the E1 gene (Morin et al., 1987; Johnson et al., 1988; Schneider et al., 1989). Johnson et al. (1988) were unable to detect herpes simplex virus (HSV) gB-related transcripts initiated from the SV40 early promoter. Instead, gB-related transcripts were initiated from one of several promoters upstream in the Ad5 genome and involved multiple splicing events. Similar observations were made by Schneider et al. (1989) after cloning the glycoprotein gene from vesicular stomatitis virus linked to the HSV thymidine kinase promoter. Cloning in the opposite orientation (i.e. right to left) of E3 transcription led in these two cases to a low level of expression of the inserted gene, and control of transcription by the foreign promoter was not demonstrated. As we have no promoter sequences upstream from the foreign MLP inserted into the left end of the linear Ad5 genome, a contribution of Ad5 promoters to the transcription of the foreign genes is unlikely in the recombinant Ad obtained.

An interesting aspect already shown by Alkhatib et al. (1988) is that expression of the cloned genes was not strictly restricted to cells complementing the E1-defective recombinant viruses. These results are different from those published by Johnson et al. (1988), who were unable to detect expresssion of HSV gB in HeLa cells early (24h) after infection. This difference could be explained by the use of a strong promoter (MLP) with the E1A enhancer in the constructions instead of the SV40 early promoter, and by longer incubation times. In the experimental conditions used, expression of PRV gp50 or EBV gp340/220 in HeLa cells were much higher than in 293 cells. Furthermore, expression of PRV gI was obtained in porcine, canine and hamster cells, confirming and extending previous results obtained by Prevec et al., (1989) in bovine, canine and murine cells. This wide host range of expression is promising for the future development of animal vaccines.

Development of recombinant Ad as live vaccine.
We have shown that recombinant Ad5 deleted in the E1 region were very efficient for in vitro expression of foreign gene products and could induce a good antibody response and protection from virulent challenge in mice and rabbits. These results confirm previous ones obtained in rabbits and chimpanzees with HBsAg recombinant E1A-defective Ad5 (Levrero et al., 1988). This kind of result has been previously demonstrated only for non-defective recombinant Ad5 which used a cloning site in the E3 region (Morin et al., 1987; Dermott et al., 1989; Prevec et al., 1989; Dewar et al., 1989, Prevec et al., 1990). In these constructions, transcription of foreign genes were initiated from E3 or MLP endogenous promoter Thus, while mouse cells are considered semi-permissive for Ad5 replication (Prevec et al., 1989), and in spite of the E1A deletion in recombinant Ad, the levels of glycoprotein produced in mice and rabbits were high enough to stimulate an antibody response. This result was not unexpected in view of the demonstration of the synthesis of glycoproteins in cells which could not complement the E1A-defective Ad5. We anticipate that cloning in the E1 region may have some advantages, such as lowering levels of replication in vivo and thus limiting the risks of dissemination of recombinant virus and making the transcription of genes, the expression of which must be regulated, more controllable. It has been reported that E3-deleted Ad titers fall quicker than wild-type Ad, consistent with the role of the E3 region in

immunosurveillance. We have found that rabbits immunized with our recombinant Ad elicited antibody production against both Ad and the recombinant protein as Morin et al. (1987) have observed in hamster. Moreover, relatively high levels of anti-gp340 antibodies have been found to persist 30 weeks after last Ad injection in rabbits. Pereira and Kelly (1954) have shown that latent infection of rabbit by Ad5 could occur with among others virus persistence into the spleen.
The ability to deliver adenoviruses via several routes of administration, such as i.m., i.n., i.p., subcutaneously, orally or intestinally from encapsulated vaccine (this paper; Sumner et al., 1988; Prevec et al., 1989; Baer et al., 1989; Lubeck et al., 1989; Dewar et al., 1989, Prevec et al.,1990) makes them powerful tools for in vivo expression of foreign genes. In particular, the possibility of obtaining an equally effective response with intranasal or oral introduction of the virus is promising for using adenoviruses to express foreign antigens in animals. The Ad-based vaccines may be easier to deliver than conventional vaccines and should be more adapted for large scale vaccination programs of wildlife or domestic animals and eliminating certain risks such as reversion to virulence. Adenovirus replicates in the gastrointestinal and upper respiratory tracts, in tonsils and salivous glands of man and some vertebrates and thus may be advantageous for vaccination against viruses which also replicate at these sites. Moreover, an IgA and secretory IgG responses could be induced with these last routes of injection which protect mucous membranes.

Perspectives.
As PRV is pathogenic for all species of mammals except primates, Ad-gp50 can easily be used to study the ability of recombinant Ad to protect a large number of animals species (particularly pigs). Previous experiments have been carried out using gp340 recombinant vaccinia (Mackett and Arrand, 1985) and Varicella-Zoster (Lowe et al., 1987) viruses. Protection against EBV-induced lymphoma was achieved using a vaccinia strain but not a vaccine strain (Morgan et al., 1988a). As persistent EBV-neutralizing antibody response was obtained in rabbits vaccinated with recombinants producing membrane gp340/220, we intend to test Ad-gp340/220 for their ability to protect cottontop tamarins against EBV-induced lymphomas.
It seems that Ad expression vectors will continue to be improved both with regard to efficiency of expression and convenience of construction. Increased expression may be achieved by using stronger exogonous promoters. An enhancement of expression can be obtained when a viral regulator gene is also inserted into recombinant Ad as in results reported by Chanda et al., (1990) where HIV rev and envelope genes were both expressed into the recombinant Ad. It is now possible to substitute up to 7,5 Kbp of heterologous DNA into Ad. Potential deletions in the E4 region may permit insertion of several genes coding for immunogenic proteins into unique recombinant Ad. Enhancement of immunological response (particularly cell mediated immunity) through antigen presentation or immune modulation must be also considered. The insertion of genes for interferon gamma, interleukin-2 or interleukin 4 into Ad genome would represent attempts at the latter approach.

REFERENCES

Alkhatib, G. & Briedis, D.J. (1988): High-level eucaryotic in vivo expression of biologically active measles virus hemagglutinin by using an adenovirus type 5 helper-free vector system. J. Virol. 62, 2718-2727.

Alkhatib, G., Richardson, C. & Shen, S-H. (1990): Intracellular processing, glycosylation and cell-surface expression of the measles virus fusion protein (F) encoded by a recombinant adenovirus. Virology 175, 262-270.

Baer, G.M., Brooks, R.C. & Foggin, C.M. (1989): Oral vaccination of dogs fed canine adenovirus in baits. Am. J. of Vet. Res. 50, 836-837.

Ballay, A., Levrero, M., Buendia, M.A., Tiollais, P. & Perricaudet, M. (1985): In vitro and in vivo synthesis of the hepatitis B surface antigen and of the receptor for polymerised human serum albumin from recombinant human adenovirus. EMBO J. 4, 3861-3865.

Berkner, K.L. (1988): Development of adenovirus vectors for the expression of heterologous genes. Biotechniques 6, 616-629.

Chanda, P.K., Natuk, R.J., Mason, B.B., Bhat, B.M., Greenberg, L., Dheer, S.K., Molnar-Kimber, K.L., Mizutani, S., Lubeck, M.D., Davis, A.R. & Hung, P.P (1990): High level expression of the envelope glycoprotein of the human immunodeficiency virus type 1 in the presence of rev gene using helper-independant adenovirus type 7 recombinants. Virology 175, 535-547.

Davis, A.R., Kostek, B., Mason, B.B., Hsiao, C.L., Morin, J., Dheer, S.K. & Hung, P.P. (1985): Expression of hepatitis B surface antigen with a recombinant adenovirus. Proc. Natl. Acad. Sci. USA 82, 7560-7564.

Dermott, M.R., Graham, F.L., Hanke, T., & Johnson, D.C. (1989): Protection of mice against lethal challenge with herpes simplex virus by vaccination with an adenovirus vector expressing HSV glycoprotein B. Virology 169, 244-247.

Dewar, R.L., Natarajan, V., Vasudevachari, M.B. & Salzman, N.P. (1988): Synthesis and processing of human immunodeficiency virus type 1 envelope proteins encoded by a recombinant human adenovirus. J. Virol. 63, 129-136.

Eloit, M., Fargeaud, D., L'Haridon, R. & Toma, B. (1988): Identification of the pseudorabies glycoprotein gp50 as a major target of neutralizing antibodies. Arch. Virol. 99, 45-46.

Eloit, M., Fargeaud, D., Vannier, P., and Toma, B. (1989): Development of an ELISA test to differentiate between animals either vaccinated with or infected by Aujeszky's disease virus. Vet. Record 124, 91-94.

Eloit, M., Gilardi-Hebenstreit, P., Toma, B. & Perricaudet, M. (1990): Construction of a defective adenovirus expressing the pseudorabies virus glycoprotein gp50 and its use as a live vaccine. J. Gen. Virol. 71, 2425-2431.

Epstein, M.A., Morgan, A.J., Finerty, S., Randle, B.J. & Kirkwood, J.K. (1985): Protection of cottontop tamarins against Epstein-Barr virus-induced malignant lymphoma by a prototype subunit vaccine. Nature 318, 287-289.

Gilardi, P., Courtney, M., Pavinari, A. & Perricaudet, M. (1990): Expression of human alpha 1-antitrypsine using a recombinant adenovirus vector. FEBS Lett. 267, 60-62.

Graham, F.L., Smiley, J., Russell, W.C. & Nairn, R. (1977): Characteristics of a human cell line transformed by DNA from human adenovirus type 5. J. Gen. Virol. 36, 59-72.

Ishii, H., Kobayashi, Y., Kuroki, M. & Kodame, Y. (1988): Protection of mice from lethal infection with Aujeszky's disease virus by immunization with purified gVI. J. Gen. Virol. 69, 1411-1414.

Johnson, D.C., Ghosh-Choudhury, G., Smiley, J.R., Fallis, L. & Graham, F.L. (1988): Abundant expression of herpes simplex virus glycoprotein gB using an adenovirus vector. Virology 164, 1-14.

Levrero, M., Ballay, A., Schellekens, H., Tiollais, P. & Perricaudet, M. (1988): Hepatitis B adenovirus recombinant as a potential live vaccine. In processings of the 8th International Biotechnology Symposium, Paris, pp. 702-712. Edited by G. durand, L. Bobichon, & J.Florent.

Lowe, S.R., Keller, P.M., Keech, B.J., Davison, A.J., Whang, Y., Morgan, A.J., Kieff, E. & Ellis, R. (1987): Varicella-zoster virus as a live vector for the expression of foreign genes. Proc. Natl. Acad. Sci., USA 84, 3896-3900.

Lubeck, M.D., Davis, A.R., Chengalva, M., Natuk, R.J., Morin, J.E., Molnar-Kimber, K., Masson, B.B., Bhat, B.M., Mizutani, S., Hung, P.P. & Purcell, R.H. (1989): Immunogenicity and efficacy testing in chimpanzees of an oral hepatitis B vacine based on live recombinant adenovirus. Proc. natl. Acad. Sci., USA 86, 6763-6767.

Mackett, M., and Arrand, J. (1985) : Recombinant vaccinia virus induces neutralising antibodies in rabbits against Epstein-Barr virus membrane antigen gp340. EMBO J. 4, 3229-3234.

Marchioli, C.C., Yancey, R.J., Petrovskis, E.A., Timmins, J.G. & Post, L.E. (1987): Evaluation of pseudorabies virus glycoprotein gp50 as a vaccine for Aujeszky's disease in mice and swine: expression by vaccinia virus and Chinese hamster ovary cells. J. Virol. 61, 3977-3982.

Morgan, A.J., Mackett, M., Finerty, S., Arrand, J.R., Scullion, F.T. & Epstein, M.A. (1988a): Recombinant Vaccinia virus expressing glycoprotein gp340 protects cottontop tamarins against EB virus-induced malignant lymphomas. J. Med. Virol. 25, 189-195.

Morgan, A.J., Finerty, S., Lovgren, K., Scullion, F.T., & Morein, B. (1988b): Prevention of Epstein-Barr (EB) virus-induced lymphoma in cottontop tamarins by vaccination with the EB virus envelope glycoprotein gp340 incorporated into immune-stimulating complexes. J. Gen. Virol. 69, 2093-2096.

Morgan, A.J., Allison, A.C., Finerty, S., Scullion, F.T., Byars, N.E. & Epstein, M.A. (1989): Validation of a first-generation Epstein-Barr virus vaccine preparation suitable for human use. J. Med. Virol. 25, 74-78.

Morin, J.E., Lubeck, M.P., Barton, j.E., Conley, A.J., Davis, A.R. & Hung, P.P. (1987): Recombinant adenovirus induces antibody response to hepatitis B virus surface antigen in hamsters. Proc. Natl. Acad. Sci, USA 84, 4626-4630.

Pereira, H.G. & Kelly, B. (1957): Latent infection of rabbit by adenovirus type 5. Nature 180, 615-616.

Petrovskis, E.A., Timmins, J.G., Armentrout, M.A., Marchioli, C.C., Yancey, R.J. & Post, L.E. (1986): DNA sequence of the gene for pseudorabies virus gp50, a glycoprotein without N-linked glycosylation. J. Virol. 59, 216-223.

Prevec, L., Schneider, M., Rosenthial, K.L., Belbeck, L.W., Derbyshire, J.B. & Graham, F.L. (1989): Use of human adenovirus-based vectors for antigen expression in animals. J. Gen. Virol. 70, 429-434; erratum 2539.

Prevec, L., Campbell, J.B., Christie, B.S., Belbeck, L. & Graham, F. (1990): A recombinant human adenovirus vaccine against rabies. J. Inf. Dis. 161, 27-30.

Ragot,T., Tosoni-Pittoni, E., De Mazancourt, A., Finerty, S., Morgan, A.J. & Perricaudet M. : Recombinant adenoviruses which express the Epstein-Barr virus major membrane antigen gp340/220 induce persistent EBV-neutralising antibodies in rabbits. (1991, submitted to Journal of General virology).

Schneider, M., Graham, F.L. & Prevec, L. (1989): Expression of the glycoprotein of vesicular stomatitis virus by infectious adenovirus vectors. J. Gen. Virol. 70, 417-427.

Sumner, J.W., Shaddock, H.H., Wu, G. & Baer, G.M. (1988) : Oral administration of an attenuated strain of canine adenovirus (type 2) to raccoons, foxes, skunk, and mongoose. Am. J. Vet. Res. 49, 169-171.

Tanner, J., Whang, Y., Sample, J., Sears, A. & Kieff, E. (1988): Soluble gp350/220 and deletion mutant glycoproteins block Epstein-Barr virus adsorption to lymphocytes. J. Virol. 62, 4452-4464.

Thumell, C., Tjian, R., Hu, S.H. & Grodzicker, T. (1983): Translational control of adenovirus late promomter. Cell 33, 455-464.

Thorley-Lawson, D.A & and Geilinger, K. (1980): Monoclonal antibodies against the major glycoprotein (gp350/220) of Epstein-Barr virus neutralize infectivity. Proc. Natl. Acad. Sci. USA 77, 5307-5311.

Tosoni-Pittoni, E., Joab, I., Nicolas, J.C. & Perricaudet, M. (1989): Complete characterization of the gene coding for the Epstein-Barr virus membrane antigen gp220/340 and selective expression of secreted form of gp220. Biochem. Biophys. Res. Commun. 158, 676-684.

Wang, Y., Silberklang,M., Morgan, A., Munshi,S., Lenny, A.B., Ronald, W.E. & Kieff, E. (1987): Expression of the Epstein-Barr virus gp350/220 gene in rodent and primate cells. J. Virol. 61, 1796-1807.

Wathen, L.M.K., Plat, K.B., Wathen, M.W., Van Dense, R.A., Wheston, C.A. & Pirtle, E.C. (1985): Production and characterization of monoclonal antibody directed against pseudorabies virus. Vir. Res. 4, 19-29.

Résumé

Les gènes des glycoprotéines membranaires gp50 et gI du virus de la maladie d'Aujeszky (pseudorage) et gp340/220 du virus d'Epstein-Barr ont été insérés dans des vecteurs adénovirus défectifs pour la région E1A. Les virus recombinants ainsi construits permettent une expression importante et une maturation correcte des protéines après infection de différents types cellulaires. Des anticorps neutralisants spécifiques sont obtenus après injection du virus chez le lapin et la souris et une protection partielle contre le virus de la maladie d'Aujeszky est observée. A partir de ces résultats, les statégies employées dans la construction des Ad recombinants pour permettre une expression efficace in vitro et in vivo sont analysées. Le développement de tels Ad recombinants comme vaccins vivants dans les domaines vétérinaire, médical et en immunologie fondamentale est ensuite envisagé.

Selected posters

Communications sélectionnées

Direct gene transfer and expression into rodent striated muscle *in vivo*

Jon A. Wolff*, Gyula Acsadi, Shoshou Jiao, Agnes Jani, David Duke [1], Phillip Williams and Wang Chong

Departments of Pediatrics and Genetics, Waisman Center, University of Wisconsin, Madison, WI 53706;
[1] *Department of Surgery, University of Wisconsin, 1500 Highland avenue, Madison, WI 53706, USA*
* *Author for correspondence*

Genes for the reporter genes chloramphenicol acetyltransferase, luciferase, and β-galactosidase within RNA and DNA expression vectors were injected into mouse and rat skeletal or cardiac muscle *in vivo*. The naked genes were injected in physiologic solutions without any special delivery system. Evidence of expression of the reporter genes were found in all cases (Wolff et al., 1990; Acsadi et al., 1991). The levels of expression from either the RNA or DNA constructs were comparable to levels of expression obtained from fibroblasts transfected *in vitro* under optimal conditions. Gene expression was localized to the skeletal and cardiac muscle cells by finding blue muscle cells on histochemical staining following injection with an E. coli β-galactosidase expression vector (pRSVLac-Z or pCMVLac-Z). In the rectus femoris part of the quadriceps, approximately one percent of the myofibers were expressing E. coli β-galactosidase.

In both injected skeletal muscle *in vivo* and transfected fibroblasts *in vitro*, RNA expression was maximal at 18 hours and then rapidly decreased. After injection of pRSVL plasmid DNA into skeletal muscle, expression was stable for at least one year in mice and for at least four months in rats. However, after injection of pRSVL into rat cardiac muscle, expression decreased dramatically between 14 and 21 days. Perhaps an inherent cellular property that is different between skeletal and cardiac tissues explains why expression is stable in skeletal but not cardiac muscle. For example, the persistence of foreign plasmid DNA in skeletal fibers may be related to their ability to maintain multiple nuclei. However this is unlikely because pUC19 as assayed by PCR persisted in both cardiac and skeletal muscle for at least two months. This suggests that cardiac muscle does not have some immutable property that prevents persistence of plasmid DNA. This results also suggests that if a plasmid such as pUC19 does not express any protein then it could persist. Thus, this implicates the immune system as a cause of the unstable luciferase expression after pRSVL cardiac injection.

In order to perform further studies to determine if the immune system is involved in the unstable luciferase expression in cardiac muscle, the stability of expression was determined in immunocompromised rats. Luciferase activity persisted for at least two months in hearts injected with pRSVL in cyclosporin-treated rats and nude rats that have hereditary absence of thymus. These results are consistent with the hypothesis that unstable cardiac expression is due to immunological effects. The death of pRSVL transfected cells from an immune response would explain why both luciferase activity and pRSVL DNA disappeared two to three weeks after injection. Perhaps a humoral or cellular immune response is induced by foreign gene expression in cardiac muscle but not in skeletal muscle. Alternatively, an immune response is induced in both but skeletal fibers are more resistant to its toxic effects.

A better understanding of the mechanism of gene uptake by skeletal muscle cells would be gained by determining if other tissues can also take up and express genes introduced by direct injection. Therefore, the levels of luciferase expression were determined in several tissues that were surgically exposed and injected with pRSVL under direct visualization. No significant levels of luciferase expression were detected in brain, liver, spleen, uterus, stomach, lung or kidney after they were injected. In order to reduce the chance that the lack of expression was due to non-function of the RSV promoter in these other tissues, a variety of other promoters were evaluated. For the liver, the mouse albumin promoter was used. For the brain, the SV40, MSV, CMV, and phosphoglycerate kinase promoters were used. Again, no luciferase expression was detected after these tissues were injected with luciferase constructs containing these promoters. These results suggest that lack of expression was not due to inability of the promoter to express. Further experiments using DNA PCR showed that the tissues contained significant quantities of pRSVL DNA at seven days after injection. This indicates that nonexpression is not due a problem in the injection technique. In summary, striated muscle appears to contain the unique property of expressing naked genes injected by a simple needle into the extracellular space.

The direct transfer of genes into muscle *in situ* has several potential applications. The treatment of genetic diseases of muscle, such as Duchennes muscular dystrophy could benefit from expression of the normal gene within muscle cells. Muscle could also be used as a target tissue for the heterologous expression of a transgene that would remove a circulating toxic metabolite (e.g. many inborn errors of metabolism such as phenylketonuria or propionic acidemia). Muscle could also be used as a "platform" for the secretion of a protein (e.g. α1-antitrypsin deficiency). The expression of genes encoding antigens within muscle cells might induce a more protective immune response than injected proteins or peptides since the antigen could be presented in association with the muscle's major histocompatibility complex (MHC).

Skeletal muscle comprises approximately 40% of the body and can probably be easily, safely and repetitively injected making it a particularly attractive target tissue for such applications. However, the level of expression achieved by this technique would have to be increased for many of these applications.

REFERENCES

Acsadi, G. et al., (1991): Direct gene transfer and expression into rat heart in vivo. *The New Biologist* 3, 71-81.
Wolff, J.A. et al., (1990): Direct gene transfer into mouse muscle in vivo. *Science* 247, 1465-1468.

RESUME : Les gènes reporters de la chloramphénicol-acétyltransférase, de la luciférase et de la bêta-galactosidase introduits dans des vecteurs d'expression d'ARN et d'ADN ont été injectés en solution physiologique in-vivo directement dans les muscles squelettiques ou cardiaques de souris et de rats. Avec le plasmide pRSVL, une expression stable a pu être obtenue dans le muscle squelettique pendant au moins un an chez la souris et au moins quatre mois chez le rat. Cependant, après injection du même plasmide dans le muscle cardiaque de rat, une importante diminution de l'expression a été notée entre les 14ème et 21ème jours. Un mécanisme de rejet immunitaire des cellules transfectées est évoqué.

Determination of DNA-elements necessary for macrophage specific and position independent expression of the chicken lysozyme gene in transgenic mice

C. Bonifer [1]*, N. Yannoutsis [2], F. Grosveld [2] and A.E. Sippel [1]

[1] Universität Freiburg, Institut für Biologie III, Schänzlestrasse 1, D7800 Freiburg, Germany; [2] Laboratory of Gene Structure and Expression, National Institute for Medical Research, The Ridgeway, Mill Hill, London NW/1AA, UK
* Author for correspondence

Summary

We are analyzing the chicken lysozyme gene region as a marker locus for macrophage differentiation. In order to investigate the regulatory function of different, previously identified cis-acting elements . during development, we have introduced the complete gene locus as well as a deletion mutant into the germ line of mice. Transgenic mice carrying the entire locus expressed lysozyme mRNA at high levels specifically in macrophages, as it is the case in the donor species. Expression levels were dependent on the copy number of integrated genes. Transgenic mice carrying a construct, in which an upstream enhancer region plus the domain border sequences (A-elements) were deleted, showed a drastic decrease as well as a loss of tissue specific and copy number dependent expression of the transgene.

Results

Nuclear DNA is organized in topologically constrained loop domains defining basic units of higher-order chromatin structure. In an effort to investigate the relevance of chromatin structure for the control of gene expression, we mapped the chromatin organization of the chicken lysozyme gene locus. The lysozyme gene is expressed in the tubular gland cells of the oviduct under the control of steroid hormones (Schütz et al., 1978). Expression of the same gene in macrophages is constitutive, the gene is progressively and selectively activated only in late stages of macrophage differentiation (Sippel et al., 1987). The active chicken lysozyme gene is located within a 20 kb chromatin domain of elevated DNAseI sensitivity of DNA. The oviduct and macrophage modes of regulation can be correlated to alternative sets of DNAseI hypersensitive chromatin sites which develop in oviduct and myeloid cells, each site marking the position of multifactorial regulatory elements (Fritton et al., 1984). The domain of general DNAse sensitivity terminates at both ends in specific DNA elements (A-elements), which are attached to the nuclear matrix. A-elements stimulate transcription of stably reinserted reporter gene ' mini-domains' in the genome of premacrophage cells in culture and protect them from chromosomal position effects (Stief et al., 1989).
In order to study the precise role of the various cis-acting elements in the developmentally controlled activation of the lysozyme locus during macrophage differentiation, we generated transgenic mice carrying the entire structurally defined wild type domain including 5' and 3' A-elements (Fig.1). We additionally wanted to know, whether our previous studies of chromatin structure had provided sufficient information to define an independent regulatory chromosomal locus rather than a gene with a subset of regulatory elements. Synthesis of mRNA from the chicken lysozyme transgene locus in the hematopoietic system of the mouse is restricted to macrophage cells. Expression ocurred at high level and independent of the chromosomal position in the host genome (Bonifer et al., 1990). The same cis acting elements as in chicken macrophages are active in the mouse, their functioning is indicated by the presence of the same hypersensitive chromatin sites. In an analysis of a series of deletion mutants we

first examined mice carrying a construct, where an upstream enhancer region as well as the A-elements were deleted (Fig.1). Expression levels in mouse macrophages dropped dramatically and copy number dependent expression was lost. Surprisingly, also tissue specific expression was abolished, while

DHS A		copy no. dep.	tissue spec. expr	expr. level
wt		+	+	+++++
ks		−	−	var.

Fig.1 Schematic map of the chicken lysozyme gene locus, indicating the gene with its exon-intron structure and the transcription start (horizontal arrow). The vertical bars mark the position of the nine DNAseI hypersensitive chromatin sites (DHS). The position of the A-elements is indicated by a horzontal line above the map (A). The lines below the map indicate the two constructs analyzed in transgenic mice. Restriction sites: k= KpnI, S= SmaI, X= XbaI.

different cell specificities of expression appeared in every independent transgenic line, indicating a strong chromosomal position effect. These experiments suggest a crucial function of the deleted region in the cell specific activation of the chicken lysozyme locus during macrophage differentiation.

References
Bonifer,C., Vidal,M., Grosveld,F. and Sippel,A.E. (1990): *Tissue specific and position independent expression of the complete gene domain for chicken lysozyme in transgenic mice.* EMBO J.9,,2843 - 2848.
Fritton,H.P., Igo-Kemenes,T., Strech-Jurk,U., Theisen,M. and Sippel,A.E. (1984): *Alternative sets of DNAseI hypersensitive sites characterize the various functional states of the chicken lysozyme gene,* Nature 311, 163 - 165
Schütz,G., Nguyen-Huu,M.C., Giesecke,K., Hynes,N.E., Groner,B., Wurtz,T., and Sippel,A.E. (1978): *Hormonal control of egg-white protein messenger RNA synthesis in the chicken oviduct,* Cold Spring Harbour Symp.Quant.Biol. 42, 617 - 634
Sippel,A.E., Borgmeyer,U., Püschel,A.W., Rupp,R.A.W., Stief,A., Strech-Jurk,U., and Theisen,M. (1987): *Multiple non-histone protein-DNA complexes in chromatin regulate the cell and stage specific activity of a eucaryotic gene,* in: Structure and function of eucaryotic chromosomes (ed.: Hennig,W.H.), Results and problems in cell differentiation, 14, Springer Verlag, Berlin, 255 - 269
Stief,A., Winter,D., Strätling,W.H. and Sippel,A.E. (1989): *A nuclear DNA attachment element mediates elevated and position independent gene activity,* Nature 341, 343 - 345

RESUME : Nous analysons actuellement la région génique du lyzozyme chez le poulet en tant que marqueur génétique de la différenciation macrophagique. Afin d'étudier les fonctions régulatrices respectives de différents éléments agissant en cis pendant le développement, nous avons introduit le locus génique complet ainsi qu'un mutant de délétion à l'intérieur de la lignée germinale de la souris. Les souris transgéniques portant l'intégralité du locus expriment l'ARN messager de lysozyme à des taux élevés et de manière spécifique dans les macrophages à l'image de ce qu'il se passe dans l'espèce dont le transgène est issu. Les niveaux d'expression sont corrélés au nombre de copies intégrées. Les souris transgéniques incluant une construction dans laquelle un enhancer d'amont ainsi que les séquences bordantes du domaine (A-elements) ont été délétées, présentent une diminution drastique de l'expression du transgène qui s'accompagne d'une perte à la fois de la spécificité tissulaire et de la corrélation avec le nombre de copies.

Adenovirus as an expression vector in muscle cells. Application to dystrophin

Béatrice Quantin [1], Michel Perricaudet [2], Shahragim Tajbakhsh [3], Margaret Buckingham [3] and Jean-Louis Mandel [1]

[1] LGME/CNRS-INSERM U184, Institut de Chimie Biologique, 11, rue Humann, 67085 Strasbourg Cedex, France; [2] CNRS UA1301, Institut Gustave Roussy, PRII, 39, rue Camille Desmoulins, 94805 Villejuif Cedex, France; [3] CNRS UA041149, Unité de Génétique du Développement, Département de Biologie Moléculaire, Institut Pasteur, 25, rue du Docteur Roux, 75724 Paris Cedex, France

SUMMARY
A recombinant adenovirus was constructed to target gene expression in muscle cells. Using β-galactosidase as a reporter gene, we were able to detect its expression in myotubes after infection of established cell lines and muscles of newborn mice.

INTRODUCTION
Adenovirus has been shown to be a candidate vector for gene therapy (1,2). We are investigating its potential for muscle diseases. Its advantages include a large host range (and thus the possibility to use the animal models available for Duchenne Muscular Dystrophy), the capacity of the vector for foreign DNA (at present 7 kbp, but in principle >30 kbp, thus compatible with the size of the dystrophin coding sequences), and a low pathogenicity in man.

METHODS
The recombinant virus was obtained as shown in Fig.1, and assayed on myogenic cell lines from mouse (C2.7) and rat (L6).
Newborn mice were infected by the intramuscular route; muscles were embedded in paraffin and sectioned after β-galactosidase detection (3).

RESULTS AND DISCUSSION
We have constructed a recombinant adenovirus where β-galactosidase is under the control of a mouse skeletal α-actin promoter reinforced by an enhancer from a mouse myosin light chain gene (MLC1-3F).
β-galactosidase expression was detected in infected myogenic cells and in mice muscle (Fig.2), but not in NIH3T3 fibroblasts. An expression was obtained even when fused myoblasts cultures were infected, suggesting that myotubes themselves can be infected.
The regulatory sequences we used should be suitable to direct muscle specific expression of a "minidystrophin" resembling that described in a family with mild Becker Muscular Dystrophy (4).

REFERENCES
1. Chasse J.F., et al.,(1989), Medecine/Sciences, $\underline{5}$, 331-337.
2. Stratford-Perricaudet L.D., et al., (1990), Human Gene Therapy, $\underline{1}$, 241-256.
3. England S.B., et al., (1990), Nature, $\underline{343}$, 180-182.
4. Sanes J.R., Rubenstein J.L.R., and Nicolas J.F., (1986), EMBO J., $\underline{5}$, 3133-3142.

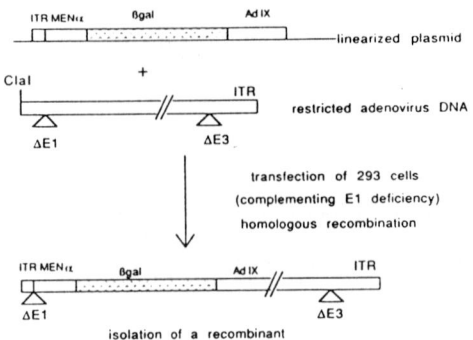

Fig.1: Obtention of a recombinant adenovirus.
  MEN : enhancer of the mouse MLC1-3F gene
  α   : mouse skeletal α-actin promoter
  βgal: β-galactosidase gene of *E.coli*
  AdlX: sequences coding for peptide IX of adenovirus, with 3' flanking region
  ITR : inverted terminal repeat.

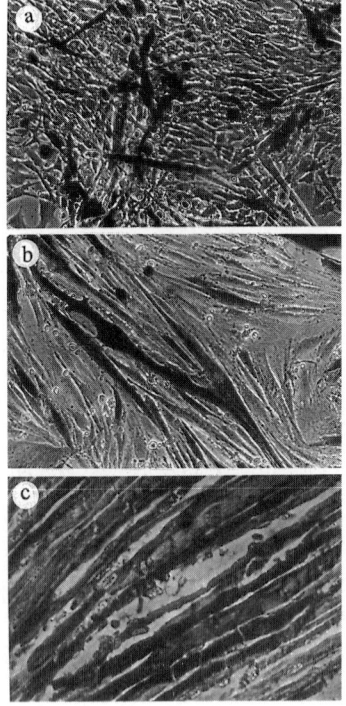

Fig.2: Expression of β-galactosidase following infection of:
  a. C2.7 myotubes (24h infection)
  b. L6 myotubes   (24h infection)
  c. newborn mice (12 days infection)

RESUME
Nous avons utilisé l'adenovirus comme vecteur d'expression dans les cellules musculaires. En utilisant le gène β-galactosidase comme "reporter", nous avons obtenu une expression après infection de myotubes de lignées myogéniques et de muscles de souris.

Highly efficient retroviral vectors derived from Harvey and Friend murine viruses

Thierry J. Velu [1, 3*], Ricardo A. Feldman [1, 4], Eva M. Valverius [2, 5], Pierre E. Tambourin [1, 6] and Douglas R. Lowy [1]

[1] *Laboratory of Cellular Oncology, and* [2] *of Tumor Immunology and Biology, NIH, Bethesda, USA;* [3] *Department of Medical Genetics, Hôpital Erasme, Bâtiment C, Route de Lennik 808, 1070 Brussels, Belgium;* [4] *Department of Microbiology and Immunology, University of Maryland, Baltimore, USA;* [5] *Department of Pathology, Academic Hospital, Uppsala, Sweden;* [6] *Institut Curie, Paris, France*

* Author for correspondence

SUMMARY: We have developed a highly efficient retroviral vector by cloning the full-length Harvey murine sarcoma virus (Ha-MuSV) genome in pBR322, and have identified a segment with enhancer activity outside the LTRs. High expression of a gene inserted in this vector was stable, even in human cells. By replacing the U3 region of both LTRs from this Ha-MuSV vector with the homologous region of the Friend murine leukemia virus, we generated an even more efficient retroviral vector which resulted in 3- to 10-times higher levels of gene expression and in a virus whose titer was up to 2 orders of magnitude greater. Compared with the Ha-MuSV derived virus, this potent virus should mediate gene expression in more differentiated primary hematopoietic cells and might therefore be useful in the design of gene therapy experiments.

The Harvey murine sarcoma virus (Ha-MuSV) was isolated following multiple passages of Moloney murine sarcoma virus (Mo-MuLV) in rats. Ha-MuSV contains a *ras* oncogene activated by two missense mutations. It is flanked by about 3.5 kb of rat-derived retroviruslike sequences called VL30 (VL: "viruslike") or 30S DRV (DRV: "defective retrovirus") because they migrate as 30S RNA. 1.5 kb of Mo-MuLV derived sequences form the viral long terminal repeats (LTR) as well as sequences just upstream from the LTR. By cloning in pBR322 the full-length Ha-MuSV genome, with one LTR at both 5' and 3' ends as found in its provirus form, we generated a highly efficient retroviral vector (pCO20-A) (Velu et al., 1989). Superinfection of mouse fibroblastic NIH 3T3 cells transformed by pCO20-A with a helper virus (amphotropic MuLV or Mo-MuLV) yielded a very high titer virus: 10^8 ffu [focus forming units] per ml. 5' noncoding rat c-*ras*H sequences were found to increase even higher the titer when substituted for the corresponding segment of v-*ras*H (10^9 ffu/ml). Very high titers were also obtained when various cDNA (c-*erb*B, v-*fes*/*fps*, cDNA coding for TGFa) were placed in pCO20-A from which the viral oncogene v-*ras*H has been deleted (10^7 ffu/ml) (Velu et al., 1987; Feldman et al., 1989). The high titers obtained with this Ha-MuSV based retroviral vector was at least partially related to the presence of a VL30-derived segment with enhancer activity. This segment is located outside the LTRs and downstream from v-*ras*H. Its deletion resulted in a decrease of the titer by about 2 orders of magnitude.

High expression of gene inserted in this Harvey vector was stable, even in human cells. The human c-*erb*B proto-oncogene [encoding the epidermal growth factor receptor (EGFR)] inserted in that vector was studied in the human breast cancer ZR 75-1 cell line: cells containing the EGFR vector expressed up to 10^6 EGFR, while control cells expressed 2×10^4 EGFR. Binding experiments demonstrated that EGFR overexpression, although apparently not confering any growth advantage, was phenotypically stable for at least 5 months in continuous culture.

Since successful gene therapy may require that the transferred gene be stably expressed in the differentiated progeny of multipotential hematopoietic progenitors and since the Friend-MuLV (Fr-MuLV) enhancer is more potent and more effective than the Mo-MuLV enhancer in mediating gene expression in more differentiated primary hematopoietic cells (Holland et al., 1987), we replace the U3 region of both LTRs from Ha-MuSV vector with the homologous region of the Fr-MuLV [the U3 region contains the enhancer, transcriptional promoter, and disease specificity sequences (Li et al., 1987)]. To have a suitable group of cells from which a high titer virus might be obtained, we cotransfected this "Friend" vector in NIH 3T3 cells with an antibiotic resistance gene (neoR) as a selectable marker to derive individual colonies of cells. Compared with the Ha-MuSV based vector, this Friend vector

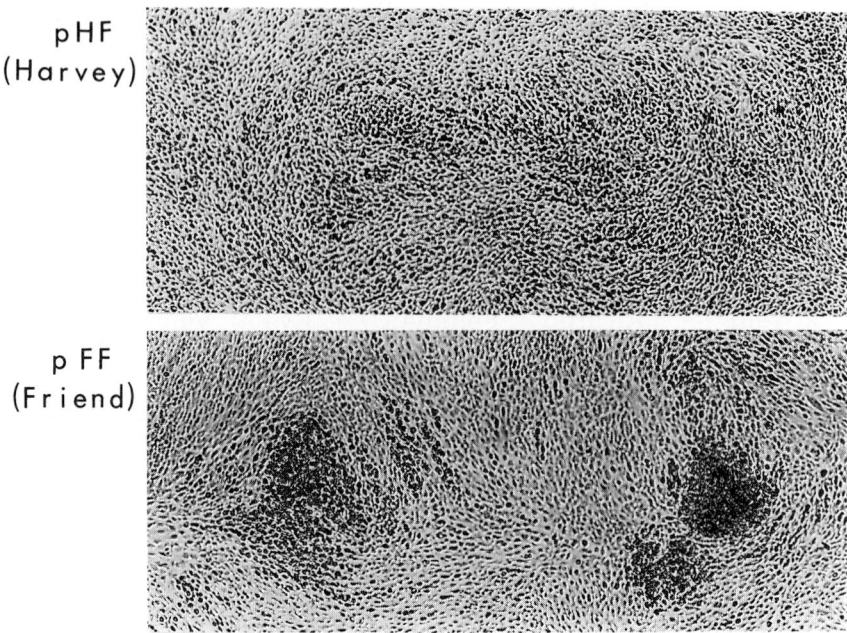

Fig. 1. Foci of morphologically transformed NIH 3T3 cells after transfection with the c-fes/fps proto-oncogene inserted in either the "Harvey" vector (pHF) or the "Friend" vector (pFF). These DNAs were cotransfected with pSV2neo into NIH 3T3 cells and transfectants were selected for G418 resistance. Mass cultures of pFF transfectants expressed 10-times-higher levels of NCP92 (encoded by c-fes/fps) than did mass cultures of pHF transfectants. pFF transfectants exhibited foci of transformed cells within 2 to 3 weeks of transfection. In the case of pHF transfectants, foci were also observed, but they took longer to appear and were weaker and less numerous.

resulted in 3- to 10-times-higher levels of gene expression and in a virus whose titer was 2 orders of magnitude greater (Fig. 1).

These data suggest that Harvey- and Friend-viruses based retroviral vectors are highly efficient and might be useful in the design of gene therapy experiments.

REFERENCES

Feldman, R.A., Lowy, D.R., Vass, W.C., Velu, T.J. (1989): A highly efficient retroviral vector allows detection of the transforming activity of the human c-fps/fes proto-oncogene. *J. Virol.* 63: 5469-5474.

Holland, A., Anklesaria, P., Sakakeeny, M.A., Greenberger, S. (1987): Enhancer sequences of a retroviral vector determine expression of a gene in multipotent hematopoietic progenitors and commited erythroid cells. *Proc. Natl. Acad. Sci. U.S.A.* 84, 8662-8666.

Li, Y., Golemis, E., Hartley, J.W., Hopkins, N. (1987): Disease specificity of nondefective Friend and Moloney murine leukemia viruses is controlled by a small number of nucleotides. *J. Virol.* 61: 693-700.

Velu, T.J., Beguinot, L., Vass, W.C., Willingham, M.C., Merlino, G.T., Pastan, I., Lowy, D.R. (1987): Epidermal growth factor-dependent transformation by a human EGF receptor proto-oncogene. *Science* 238: 1408-1410.

Velu, T.J., Vass, W.C., Lowy, D.R., Tambourin, P.E. (1989): Harvey murine sarcoma virus: influences of coding and noncoding sequences on cell transformation in vitro and oncogenicity in vivo. *J. Virol.* 63: 1384-1392.

RESUME: Nous avons construit un vecteur rétroviral très efficient en clonant l'intégralité du génome du virus du sarcome murin de Harvey (Ha-MuSV), dans pBR322, et avons identifié une séquence possédant une activité "enhancer" en dehors des LTRs. L'expression élevée d'un gène inséré dans ce vecteur fut stable, même dans des cellules humaines. En remplaçant la région U3 des deux LTRs de ce vecteur Ha-MuSV par la région homologue du virus de la leucémie murine de Friend, nous avons généré un vecteur rétroviral encore plus efficient, qui résulte en des niveaux d'expression 3 à 10 fois plus élevés et en un virus dont le titre est jusque 2 ordres de grandeur plus élevé. Par rapport au virus dérivé de Ha-MuSV, ce virus puissant devrait permettre d'induire l'expression de gène dans des cellules hématopoïétiques primaires plus différenciées et pourrait servir de base dans le développement de certaines thérapies géniques.

Gene transfer into birds using ALV-based retrovirus vectors

F.L. Cosset, J.L. Thomas, M. Afanassieff, C. Legras, R.M. Molina, C. Faure, Y. Chebloune, A. Drynda, C. Ronfort, S. Valsésia, V.M. Nigon and G. Verdier

Laboratoire de Biologie Cellulaire, INRA, CNRS UMR 106, Université Claude Bernard Lyon-I, 43, boulevard du 11 Novembre 1918, 69622 Villeurbanne Cedex, France

The difficult access to fowl oocyte nucleus leads to consider retrovirus vectors as appropriate vehicles for gene transfer into avian germinal cells. Although replication-competent vectors have been tested with success, they are endowed with major drawbacks related in particular to their replicative potencies. Such problems can be avoided by using defective retrovirus vectors. We report here our approach to generate and to improve retrovirus vectors derived from the genome of Avian Leukosis Viruses (ALV), and preliminary studies of expression following their inoculation into chick embryos.

I-RETROVIRUS VECTORS AND PACKAGING CELL LINES

Vectors. Starting with the genome of the oncogenic retrovirus AEV (Avian Erythroblastosis Virus) [1], we have constructed a set of double expression (DE) vectors carrying and expressing two genes under control of the cis-acting sequences contained in the AEV LTR; one of the gene being represented by the neo selectable gene, and the other one being the gene of interest [2,3]. These DE vectors have been recently improved by exchanging the most part of cis-acting sequences of AEV by the ones from other ALVs (fig 1). We have shown (Table 1) that we could obtain a gain of one log of virus production (more than 10^6 helper-free particles/ml in the supernatants of some clonal producer cell lines) when the cis-acting sequences were originated from Rous Associated Viruses type 1 or 2 (RAV-1 or 2) compared to vectors bearing sequences from AEV [2]. Moreover, these new types of vectors could be characterized by an increased expression and stability of the reporter gene (i. e. lacZ gene) in the QT6 avian cell line commonly used as target cells for in vitro studies [2,3].

Helper cells. We have constructed plasmids expressing the retroviral structural genes gag-pol and env. These packaging vectors derived from the genome of RAV-1, from which both the packaging sequence located into the leader region and the 3' terminal regions (3' non coding region and LTR) had been deleted, this latter being replaced by an heterologous polyadenylation sequence. These plasmids allowed us to generate helper cell lines from which AEV-based vectors could be produced at titers of about 10^4 RFU/ml [4]. As an improvment of these cell lines, we have generated a second set of helper plasmids in which the viral coding sequences were expressed from two different plasmids and were linked to selectable markers which were expressed from the same transcriptional unit (either gag-pol/hygro or phleo/env) [5]. Compared to previous packaging cell [4], we have shown that helper cell lines generated with these two complementary plasmids could be characterized by an enhancement in vector titers [5], and by an increased stability of both expression of helper functions and of vector production (Table 1), [2]. No replication competent viruses could be detected in the supernatants of all of our helper cell lines, even if grown during continuous long-term culture.

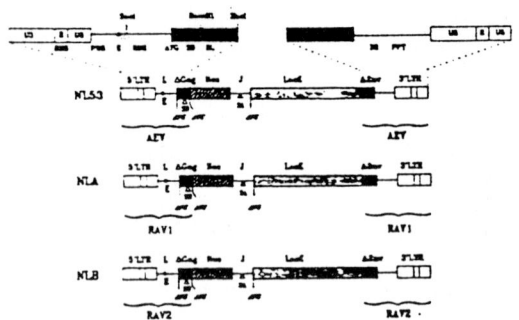

Fig. 1. Structure of NL retrovirus vectors. RBS, ribosome binding site; PBS, primer binding site; E, encapsidation sequence; ATG, gag gene initiator codon; SD & SA, splice donor & acceptor sequences; DL, dimer linkage sequence; DR, direct repeat sequence; PPT, polypurine track; LTR, long terminal repeat; L, leader region; J, junction fragment.

TABLE 1. Titers obtained with NL retrovirus vectors transfected into Isolde packaging cell line

Vector[a]	Neo (RFFU/ml[b])	Titers lacZ (CFU/ml[c])			
		Initial	1 mo	4 mo	5 mo
NL53	2×10^4	3×10^4	2×10^4	1.5×10^4	1×10^4
NLA	2×10^5	2×10^5	2×10^5	1.4×10^5	1×10^5
NLB	2×10^5	3×10^5	1×10^5	2×10^5	2×10^5

[a] Vector structures are depicted in Fig. 1. NL vectors were introduced into Isolde packaging cells by lipofection according to the standard procedure recommended by the supplier (Lipofectin, Gibco-BRL);
[b] RFFU are per milliliter of supernatant collected from pools of stable producer Neo+ clones of Isolde cells;
[c] Viral supernatants were harvested after different growth periods (up to 5 months) of NL vector producer cells. ND, not determined. Fewer than 1 helper virus was detected at each titration per 5 ml of viral supernatants, as previously described.

II-IN VIVO GENE TRANSFER

Viral supernatants of three neo-lacZ vectors (NLA, NLB, and NL53, Fig. 1) were collected and were concentrated 50-100 times by ultracentrifugation. These viral stocks were inoculated to early chick embryos (before incubation) by injection with a capillary glass pipette into the germinal cavity through the blastodisc at its periphery. About 10^5 lacZ-CFU were inoculated per embryos, thus giving a multiplicity of infection of about 2 infectious NL virus per embryo cell. Injected eggs were incubated, and embryos were recovered at different stages of development: 18 h, 72 h, or 5-6 days of incubation. Some embryos were analysed by Southern blot to detect the exogenous lacZ gene, and other embryos were fixed and stained with X-GAL to study the in situ expression of the NL vectors.

Compared to the number of infectious NL particles injected into the embryos, the number of expression foci was very low since no more than about 30 lacZ positive foci could be observed in embryos stained at stage 18 h. By comparison, we have found that NL proviruses could be detected by Southern blots in the DNA of marked embryos, since NL proviruses could be detected above the limit of detection (1/75 cell) for 30% of the embryos; one strongly positive embryo displaying NL proviruses in about 5% of its cells. Hence, only a small proportion of proviruses could give rise to lacZ expression (no more than 0.6 %, [Thomas et al., in preparation]).

From observations of either whole-mounts or serially sectioned X-GAL stained embryos, we have localized precisely the sites of expression of the helper-free vectors. No evidences for tissue-restriction were observed (Fig. 2). However, slight differences of behaviour between the 3 NL vectors were found regarding the staining of specific organs like the heart and the neural tube. Compared to the vector NLB (in which the regulating sequences originated from RAV-2), the NLA vector (carrying cis-acting sequences from RAV-1) was more often expressed in the heart (3 times) and less often in the neural tube (2 times). The vector NL53 in which the cis-acting sequences originated from AEV did not display such a preferential tropism of expression. Since variabilities can be found between the sequences of enhancer parts of the U3 regions of these different LTRs, our results suggest that the discrepancies observed between the vectors might be related to specific cellular factors interacting with the LTRs, thus regulating their activities in specific embryo cell types.

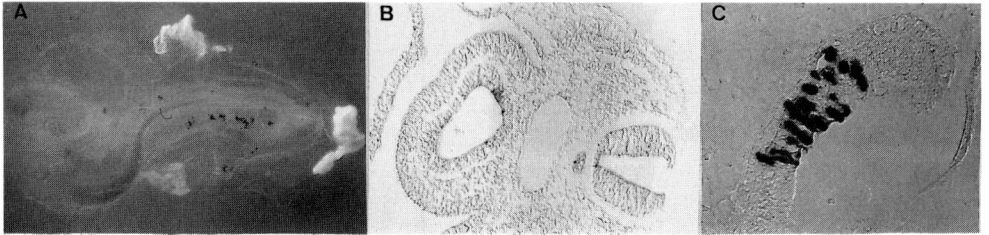

Fig. 2. X-GAL stainings of NL infected chick embryos.
NLB-infected embryos, stained at 72 h (A, B) or at 5 days (C), and observed either as whole-mount (A), or after serial sections in the region of the trunck (B) or in the eye (C).

III-CONCLUSIONS AND PROSPECTS

These preliminary results demonstrate that ALV-based vectors can be usefull tools for gene transfer into birds. We are currently working on two major fields of interest: germinal transgenesis and use of our vectors as vaccine vectors [Chebloune et al., Cosset et al., in preparation].

Experiments are in progress to improve both retrovirus vectors and packaging cell lines. We are trying to construct vectors with internal promoters able to integrate into target cell DNA as a disorganized proviral structure because of the presence of an internal retroviral attachment sequence within the vector. Such integrations would result in a specific expression of the internal promoter, and in the inability to obtain further virus production [Drynda et al., in preparation].

To develop packaging cell lines, we are constructing helper cells able to produce retroviral vectors pseudotyped by different retroviruses envelopes. We are also trying to modify envelopes proteins in order to increase the affinity of attachment between the virion and its receptor.

[1] BENCHAIDI M., MALLET F, THORAVAL P., SAVATIER P., XIAO J. H., VERDIER G., SAMARUT J. and NIGON V. M. 1989. Virology 169:15-26.
[2] COSSET F. L., LEGRAS C., THOMAS J. L., MOLINA R. M., CHEBLOUNE Y., FAURE C., NIGON V. M. and VERDIER G. 1991. J. Virol. In press.
[3] LEGRAS C., COSSET F. L., CHEBLOUNE Y., MOLINA R. M., THOMAS J. L., FAURE C., NIGON V. M. and VERDIER G. 1991 Submitted to J. Virol.
[4] SAVATIER P., BAGNIS C., THORAVAL P., PONCET D., BELALEBI M., MALLET F., LEGRAS C., COSSET F. L. THOMAS J. L., CHEBLOUNE Y., FAURE C., VERDIER G., SAMARUT J. and NIGON V. M. 1989. J. Virol. 63:513-522.
[5] COSSET F. L., LEGRAS C., CHEBLOUNE Y., SAVATIER P., THORAVAL P., THOMAS J. L. SAMARUT J., NIGON V.M. and VERDIER G. 1990. J. Virol. 64:1070-1078.

RESUME : Les difficultés d'accès au noyau d'oocytes de volaille nous ont conduit à envisager les vecteurs rétroviraux pour transférer des gènes dans les cellules germinales aviaires. Bien que des vecteurs compétents pour la réplication aient été testés avec succès, leur utilisation est nuancée par des inconvénients majeurs et, en particulier, leur potentiel de réplication. De tels problèmes peuvent être contournés par l'utilisation de vecteurs rétroviraux défectifs. Nous présentons ici une autre approche qui consiste à générer et à améliorer les vecteurs rétroviraux dérivés du génome de virus de la leucose aviaire (ALV), ainsi que l'analyse préliminaire de l'expression consécutive à leur inoculation dans les embryons de poulet.

Fatal polycythemia induced in mice by dysregulated erythropoietin (Epo) production by hemopoietic cells

Jean-Luc Villeval [1], Donald Metcalf [2] and Gregory R. Johnson [2]

[1] *INSERM U 91, Hôpital Henri Mondor, 94010 Créteil, France;* [2] *Cancer Research Unit, the Walter and Eliza Hall Institute, PO Royal Melbourne Hospital, 3050 Victoria, Australia*

Murine bone marrow cells from C57BL/6 mice were infected with a retroviral vector (MP Zen) carrying a monkey Epo cDNA (Fig. 1). Cells were transplanted into lethally-irradiated recipients to study the effect of Epo production by hemopoietic cells.

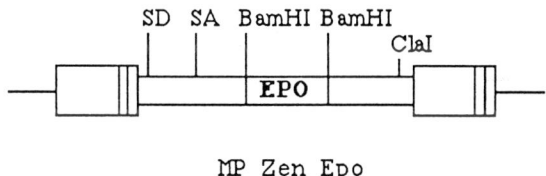

Fig. 1. Structure of the MP Zen Epo retrovirus. The vector MP Zen has been previously described (Johnson et al., 1989). SD and SA indicate the position of splicing donor and acceptor site. The Epo cDNA (~ 600 bp) was ligated into the BamH1 polylinker site of the vector.

High levels of Epo were recorded in the plasma (median value: 1.2 units/ml) and in media conditioned by peritoneal, spleen and bone marrow cells from recipient mice. The hematocrit was elevated (90±5%) (Fig. 2A) and the mice died at a mean of 71 days after transplantation (Fig. 2B). In the blood, platelet counts were usually low and nucleated blood cells slightly elevated. Spleen weight increased 5-fold and bone marrow cellularity decreased slightly. There was a 10-fold increase in erythroblast numbers, a 2-fold reduction of lymphocytes and no variation of the myeloid cells when the total cellularity of bone marrow, spleen, peripheral blood and peritoneal cells were considered.

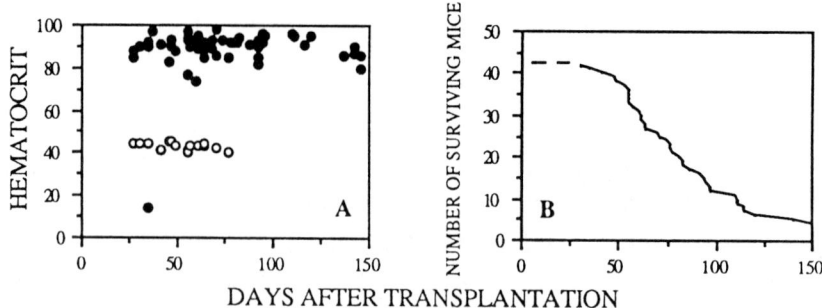

Fig. 2. Hematocrit levels (**A**) in mice transplanted with MP Zen Epo (closed circle) or the control, MP Zen Neo, (open circle) virus-infected bone marrow cells and survival curve (**B**) for mice transplanted with MP Zen Epo virus infected bone marrow cells (no deaths occurred in control transplanted mice during this period of the survey). The lowest hematocrit was observed in a case of hemorrhage.

Calculation of the total numbers of progenitor cells in these organs revealed an 18-fold increase in CFU-E but no significant variation of the BFU-E and myeloid progenitor cell numbers. A variable proportion of CFU-E, (12% or 24% in bone marrow or spleen, respectively) was able to proliferate in unstimulated cultures. Erythropoietic amplification occurred in the spleen and there was a redistribution of the BFU-E and myeloid cells from the bone marrow to the spleen. No significant extramedullary erythropoiesis was seen. The blood vessels were enlarged.

In conclusion, this study emphasizes the erythroid specificity of Epo and shows that elevated dysregulated Epo production by hemopoietic cells leads to a fatal polycythemia. We showed recently (Mitjavila et al., in press) that some primary human erythroleukemic cells transcribe the Epo gene, suggesting that activation of this gene in erythroid cells may be implicated in an autocrine process of transformation. No leukemia or disturbance of the erythroid differentiation was observed in the mice studied. This suggests that perturbed Epo production alone is insufficient to induce erythroleukemia and that other molecular events are required. Finally, in contrast to recent data (Hoatlin et al., 1990), we did not observe an attenuated erythroproliferative disease in our C57 BL/6 Fv-2r mice.

REFERENCES

Hoatlin M.E., Kozac S.L., Lilly F., Chakraborti A., Kozac C.A., Kabat D. (1990): Activation of erythropoietin receptors by Friend viral gp55 and by erythropoietin and down-modulation by the murine Fv-2r resistance gene. *Proc. Natl. Acad. Sci. USA* 87, 9985-9989.

Johnson G.R., Gonda T.L., Metcalf D., Hariharan I.K., Cory S. (1989): A lethal myeloproliferative syndrome in mice transplanted with bone marrow cells infected with a retrovirus expressing granulocyte-macrophage colony stimulating factor. *EMBO J.* 8, 441-448.

Mitjavila M.T., Le Couedic J.-P., Casadevall N., Navarro S., Villeval J.-L., Dubart A., Vainchenker W.: Autocrine stimulation by erythropoietin and autonomous growth of human erythroid leukemic cells in vitro. *J. Clin. Invest.*(in press).

RESUME : Des cellules de moelle osseuse dérivées de la souris C57BL/6 ont été infectées avec un vecteur rétroviral (MPZen) contenant un ADN complémentaire d'érythropoïétine de singe. Les cellules ont été transplantées sur des receveurs léthalement irradiés afin d'étudier les effets de la production d'érythropoïétine par les cellules hématopoïétiques. Cette étude vérifie la spécificité érythroide de l'érythropoïétine et démontre que la production dérégulée de celle-ci à un niveau élevé par les cellules hématopoïétiques conduit à une polyglobulie fatale. Aucune anomalie de la différenciation érythroide et aucune apparition de leucémie n'ont été observées chez les souris étudiées.

Gene transfer of adenosine deaminase into primitive human hematopoietic progenitor cells

Denis Cournoyer [1, 3*], Maurizio Scarpa [1, 4], Kohnosuke Mitani [2], Kateri A. Moore [1], John W. Belmont [1, 2] and C. Thomas Caskey [1, 2]

(1) Institute for Molecular Genetics and (2) Howard Hughes Medical Institute, Baylor College of Medicine, Houston, Texas, USA; (3) Montreal General Hospital, Division of Hematology and Centre for Host Resistance, 1650 Cedar Avenue, Room 7129, Montreal, Quebec H3G 1A4, Canada; (4) Department of Pediatrics, University of Padova, Padova, Italy

* Author for correspondence

Abstract. We have used a combination of recombinant human interleukins (IL) 3 and 6 to stimulate the proliferation of primitive human hematopoietic progenitor cells during a period of co-cultivation with irradiated cells producing an ADA-transducing retroviral vector packaged in amphotropic particles. In a series of nine experiments, 73 to 78 % of the clonogenic progenitors (CFU-E and CFU-GM) were found to have acquired the transferred sequence as determined by polymerase chain reaction analysis. In addition, 24 to 44 % of the clonogenic progenitors derived from long-term myeloid cultures nine weeks post-infection were found to contain vector sequence. Moreover, the transduced ADA enzyme was found to be expressed in both normal and ADA deficient erythroid colonies, and in the non-adherent cells of long-term bone marrow culture for at least two weeks at levels which approximate to the endogenous ADA levels of normal erythroid cells. These results indicate that the ADA coding sequence can efficiently be introduced by retroviral gene transfer into both committed and primitive human hematopoietic progenitor cells, and that this will result in adequate expression of the transduced enzyme in the progeny of committed hematopoietic progenitors.

We are using retroviral vectors to develop a gene transfer system applicable to human gene therapy by means of the modification of hematopoietic stem cells (HSC). The model disease that we have selected is the inherited deficiency of adenosine deaminase (ADA). This defect is responsible for 15% of all cases of Severe Combined Immunodeficiency (SCID) and has been widely investigated as a model disorder to develop human somatic gene therapy.

Gene transfer into clonogenic human hematopoietic progenitor cells. Light density mononuclear bone marrow cells (BMC) ($d \leq 1.077$) were cocultivated for 48 to 60 hours with GP+envAm-12 amphotropic packaging cells (Markowitz et al., 1988) producing the vector ΔN2stADA at 10^6 viral particles/ml (Scarpa et al., 1991) in presence of recombinant human IL 3 10 U/ml and IL-6 200 U/ml. These growth factors were selected for their known synergistic effect on the proliferation of primitive human hematopoietic progenitors. Following cocultivation, a fraction of the cells were grown in methylcellulose for colony-assay (Fauser et al., 1979). The presence of vector sequence in individual colonies was detected by polymerase chain reaction. In a series of nine experiments, the overall infection efficiency of human clonogenic hematopoietic progenitor cells varied between 45 to 100% (mean 73%) in erythroid progenitors (CFU-E) and 40-100% (mean 78%) in granulocyte/macrophage progenitors (CFU-GM).

Gene transfer into hematopoietic progenitors derived from long-term culture (LTC). We have used the myeloid LTC system (Dexter et al., 1984) to evaluate the efficiency of gene transfer into more primitive cells. The clonogenic cells grown from human LTC after five weeks appear to be derived from more primitive hematopoietic progenitors which were not in themselves clonogenic at the time of initiation of the culture (Sutherland et al., 1989). In two cases where hematopoietic progenitors could be maintained for more than five weeks in LTC, efficient gene transfer (24 and 44% respectively) could be demonstrated into progenitor cells that gave rise to CFU-GM nine weeks after cocultivation.

Expression of the transduced ADA. A microradioassay (Aitken et al., 1980) was used to measure the ADA activity in pools of CFU-E submitted or not to retroviral gene transfer. The ADA activity was normalized to the activity of an independent enzyme of purine metabolism, purine nucleoside phosphorylase. There was an increase of 1.7- to 1.8-fold in the normalized ADA activity of normal cells following gene transfer, and a 22.5- to 27-fold increase in the ADA deficient cells. Moreover, the ADA activity of erythroid cells derived from the deficient marrow following infection was in the same range as those derived from normal cells. Increase in ADA activity was also detectable in the non-adherent cells of LTC for two weeks following infection of BMC from ADA deficient patients with virus-containing supernatant.

Conclusion. Although a clinical trial of gene therapy for ADA deficiency involving retrovirus-mediated gene transfer into peripheral blood T-cells has been initiated, the optimal target for gene therapy in this and many other disorders affecting the hematopoietic system remains, in our opinion, the primitive lympho-hematopoietic stem cell with long term repopulating ability. Several groups, including ours, have developed efficient and safe retrovirus-mediated gene transfer systems with which to introduce vector-encoded human ADA into mouse hematopoietic stem cells. We have also obtained preliminary evidence that similar results can be reproduced in the human system. The results obtained to date support the feasibility of somatic gene therapy of ADA deficiency *via* the introduction of a retroviral vector into human HSC.

Acknowledgements. This work has been supported by U.S.P.H.S. grants P01 HD21452 (C.T.C.) and R29 HD22880 (J.W.B.), Cystic Fibrosis Foundation grant MR004-9 (J.W.B.) and the Howard Hughes Medical Institute (C.T.C. and J.W.B.). D.C. was the recipient of a senior fellowship from the National Cancer Institute of Canada. M.S. was the recipient of a Cystic Fibrosis Foundation Post-doctoral Fellowship F054-9. K.A.M. is the recipient of U.S.P.H.S. Individual National Research Service Award F32 RR05034.

References

Aitken, D. A. *et al.* (1980). Prenatal detection of a probable heterozygote for ADA deficiency and severe combined immunodeficiency disease using a microradioassay. *Clin. Genet.* 17, 293-298.
Belmont, J. W. *et al.* (1988). Expression of human adenosine deaminase in murine hematopoietic cells. *Mol. Cell. Biol.* 8, 5116-5125.
Dexter, T. M. *et al.* (1984). Long-term marrow culture: an overview of technique and experience. In *Long-term bone marrow culture*, eds. D. G. Wright and J. S. Greenberger, pp. 57-96. New York: Alan R. Liss Inc.
Fauser, A. A. and Messner, H. A. (1979). Identification of megakaryocytes, macrophages, and eosinophils in colonies of human bone marrow containing neutrophilic granulocytes and erythroblasts. *Blood* 53, 1023-1027.
Markowitz, D. *et al.* (1988). Construction and use of a safe and efficient amphotropic packaging cell line. *Virology* 167, 400-406.
Scarpa, M. *et al.* (1991). Characterization of recombinant helper retroviruses from Moloney-based vectors in ecotropic and amphotropic packaging cell lines. *Virology* 180, 849-852.
Sutherland, H. J. *et al.* (1989). Characterization and partial purification of human marrow cells capable of initiating long-term hemopoiesis in vitro. *Blood* 74, 1563-1570.

Résumé. La déficience en "adenosine deaminase" (ADA) résulte en immunodéficience combinée sévère et nous sert de modèle pour développer un système de thérapie génique *via* la modification de cellules souches hématopoïétiques. Nous démontrons ici qu'une combinaison d'interleukines 3 et 6 permet d'obtenir une haute efficacité de transfer du gène de l'ADA par rétrovirus dans les cellules qui forment des colonies hématopoïétiques (73 à 78 %), ainsi que dans les cellules qui initient la culture à long terme. Le gène transféré paraît aussi être exprimé adéquatement. Ces résultats constituent d'importantes données préliminaires au développement de la thérapie génique *via* les cellules souches hématopoïétiques.

Transfer and selective expression of interleukin genes in neoplasic cells by means of recombinant parvoviruses

Annick Brandenburger [1]*, Stephen J. Russel [2,3], Mary K.L. Collins [3], Jean Rommelaere [1,4]

(1) Université Libre de Bruxelles, Département de Biologie Moléculaire, Laboratoire de Biophysique et Radiobiologie, rue des Chevaux 67, B1640, Rhode Saint-Genèse, Belgium; (2) MRC Centre Cambridge, Cambridge Centre for Protein Engineering, Cambridge, UK; (3) The Institute of Cancer Research, Chester Beatty Laboratories, Cambridge, UK; (4) INSERM U 186, Oncologie Moléculaire, Institut Pasteur de Lille, 1, rue Calmette, 59000 Lille, France

* Author for correspondence

Summary. We could show that the autonomous parvovirus MVM is a very efficient expression vector in transformed eucaryotic cells. The fact that this expression is dependent on the transformed phenotype of recipient cells makes parvoviruses a tool of choice for cell targeted gene therapy of cancer. We have cloned the human IL2 gene into the parvovirus capsid-coding region. Recombinant MVM-IL2 viruses were obtained in the presence of a helper and used to transfer the IL2 gene to cells in culture.

Autonomous parvoviruses have a number of properties that render them particularly interesting for the construction of eucaryotic expression vectors. Most of these viruses provoke an asymptomatic infection in adults. In vitro they infect a large variety of animal (including human) cell types, although parvoviral proteins are preferentially expressed in transformed cells. Non-transformed cells usually resist their lytic action. The genetic organization of parvoviruses is well understood (Berns, 1990). The genome of the prototype strain of Minute Virus of Mice (MVM(p)) has been entirely cloned into pBR322 to give plasmid pMM984 (Merchellinsky et al. 1983). When transfected into permissive cells, this plasmid generates free, infectious virus. MVM DNA contains 2 promoters, P4 and P38, that control the expression of 2 groups of overlapping genes coding for non-structural (NS) and capsid (VP) proteins, respectively. NS-1 is involved in the replication and the toxicity of MVM(p) and transactivates the P38 promoter (Rhode, 1985).
We would like to use the oncotropic properties of parvoviruses to obtain targeted expression of interleukin genes in tumor cells and, in this way, to localy stimulate antitumor immune responses mediated by specific lymphocytes and non-specific lymphokine- activated killer cells (LAK)(Russell, 1990). Therefore, we have replaced part of the capsid protein coding genes of MVM(p) by cDNAs coding for human IL2 or murine IL4, thereby placing the interleukin gene under the control of the P38 promoter.
pMVM-IL2 was either transfected alone or cotransfected with a "helper plasmid" into permissive cells to check (1) the expression of the IL2 gene, (2) the excision of MVM-IL DNA and its replication, (3) the encapsidation of MVM-IL DNA into recombinant virions. Helper plasmids were either intact pMM984 (w.t. MVM) or the replication defective mutant pULB3235 (rep-), both of which can provide capsid proteins in trans.
Expression of the IL2 gene in transformed cells. IL2 production was measured in supernatants from human SV40-transformed NB-K fibroblasts, 3 days after transfection with pMVM-IL2 (Tab. 1). Supernatants from cells co-transfected with wt or rep-MVM contained infectious MVM-IL2 recombinant virions (see below) and were used to infect two pairs of normal and transformed fibroblasts : (i) the human MRC-5 cell strain and its SV40 transformed MRC-V1 derivative (Huschtscha and Holliday, 1983), (ii) the rat FR3T3 cell line and its ras-transformed FREJ4 counterpart (van Hille et al., 1989). Significant IL2 production was only observed in the transformed line of each pair (Tab. 2), confirming the transformation-dependent expression of MVM.

Tab. 1 - IL2 secretion and release of wild type MVM(p) during serial passage of MVM-IL2 virus stocks. IL2 activity was measured in the CTLL-bioassay and is expressed as U/ml. Figures in brackets represent infective centres of wt MVM/ml.

	Imput plasmids					
	pMVM-IL2 pMM984		pMVM-IL2 pULB3235		pMVM-IL2	
Transfected NB-K	122	(2.5×10^4)	108	(5)	50	(0)
1st infection	85	(1.3×10^6)	83	(7)	0	(0)
2nd infection	126	(1.3×10^6)	0	(1.6×10^3)	0	
3rd infection	35	(5.0×10^5)	0	(6.0×10^6)	0	
4th infection	0.2	(3.0×10^4)	0	(1.6×10^6)	0	
5th infection	0	(5.5×10^4)	0	(1.3×10^6)	0	

Tab.2 - Transformation-dependent induction of IL2 secretion by MVM-IL2 vector (IL2 U/ml).

Helper plasmid	Cells			
	MRC-5	MRC-5V1	FR3T3	FREJ4
pMM984	0.29	210	<0.1	19
pULB3235	0.11	170	<0.1	21

Excision and replication of MVM-IL2 DNA. Both helper (w.t.) and recombinant parvoviral genomes are excised from their respective plasmids and replicate autonomously. Indeed, Hirt's extracts of transfected NB-K cells contained MVM 5 (kb) and MVM-IL2 (4 kb) DNA replicative forms, as shown by Southern blotting with probes specific for the helper (part of the VP gene) or recombinant (IL2 gene) virus, respectively.

Generation of infectious recombinant virions. The IL2 gene could be transferred to new NB-K monolayers through the inoculation of treated culture supernatants. This transfer required the inclusion of a helper genome in the initial transfection, indicating the involvement of MVM-IL2 recombinant viruses. Consistenly, 2 to 3 serial infections were achieved, when w.t. helper plasmids were present in the transfection (Tab. 1). The efficiency of transfer diminished rapidly after the third infection, parallel to a decrease in.the titer of w.t. helper virus. This is probably due to the generation of defective interfering (DI) particles that appear after high multiplicity infection with wild-type MVM stocks (Rhode 1978). When rep- helper plasmids were used, the IL2 gene was only transferred in the first infection, as expected; yet, w.t. MVM appeared when supernatants were passaged, indicating the occurrence of recombination between pMVM-IL2 (VP-) and helper (VP+) genomes.

From our results we can conclude that MVM is a very efficient vector for the expression of heterologous genes in transformed human and rodent cells. Recombinant particles can be obtained in the presence of a suitable helper, although the packaging system needs to be improved, in order to increase the titre of recombinant virus stocks and to minimize recombination between helper and recombinant DNA. It should then be possible to determine whether infections with recombinant parvoviruses may find a place in the gene therapy of cancer.

References
Berns, K. (1990). Microbiol. Rev. 54 : 316-329.
Huschtscha, L.I., Holliday, R. (1983). J. Cell Sci 63 : 77-99.
Merchellinsky, M.J., Tattersall, P.J., Leary, J.J., Cotmore, S.F., Gardiner, E.M., Ward, D.C. (1938). J. Virol. 47 : 227-232.
Rhode, S.L. (1978). J. Virol. 27 : 347-356.
Rhode, S.L. (1985). J. Virol. 55 : 886-889.
Russell, S. (1990). Immunol. Today 11 : 196-200.
van Hille, B., Duponchel, N., Salomé, N., Spruyt, N., Cotmore, S.F., Cornelis, J.J., Rommelaere, J. (1989). Virol. 171 : 89-97.

Résumé. Nous avons montré que le parvovirus autonome MVM est un vecteur d'expression très efficace, spécifique des cellules transfomées. Cette spécificité en fait un vecteur de choix pour la thérapie de gène du cancer. Dans ce but nous avons cloné le gène IL2 humain dans la région d'ADN du parvovirus codant pour les protéines de capside. Des virus recombinants MVM-IL2 ont été produits en présence d'un virus assistant produits et utilisés pour transférer le gène IL2 dans des cellules transformées en culture.

Targeted disruption of the murine CD4 gene in the germ-line by homologous recombination

A. Rahemtulla*, A. Arabian, W.P. Fung-Leung, M. Schilham, A. Wakeham and T.W. Mak

Department of Bioresearch, Ontario Cancer Institute, 500 Sherbourne Street, Toronto, Ontario, M4X 1K9, Canada

*Author for correspondence

The CD4 molecule is known to be involved in the process of MHC Class II restricted antigen recognition by the T-cell receptor (Schwartz,1985; Parnes,1989). The precise role of the CD4 molecule in antigen recognition is not well understood and the influence that it has on T-cell development even less so.

T cell precursors entering the thymus express CD4 at a low level. They go through a stage in their development when the thymocytes express neither CD4 nor CD8 (double negative). They then express both CD4 and CD8 (double positive) and low levels of CD3 and TcR. It is at this stage of development that the T cells undergo positive and negative selection and eventually emerge as mature $CD4^+8^-$ or $CD4^-8^+$ (single positive) T cells. Preliminary evidence from studies using antibodies to the CD4 molecule suggest that the CD4 molecule is involved in the thymic selection of the T-cell repertoire (Fowlkes et al.,1988; MacDonald et al.,1988). This role of the CD4 molecule would become more clear if we were to mutate the CD4 gene such that the T-cells did not express the CD4 molecule on their surface. To this end, we have disrupted the CD4 gene in the pluoripotent embryonic stem (ES) cells (Evans and Kaufman,1981) through a targeted mutation by homologous recombination (Smithies et al.,1985; Thomas and Capecchi,1987). Germ-line transmission of the mutation has resulted in the generation of a mutant mouse strain that does not express the CD4 molecule on the cell surface.

Gene targeting of CD4   The CD4 molecule is a 55kd cell surface glycoprotein found on a sub-population of lymphocytes, and exists on the cell surface as a monomeric structure. The CD4 gene in the mouse is 26kb long and has 10 exons and 9 introns (Gorman et al.,1987). For homologous recombination, a replacement-type vector was designed to create a mutant CD4 gene. This was a 2.8 kb genomic fragment containing exon 5 and exon 6. Exon 5 was disrupted by insertion of the bacterial neomycin resistance gene. This DNA construct was introduced into D3 ES cells by electroporation. Eight independent lines of ES cells with one of the alleles at the CD4 locus disrupted were generated. Southern blot analysis confirmed the replacement of the endogenous CD4 gene by single copy insertions of the construct by homologous recombination. Six of these clones were injected into pre-implantation embryos from C57Bl/6J mice. Mice with germ-line transmission representing four of the six independent clones were obtained.

Phenotypic analysis   Mice lacking surface expression of CD4 were healthy, fertile and indistinguishable from heterozygous or wild-type littermates on gross physical inspection. The numbers of cells in the lymphoid organs were similar to those in heterozygous or wild-type mice. Surface expression of CD4, however, was not detected on thymocytes or lymph node cells from mice homozygous for the mutant CD4 alleles. Staining of the thymocytes in the CD4⁻ homozygous mice shows that CD8⁺ cells are present in normal numbers in the thymus but expand in the periphery to occupy the compartment that would otherwise have been occupied by CD4⁺ cells. Analysis using antibodies against CD3 and $TcR_{\alpha\beta}$ showed that the expression of these molecules is normal in thymocytes of the mutant mice. There is no difference in the proportion of cells with high and low levels of $TcR_{\alpha\beta}$ on the surface, between the wild-type mice, heterozygous mice and the homozygous mutant mice. This indicates normal maturation of the CD8⁺ T cells, as far as the expression pattern of $TcR_{\alpha\beta}$ on the thymocytes is concerned. These results demonstrate that the expression of CD4 on the surface of the progenitor cells and on the double positive thymocytes is not required for the normal development of CD8⁺ cells. The functional consequences of the CD4⁻ phenotype are being assessed at present.

REFERENCES

Evans, M.J. and Kaufman, M.H. (1981): Establishment in culture of pluripotential cells from mouse embryos. *Nature* 22, 154-156.
Fowlkes, B.J., Schwartz, R.H. and Pardoll, D.M. (1988): Deletion of self-reactive thymocytes occurs at a CD4⁺CD8⁺ precursor stage. *Nature* 334, 620-623.
Gorman, S.D., Tourville, B. and Parnes, J.R. (1987): Structure of the mouse gene encoding CD4 and an unusual transcript in brain. *Proc. natn. Acad. Sci. USA.* 84, 7644-7648.
MacDonald, H.R., Hengartner, H. and Pedrazzini, T. (1988): Intrathymic deletion of self-reactive cells prevented by neonatal anti-CD4 antibody treatment. *Nature* 335, 174- 176
Parnes, J.R. (1989): Molecular Biology and Function of CD4 and CD8. *Adv. Immun.* 44, 265-311.
Schwartz, R.H. (1985): T-lymphocyte recognition of antigen in association with gene products of the major histocompatibility complex.   *A. Rev. Immun.* 3, 237-261.
Smithies, O., Gregg, R.G., Boggs, S.S., Koralewski, M.A. and Kucherlapati, R.S. (1985): Insertion of DNA sequences into the human chromosomal β-globin locus by homologous recombination. *Nature* 317, 230-234.
Thomas, K.R. and Capecchi, M.R. (1987): Site-Directed Mutagenesis by Gene Targeting in Mouse Embryo-Derived Stem Cells. *Cell* 51, 503-512.

RESUME : La molécule CD4 est impliquée dans le processus de reconnaissance de l'antigène par le récepteur des cellules T soumis à la restriction allogénique par le système majeur d'histocompatibilité de classe II. Cependant le rôle précis de la molécule CD4 dans la reconnaissance antigénique n'est pas parfaitement compris ; son influence sur le développement des cellules T l'est encore moins. Les études préliminaires utilisant des anticorps contre la molécule CD4 suggèrent que celle-ci est impliquée dans la sélection thymique du répertoire des cellules T. Afin d'élucider la fonction de cette molécule, nous avons interrompu le gène CD4 dans des cellules souches embryonnaires de souris en créant une mutation ciblée par recombinaison homologue. La transmission de cette mutation à la lignée germinale a permis de générer des souris mutantes qui n'expriment pas la molécule CD4 à la surface des cellules. Les conséquences fonctionnelles de ce phénotype CD4- sont en cours d'évaluation.

Round table:
Gene transfer and human diseases

Table ronde :
Transfert de gènes en pathologie humaine

Round table:
gene transfer and human diseases*

* *Transcription : Odile Cohen-Haguenauer*

*Chairmen : Hal E. Broxmeyer (USA), Thomas Caskey (USA),
Lucio Luzzatto (UK), Bruno Varet (France)*

1) **Introduction**
   Thomas Caskey (Institute for Molecular Genetics and Howard Hughes Medical Institute, Houston, USA)

2) **Hemoglobinopathies and human gene transfer in mice**
   Yves Beuzard (INSERM U.91, Créteil, France)

3) **Severe combined immunodeficiency**
   Alain Fischer (INSERM U.132, Paris, France)

4) **Fetal medicine and cord blood**
   Eliane Gluckman (Hôpital Saint-Louis, Paris, France)

5) **Tumor suppressor genes**
   Claudine Junien (INSERM U.73, Paris, France)

6) **Gene transfer and leukemias**
   Gérard Schaison (Hôpital Saint-Louis, Paris, France)

7) **Inborn errors of metabolism**
   Arnold Munnich (INSERM U.12, Paris, France)

8) **Gene transfer and liver cells**
   Didier Houssin (Groupe hospitalier Cochin, Paris, France)

9) **Cystic fibrosis**
   Ronald Crystal (NIH, Bethesda, USA)

10) **Fragile X syndrome**
    Jean-Louis Mandel (INSERM U.184, Strasbourg, France)

11) **Duchenne muscular dystrophy**
 Thomas Caskey (Institute for Molecular Genetics and Howard Hughes Medical Institute, Houston, USA)

12) **CNS and neurons**
 Jacques Mallet (CNRS, Gif-sur-Yvette, France)

13) **Scientific and ethical points to consider for the design of clinical trials of human gene therapy**
 Pierre Lehn (Hôpital Saint-Louis, Paris, France)

14) **Concluding remarks**
 Lucio Luzzatto (National Cancer Institute, London, UK)

15) **Closing address**
 Michel Boiron (Hôpital Saint-Louis, Paris, France)

1. TOM CASKEY : Introduction

One always wonders when you come to such an international meeting, how do you measure whether that meeting is a successful one.

There is one way I look back on meetings of my experience and training, that's a fairly good measure for me : I had a post doctoral fellow at one time who was an extremely productive post-doc fellow and I travelled with him to numerous meetings and I could always tell when the science was excellent because the post-doc would never remain at the meeting more than about half a day. When the science was particularly good, he would return to the research laboratory and go back to work. That post doctoral fellow is now scientific vice president of Merck Corporation Ed Skolnick. I never had that behaviour pattern but I begin to pick up on those signals from Ed and the only thing that ever happened to me at scientific meetings when they were outstanding is I got very nervous and I'd just like to report that during this meeting I remained very nervous, and so I think the quality of the science was really excellent, the presentations were of the highest quality and I particularly enjoyed the mix of the science. I thought that we had extremely good experts in a wide variety of areas. Now, the other point I'd like to make just to give you an indication of how important I felt the science at this meeting was that I called back yesterday to my own department ; I felt that there was so many people in my own department that would profit by the knowledge that came out of this meeting that I have set up an eight o'clock meeting just to brief everybody on the science ; and in a way it's a shame that small meetings lead to the situation of many people not hearing the latest facts but I would urge all of you to return from this conference and to sit down with your colleagues and review the entire meeting with your colleagues ; there will be no quick rapid report that comes out of this meeting, but there was an awful lot of current information that many scientists would profit from.

So, the other thing that will require you to do of course is to try to read your own handwriting at least 24 or 48 hours after you've written and that will be a good examination. The final point I would like to make is that I am extremely optimistic about the possibilities for a success in the area of gene transfer therapy.

I feel that we are definitely, as reflected by the quality of the science at this meeting, in the draft to develop a therapeutic option for patients that have heritable diseases or acquired diseases that have a genetic basis.

This field will be in a very significant manner contributing to new knowledge and fundamental research.

There is just no doubt about that. We lack so much information that we have to return to very basic principles to be able to develop the technology that will be required for the implementation of a successful clinical experiment.

So regardless of whether we succeed in a short period of time in successfully treating a patient to the benefit of that patient, this field is definitely stimulating the area of fundamental science, and I think we should always keep that in mind as we make our public presentations and discussions with scientists.

The second area that I would like to point out and I think it is an important one for us to keep in mind ; we are in a new era of molecular medicine ; there is no doubt about that ; you could date it back to the early nineteen eighties when the first applications of DNA based diagnostics were applied, and that area has done nothing but accelerate since the early eighties. So in the area of molecular medicine, diagnostics is definitely an established part of the field at this point ; secondly, we have seen since the era of recombinant DNA technology, the emergence now of pharmaceutic drugs that have been produced by the methodologies of more fundamental nucleic acid recombination mechanisms and gene expression and the first drugs are on the market.

So you have seen diagnostics, and you have seen therapeutics and I would say that this conference deals with the next phase of the molecular medicine era ; and that is the development of treatment procedural activities and what we have been discussing at this conference, is a complex interaction of laboratory and scientists to arrive at the addition of this third element in the era of molecular medicine ; and so I'll come away from the conference extremely optimistic about the field, and extremely optimistic about the advances that have been made.

I have said too much ; what we will like to do this morning is to give each speaker a few minutes to discuss each of their areas, to try not to give us all new data but to try to frame major questions that they think the audience would enjoy discussing in the relatively short period of time that we have for each of the areas. And so we will start first with an area that was somewhat neglected at the conference and that is the area of the hemoglobinopathies.

2. Y. BEUZARD : "Hemoglobinopathies and human gene transfer in mice"

The mouse models of human hemoglobinopathies (beta-thalassemia, sickle cell disease) are of special interest in several complementary fields :
- The gene therapy of genetic diseases which affect a protein present in high concentration within a specific cell line.
- The relationship between the host genes and the transgene expression (transcription of regulation but also at the levels of translation, protein assembly and turnover).
- The relationships between structure, function and molecular pathology of hybrid proteins containing host and transgenic subunits (normal or variant) in comparison to host and human non hybrid molecules.
- The consequences of transgene expression at the cellular level with regard to secondary molecular defects and cellular pathophysiology.
- The expression of new human transgenic variants in order to modify a preexisting mouse model and to obtain a mouse phenotypic syndrome more relevant to the human disease, at the molecular, cellular or whole organism levels.
- The design of new therapeutic approaches.

I will try to document a little bit these animal models for human diseases. Hemoglobinopathies have a major interest which can be to follow the effect of transgene and gene therapy from genes to phenotype. In mice when you transfer the human globin genes, various molecules appear because they form hybrids. In transgenic mices, you find mouse hemoglobin, human hemoglobin and the combination of these. Changes may affect the function of the proteins and the stability of the proteins which may tremendously modify the phenotype. Two groups have published last year the expression of high level of hemoglobin S. Surprisingly 80% of hemoglobin S did not induce sickle cell disease. We thus have to work in two directions :

- first, obtain 100% of hemoglobin S in the animals which is not yet the case ;

- second, to obtain the polymerisation of super S hemoglobin and this has been published this year by Rubin's group in San-Francisco with a hemoglobin-S-Antilles transgene. We have been working to increase polymerisation of hemoglobin using a third mutant hemoglobin DPunjab and S Antilles which decrease the affinity of hemoglobin to oxygen thus making the hemoglobin polymerize at a higher oxygen tension than hemoglobin S.

The phenotype we have obtained is much closer to sickle cell disease in human, although it is not the same and this is call the SAD hemoglobin.

L. LUZZATTO : I think Y. BEUZARD's and his group's work is extremely elegant. I was involved peripherally with Frank GROSVELD's and David GREAVES' original work on making the first high expression transgenic mice (we did the hematology on them). It was quite striking that although the phenotype was in some respect quite similar to the one we have just heard, the mouse with the highest level of hemoglobin S which was 80% had a clinical phenotype which best was reminiscent of combination in human of S and hereditary persistance of fetal hemoglobin.

With 80% S the mouse had very little evidence of hemolysis although it was an excellent sickling model and we demonstrated sickling in vitro as well as in vivo in the organs.

Unfortunately this mouse turned out to be a sterile male. What is characteristic of sickle cell anemia and sickling disorders is that much of the work can be done in vitro because we have cells that we can handle. But one of the most intriguing features and clinically worrisome features has been the very complicated matter of pathophysiology and pathogenesis, for instance of bone pain crisis and on that, the handling of red cells in vitro can tell us nothing. That is why I think that this animal model is of extreme interest and of course it is quite obvious that others will want to use them for instance for testing so-called "anti-sickling agents" which until now has been a great disapointment in clinical practice ; now there is a way that they could be tested more appropriately rather than by extremely cumbersome, and for some of them, almost impossible clinical trials. So I think this is really a step forward.

T.CASKEY : I can just offer one comment at the area. I think that the models that have been developed also offer the opportunity for the development of the technology of stem cells isolation, the maintenance of stem cells and the attemps for homologous recombination in these stem cells. You have a marker system that is into the hematopoietic tissue. It is in the target gene of your interest for the adult. And so you have the opportunity to work a model system before advancing to studies in humans. I think this is a very important research tool for the development of that technology.

I would like to raise a point for discussion : I put forward the concept that if we were to select one disease entity that has a high profile in inheritable disease area where a true gene remplacement would be preferable to gene transfer is that this group of diseases would represent that example. Given the difficulties of trying to understand the regulation of transgenes I would like to draw out Doctor Capecchi, Doctor Mulligan and others that are in the audience that would perhaps have alternative technologies : homologous recombination versus gene transfer with proper regulatory elements to get some estimate of what they think the relative difficulties of the developments of these two strategies for therapy may be. Are there others that have been participating in hemoglobinopathy transfer technology and would like to make comments on that ?

O.COHEN-HAGUENAUER : Doctor CAPECCHI could you comment on the relevance of homologous recombination regarding somatic gene therapy ? Even if this will happen in the future or not.

M.CAPECCHI : I guess my comment is just directed to the last statement you made ; that is that successful science is dependent on timing : being too early is just as disastrous as being too late. Having said that, the other thing that is fairly obvious is that there is an enormous advantage to doing homologous recombination, that is correcting the endogenous gene. Because of that impetus, that is both in terms of regulation and not having to worry about packaging sizes, I think the ingenuity of man is going to come up to this challenge and allow people to do homologous recombination with respect to gene therapy.

I think what will be required is the ability at least in its current form to culture stem cells of whatever somatic type that you are interested in at least for a period of about two weeks and retain their potentiality. Once this is available, we can start seriously thinking about this type of analysis.

O.COHEN-HAGUENAUER : Regarding this, speaking of genetic defects, for example within the beta-globin locus in which the mutation can affect any of thirty or fifty kilobases in the region ; do you think that you would be able to design a standard replacement gene or donor sequence for homologous recombination in this context and have thirty kilobases replaced at once without first having to type the mutation itself very precisely ?

M.CAPECCHI : I tried to indicate that actually in a slide ; there is no indication right now that there is any limit in the types of changes that can be made. That is a single point mutation replacement goes at the same frequency than eighty kilobases deletion or replacement. We have no idea of what the upper limit is. In theory, you could make any type of change you want and not affect the frequency ; so I don't think that seems to be a limitation.

O.COHEN-HAGUENAUER : Do you think that such replacements could occur without new mutations in the donor sequence itself ?

M.CAPECCHI : We have not actually seen very much alteration of the input DNA in terms of its transfer, though obviously we do not sequence every time we do a targeting event. What we do ask is simply function ; we have several systems in which we can ask for the gene to go in and then for the gene to come out and then revert to activity. So in the process of putting something in, we had created other mutations which if they would have had a functional effect, we would have detected that. But we have not observed that since we can revert at the same frequency ; at least on our functional assays, we have not picked up any other mutations.

O.COHEN-HAGUENAUER : OK. Thank you very much.

T. CASKEY : Let's move on to the next topic.

3. A. FISCHER : "Severe combined immunodeficiency"

More than fifty immunodeficiency diseases (ID) have been identified. In most cases, the affected cells belong to the haematopoietic lineage. Some of the IDs are lethal or life threatening and justify curative therapeutic approaches. To date, ID related genes have been characterized for 7 diseases : adenosine deaminase deficiency (ADA), nucleoside phosphorylase deficiency (NP), leukocyte adhesion deficiency (B2 integrin, LAD), chronic granulomatous diseases, X-linked : p91 chain of cytochrome b, autosomal recessive : p47, p67 deficiencies and p22 chain of cytochrom b. For some other diseases, genes have been mapped (X linked SCID, XL-agammaglobulinemia, Wiskott-Aldrich syndrome (WAS), XL proliferative syndrome, ataxia telangiectasia).

Gene therapy is of potential interest and feasibility in severe combined immunodeficiency (SCID) such as ADA deficiency, WAS, CGD and LAD provided that stem cells could be targeted. However alternative therapy(ies) does exist. HLA identical allogeneic bone marrow transplantation cures more than 90% of ID patients. Patients with SCID and other immunodeficiencies transplanted with the marrow of a matched unrelated donor or a family partially mismatched donor have now a survival expectancy over 70%. In addition, ADA substitution by i. muscular infusion of PEG-ADA is partially effective in correcting the ID. Most CGD patients are doing well under prophylactic antibiotic therapy and possibly interferon gamma.

The place of gene therapy in the treatment of ID will very much depend on the potential selective advantage of transduced stem cells that could allow autologous transplantation without chemotherapy or irradiation.

T.CASKEY : I will keep raising questions until the audience warms up this morning ! You brought up one disease in which there is an alternative therapy now and that is chronic granulomatous disease (C.G.D.). I would love to hear your comments on what I consider to be a rather modern therapy.

A.FISCHER : C.G.D. I would say at this point before gene therapy has three treatments. One is antibiotics and antibiotic therapy by itself is very efficient. Prevention therapy of bacterial and fungal infection is very efficient. The outcome, the life expectancy and the quality of life of these patients has been modified significantly. Very recently there has been an international study which has proved that the addition of gamma-interferon in these patients may further reduce the frequency of infections. It is strange that it seems to be more efficient in the United States than in Europe, but anyway it works.

T.CASKEY : According to where the company is located...!

A.FISCHER : But the patients are supposed to suffer from the same disease. Anyway this disease was lethal twenty years ago and now there is hardly a single patient dying from the disease. In addition to that, bone marrow transplantation is efficient. There have been few patients all over the world who have been cured by allogeneic bone marrow transplantation. But even this therapy is no longer considered in CGD because of the high efficiency of the two other treatments.

T.CASKEY : Are there any other comments ? Michael, can I draw you out on something ? You mentioned yersterday data for something very interesting about the ADA-patients with regard to reconstitution by bone marrow transplantation. As you reconstitute you see the elements : T and B cells elements were evolving from the transplants but not the myeloid components. Could you make a general comment about whether this is true of all of the immunodeficiency states or is it just a characteristic of ADA ?

M.BLAESE : Alain is more expert with that than I am. It certainly has been an experience in ADA and some of the other forms of SCIDs. That in ADA in particular it is only the T cells, even the B cells are still ADA deficient. It depends somewhat on the property of reagents that are required. Obviously if you do late SCIDs recipient you get usually complete myelo and lymphoid reconstitution with donor type cells. But the initial SCIDs let us say ADA and other ill-defined forms of SCIDs, had primarily T cell or T cell and B cell engraftment. In Wiskott-Aldrich syndrome for instance, it has been a major problem trying to treat it by bone marrow transplantation with a haplo-identical T cell depleted donor. The survival rates at best until perhaps last year had been less than 50% and the alternative standard medical therapy gives a survival rate that is approximatively of 90% ; So the transplantation is a significant disadvantage. We should be well aware as Alain was right to point out, of the alternative therapies for things like CGD.

A.FISCHER : I slightly disagree with you Mike, because there has been a selection for the Wiskott-Aldrich patients. Those who have received haplo-identical transplants have been selected for transplantation because they had very severe complications of the disease. So they might have had more severe forms of the disease than the general Wiskott-Aldrich population of patients. I am not saying that bone marrow transplantation is definitively the solution to cure Wiskott-Aldrich syndrome. I think that the significant advances which have occurred during the last five years, in terms of bone marrow transplantation, may give the hope that if we continue to progress, even the use of an haplo-identical transplant will be able to cure this disease.

M.BLAESE : We also have considered the impact of bone marrow transplantation on the hemoglobinopathies because clearly that is another major therapeutic option for those diseases.

T.CASKEY : In fact, it amazes me in the hemoglobinopathy area in the States, that there has been a relatively low incidence of Bone Marrow Transplants and yet experiences in Italy and in Greece have been extremely promising.
Any other comments ?

O.COHEN-HAGUENAUER : Just a comment on the target for gene therapy. Doctor BLAESE, will you keep on working on lymphocytes or do you think that you will try to do bone marrow rather than lymphocytes when this will be possible ? Could you comment on this according to your data ?

M.BLAESE : I certainly think that when bone marrow becomes available it would be preferable to lymphocyte therapy at least as we envision it now. If it turns out that lymphocyte therapy is going to be effective, with relatively few treatments without consistent retreatment of a child. Then, lymphocyte therapy is certainly a simple procedure that would be justified. But I would certainly hope that bone marrow gene therapy becomes available soon, so that we can go to that round.

L.LUZZATTO : Doctor FISCHER, you showed us that map of the X chromosome and was it just because there is some gene you are interested in or do you think there is an over-representation of genes on the X in immunodeficiency syndromes in general?

A.FISCHER : Well, there are six known immunodeficiences that map to the X, so that is six out of fifty immunodeficiencies so it is probably not significant. I showed the picture of the X for two reasons. The first one is because five of these genes have been mapped quite recently, and the second is that we are working on that. But still there is one X-linked immunodeficiency in mouse which is the X^{ld} mouse ; so one may still speculate that there could be a family of gene on the X chromosome although they are not located in the same region, which might be involved in T and/or B cell differenciation. But these are obviously only speculations because we don't know anything about these genes yet.

T.CASKEY : We will move on to Doctor GLUCKMAN.

4. Eliane GLUCKMAN : "Fetal Medicine and Cord Blood"

The main thing we could discuss is the reason why we should work towards gene therapy when the results of bone marrow transplantation (BMT) are so good.

And in most of these diseases you mentioned thalassemia over non-malignant hematological diseases, we can achieve 80% long term survival. One of the main problems is the long term effect of the conditioning ; this is a study which is ongoing and we really don't know what will be the fate of these patients after ten years, after total body irradiation in the young age. This can be a first point to consider when we have to compare BMT and gene therapy.

The second point is that at the present time we are obliged to have an HLA-identical donor to achieve these results of 80% and even if there are improvements in mismatched transplants, results are not as good as they are in HLA-identical siblings. So there has been a big effort, and a very costly effort, to do bone marrow registries of normal volunteers. There is one in France, one in the United States and several in Europe, but even in the best hypothesis, we think that we will not have more than 30% chances to find a donor ; because of the heterogeneity of the HLA-typing. So 60 or 70% of the patients remain and will never benefit of an HLA-identical donor for BMT. There is thus still an open field for gene therapy or at least for finding alternative therapies for these patients.

We have been working on the use of Cord Blood for transplants together with Hal BROXMEYER (see this issue). One of the aims of this study was to have cells which were readily available; another thing that we thought could be interesting was that these very young cells might have advantages for BMT and perhaps for gene therapy. We may use in a small volume, a small number of cells appropriate for graft or any manipulation. These cells are easy to freeze ; they might have a relative immaturity of the immune system which could allow some degree of mismatch for transplant.

The first transplants we have performed are in patients with Fanconi's anemia. This disease is recessive autosomal, characterized by chromosome breakages which are increased when the cells are incubated with alkylating agents. A prenatal diagnosis can be performed before three months of pregnancy. In these two families, the mothers had both an affected child and were pregnant. Since the disease is very severe, they underwent prenatal diagnosis ; the fetuses were not affected and happened to be HLA-identical to the affected siblings.

Cord blood cells were collected at birth and were infused to the recipients after normal conditioning ; without any cell separation. The reconstitution was very good, quicker in one case where the patient received twice as many cells. The first patient is doing well two years after transplant; the second one is also well after one year following BMT. The study of chimerism shows that the recipient type is decreasing slowly ; after three months almost all cells are of donor type. We were able to obtain a complete donor reconstitution.

We have then envisaged the possibility and conditions for banking cells of this origin. We have now started to bank such samples. In addition, when a patient's mother undergoes pregnancy, we are now keeping cord blood cells at birth. This implies to perform prenatal diagnosis first and to be ready to freeze the cells ; this had been done in hereditary diseases like thalassemias.

In fact, this is very easy to do and the whole procedure is quite simple. It has no ethical constraint since cord blood is usually discarded. The mean sample size is one hundred mls ; this size varies a lot from one sample to the other : from 30 to 200 ml. The number of CFU-GM is quite acceptable, and one cord can be used for one transplant and some of them are so rich in hematopoietic stem cells that they can be used in adults. Factors affecting sample volume are both the weight of the placenta and the clamping technique. The earlier the clamping occurs, the more cells you get. Cord blood collection does not affect the newborn as testified by the hemoglobin level which do not vary significantly.

Some factors appear to affect considerably the number of CFU-GM :

1) Any attempt to separate cells decreases the number of progenitor cells;

2) the duration of pregnancy : the earlier the delivery occurs, the larger the number of cells is ; upmost results were obtained when the delivery took place two weeks before normal term ;

3) the time between blood collection and handling ;

4) Cell incubation with interleukin 3 (IL3) increases the number of CFU-GM.

As a conclusion, I will summarize the advantages of using cord blood :

1) easy collection and storage together with the reproducibility of the number of cells from one sample to the other ;

2) it can be used for both autologous and allogeneic transplants. With the aim of gene therapy, it seems easy to make prenatal diagnosis, collect cells at birth and reconstitute the child with engineered cells.

This would offer the advantage to profit from the relative neo-natal immunodeficiency to do the transplant, even before birth ;

3) this source of stem cells also appears very useful for laboratory investigation ; we plan to use cord blood for stem cell purification, study of growth factors, drug toxicity and gene transfer, since these cells might be more permissive than others to retroviral infection.

T.CASKEY : Open for discussion.

H. BROXMEYER : I will just add three comments to that. In the experiments that Eliane showed you when she said that the number of cells that she had was related to the speed of recovery, such as twice as many cells gives you faster recovery, it is not actually that simple, because we received a cord-blood of only about a fifty milliliters that was used and actually was less than the number of cells put into the recipient in which the population was low, and we observed the reconstitution just as fast as in the second. So it is not only the cellularity that is important but also the number of progenitor cells or stem cells that are in that population. So it might not be as simple as : the more you put cells in, the faster you get a reconstitution.

The second point is when we originally thought of doing the cord blood it was mainly in the context of autologous because essentially the only perfectly matched cells for a person is that person's own cells ; and that actually was highlighted by a recent report in the New England Journal of Medicine, where they show that as much as a single amino-acid difference in an HLA-type was associated with problems in the transplantation setting. I mean I personally envision a time where eventually, unless something else comes up, every child that's born will have the capability of having his cells stored away. So that they can use it for themselves ; you can laugh about it but you can't make a cell ! Okay ; and unless gene therapy or whatever gives you what you are really looking for, right now, at this time, the only perfectly matched cells are your own.

O.COHEN-HAGUENAUER : What about the banking ?

H.BROXMEYER : That's going to have to be done by companies ;

O.COHEN-HAGUENAUER : But they surely will mix names !

H.BROXMEYER : Well, you know, that's life ; when you start anything, you have problems and if we had worried about every problem that we thought about, we would never have believed in the first transplant. So you are right, there will be problems, but that doesn't mean that the concept won't eventually come about hopefully in somebodies life time.

T.CASKEY : The President for the banking is already in place. I can think of at least three locations in the United States ; there is a reasonable interest, I was quite surprised, but there is a very reasonable interest of parents in banking DNA for fingerprinting purposes ; child loss is a reasonably low frequency event, and I would guess that a low frequency event like ill-health also will be proceeded by parents at substantial risk ; I will not be too surprised at all, to see this concept accepted.
   Any other comments ?

P. LEHN : I would like to make two broad comments. The first is to think of Bone Marrow Transplantation long term consequences. The second comment concerns genetic diseases. If you have access to prenatal diagnosis then you just have to make abortion of affected fetuses ; and to my opinion, there is absolutely no reason to use cord-blood cells for gene transfer.

E.GLUCKMAN and H.BROXMEYER : Oh!

T.CASKEY : Let me be sure we can clarify what you mean. Are you saying that it is not a worthwhile venture to use normal cells that are derived following prenatal diagnosis or ...

P.LEHN : No. I am saying to use these cells for gene transfer ; because to use them you have to take them immediatly at birth, and this implies that you already have performed prenatal diagnosis ; you have to know that the fetus is affected.

T.CASKEY : I see ; so you take prenatal diagnostic option as opposed to the therapeutic option. I just want to clarify.

Dr. IOANNOU : I must say that I strongly disagree with that, because following prenatal diagnosis in my country, Cyprus, everytime we have an abortion, we consider that it is a defeat of science.

The whole point with prenatal diagnosis is not to turn out to an abortion, but to develop techniques through which you eventually will be able to do fetal medicine to help the fetus to survive ; you abort the fetus because of a single point mutation ; he could be a human beeing with tremendous capabilities why should you abort because of a single point mutation ?

E.GLUCKMAN : I absolutely agree with Dr. IOANNOU. In countries where the number of mutations in the hemoglobin is so high that some parents are subjected to repetitive abortions, it is absolutely a failure. Some parents, in addition, do not want to have an abortion, for religious reasons in particular. So I do think that there should be an alternative. If we could cure, through a single hit procedure, the fetus in utero, it would be much less expensive than to transfuse patients every month all life long.

T.CASKEY : We could start a new ethics conference and go on for several months ! I would like to make a few points here, though. I think it would be wrong if our enthousiasm for the science of gene therapy and gene transfer technology led the public to think that this in fact was going to be a realistic option for children in the near future. I heard that said by parents. I think that it is an absolute misrepresentation of the current state of the technology. So it is wrong to misrepresent the public.

The second point is I think that it is our responsability as medical geneticists to provide families with the information so that they can make their family decisions. These are very private decisions not to be made by the doctors around the table but by the parents who have to deal with problems.

H.BROXMEYER : Before we move to the next topic, I would like to ask a question : does anybody here have an information on the comparative efficiency of retroviral infection of bone marrow cells versus let's say cord blood cells or other fetal cells ; does anybody know if there is a difference in the infection rates ?

T.CASKEY : No, I would predict.

M.BLAESE : Well, the only experiment that we have, is in sheep, where if you try to do bone-marrow gene therapy in adult sheeps, we have not been successful in terms of long-term expression.

Whereas, taking these animals' fetal blood and transducing this with retroviral vectors, we do get expression in the newborn lamb. So in that one limited experience it appeared that fetal circulating progenitor cells might be a more susceptible target for gene transfer.

T.CASKEY : We're going to move on to the next speaker, **Claudine Junien.**

5. C. JUNIEN : Tumor suppressor genes

I will try to raise a few questions that came to me since yesterday when I was asked to talk about tumor suppressor genes (since John JENKINS finally could not join the meeting).

I think that especially since the beginning of this workshop, we have heard about gene transfer for monogenic disorders. The big difference with cancer is that it is not a monogenic disorder, even when it is inherited, there are so many different hits in the cancer cells that the problem is quite different and may be more complicated. The sequences of hits that have been described in colon carcinoma, which also seems to be the rule in other solid tumors, is not compulsory ; but what seems important is the accumulation of hits. So we have to face here ten different events, some of which correspond to tumor suppressor genes, but some others to ras mutation or myc overexpression, for example.

What can we think about tumor suppressor genes as candidates for therapy ?

In fact, there has been many experiments that show that they do work as tumor suppressors ; that is dealing with somatic cell hybrids, microcell transfer and retroviral transfer with cloned genes. It has been shown that changes occur either in cell morphology, growth rate, colony formation or in immortality and even in tumorigenicity. This demonstrates that one hit can be cured but what about the nine other remaining ones ? Which might be oncogenes, tumor suppressor genes and above all chromosome instability. The other point concerning these experiments is that they were done in vitro, on cell-lines without any surrounding cell which could have mimicked what the tumor environnement is really like in vivo.

So my question is : can we trust cancer cells since once one hit has been repaired, the others are still there ; and we could make some kind of present comparison with what is happening in the Gulf ; can we really trust it ?

Would it not be the best way to get rid of tumor cells namely to destroy them completely instead of letting them survive with all the damage that they still carry and might cause ?

Therefore, we can examine different types of mechanisms that are involved in tumor suppression. There are different approaches ; some of them beeing within the cells and others concerning interactions between several types of cells, surrounding the tumor. The inner part of the cell concerns chromosome stability ; how can we deal with that ? There may be ways to stabilize chromosomes and to prevent further rearrangements. These cells should then be able to terminally differenciate ; in addition, the control of the proliferation has to be perfect including operating negative and positive regulatory genes.

Another problem following the introduction of a gene is that of genomic imprinting ; since we know that some tumor suppressor genes undergo genomic imprinting, then we have to think of introducing the proper gene in order for it to be properly expressed.

As for systemic interactions, there are lots of communications between cells such as : junctional connections, steroid hormones, secreted signal peptides, the immune surveillance, angiogenesis regulation which is very important and the regulation of tumor invasion with possible interactions of matrix components and differential expression of proteases.

Another problem which also seems to be quite important is cancer cells microenvironment. This is a hypothesis which has recently been published ; considering hereditary colon cancer, the authors have shown that events that occur in hereditary cancer do not follow the same sequence ; without a perfect similarity of events. This suggests that all the cells surrounding potential malignant cells carry the same mutation in hereditary forms ; whereas in sporadic tumors, surrounding cells are normal. Therefore, the signals are different whenever you are dealing with a sporadic or a hereditary tumor. The approaches you might use for therapy might thus be quite distinct.

Finally, what should be suggested in the case of cancer ? We are facing two different situations ; cancer predisposing genes which can be assimilated to monogenic disorders ; or, could we just point out that the disease is not yet present; and we thus do not know yet where it will occur except in case of very specific cancers, which have only one very specific target. Even retiblastoma is not the safest one since osteosarcomas also arise in many young patients who have inherited the disease. Therefore, I am asking you specialists this basic question : do you have any idea of how to get to this and is it useful to do it before the tumor appears ?

Now, dealing with the tumor itself, we could target events that occur within cells ; and therefore we can envisage to act at the level of tumor suppressor genes. Towards this, is it feasible to prepare "cocktails" including all appropriate tumor suppressor genes that are altered in a very specific type of tumor ?

Following their introduction, theses genes will also have to be expressed in controlled amounts in order for cell-stability to be maintained ; since we know that after having been introduced in some cell-lines, a single copy of chromosome 3 is still to some extent compatible with cell growth, whereas two copies induce loss of tumorigenicity. But we don't know what could be the consequences of tumor suppressor genes overexpression not only for cancer cells, but also in the surrounding cells which should be able to divide. What could happen if cell-division would be inhibited ?

Another point is that, in constrast with monogenic disorders where if one introduces a gene with the aim to compensate for the endogenous gene defect, then one does not need to transfer the gene to every cell. A small percentage might be sufficient. In the context of malignancy, one cannot afford to leave a single cell alive without the therapeutic genetic manipulation. How can we get an even and complete distribution of gene-transfer ?

Although we have seen that some approaches work in vitro, if we take into account cancer complexity, it is probably wise to use complementary approaches all at the same time in order to be able to kill cancer cells and get rid of them.

T.CASKEY : Open for comment ? : On this last point, the kill characteristic, we have the whole field of medicine of hemato-oncology that has developped which has accurately measured kill rates on neoplastic cells as a preliminary test before going to clinical trial ; and I wonder if the same type of evaluation should not be applied to the introduction of recombinant DNA kill-molecules that is the standard of the practice is established in Hem-Onc before you go to clinical trials ; should we have the same principles applied in the gene-transfer kill phenomena. Mike, do you want to make any comment on that ?

M. BLAESE : Certainly, you have to have some sort of standardized approaches. Right now, I think your synthesis of what is going on in the field is very accurate ; we just do not know enough about the normal function of tumor suppressor genes in normal cells or the consequences of overexpression of those genes.

Until we really understand somewhat more about this, the development of a rational approach to treatment using gene transfer is very difficult.

D. LOWY : I just would like to echo what has been said. The treatment of cancer at the moment is basically to try to kill cancer cells whereas the notion of gene therapy is a kind of replacement therapy which would be to try to render otherwise malignant cells inoffensive. In principle, this is really conceptually quite different from the current approach ; and therefore it is going to take a long time before we would be successful.

T.CASKEY : Let's stay to the same subject area, but move on to leukemias. Dr. SCHAISON :

6. G. SCHAISON : Gene Transfer and Leukemia.

I first want to show you the results of classical treatment of acute leukemia, and secondly I shall address one or two questions dealing with gene therapy.

At present two thirds of children with acute lymphoblastic leukemia achieve long term complete remission. In contrast two thirds of children with acute myeloblastic leukemia will die of their disease. As for secondary leukemias, they are resistant to treatment. Bone Marrow Transplantation can cure half of the patients with acute myeloblastic leukemia in first complete remission ; it also rescues half of the children in second remission.

New therapeutic approaches of hematopoietic malignancies are greatly needed. There is no real progress in the treatment of leukemia since 1980. No new drug is available since 1970. But we now have identified prognostic factors which lead us to tailor the treatment according to the initial evaluation.

As for the results of bone marrow tranplantation, there has not been significant improvement in this context since ten years.

New approaches consist of :
1) Bone Marrow Transplantation in high risk leukemias ;
2) The use of hematopoietic growth factors - for example G-CSF and GM-CSF to overcome myelosuppression and perhaps allow to increase chemotherapy ;
3) The use of differenciating agents such as retinoic acid which has been administered with success in acute promyelocytic leukemia.

There are many reasons for considering gene transfer in leukemias since:

1) Bone marrow is easy to manipulate and the transfer of a gene in the pluripotent stem cell can result in a continuous expression in all hematopoietic lineages ;

2) Both dihydrofolate reductase (DHFR) mutant gene and multidrugresistance (MDR) gene have been cloned ;

3) Bone Marrow Transplantation is a well known procedure and there should be no ethical problems with relapse in patients who could not benefit of any alternative treatment. In vitro colonies of stem cells transfected with the DHFR gene are resistant to methotrexate. The same sequences have been expressed in vivo in mice and proved to confer a selective advantage to transfected cells. Recipient of transduced marrow are partially protected against methotrexate toxicity. Mice transgenic for the pleiotropic multidrug-resistance gene have also been shown to be protected against daunorubicin induced pancytopenia.

But will more intensive chemotherapy of leukemia increase cure rates ? In most instances, when one considers radiation therapy, increasing doses do not improve either relapse or cure rates. New treatments may only increase those rates in a subset of patients, others may not benefit or even have a shorter survival following increased toxicity. I personally think that a plateau has been reached since the most intensive therapy is bone marrow conditioning and after three successive grafts the incidence of relapse is similar to that following intensive chemotherapy.

If increasing chemotherapy doses is unlikely to improve cure rates, the usefulness of drug-resistance gene transfer is questionable ?

M. GOTTESMAN : I just would like to comment on the notion of introducing drug-resistance genes into bone marrows of patients who have leukemia. I think probably it is not the initial intent to do that ; the last thing you want to do is to put a drug-resistance gene into the marrow of patients with disorders of the bone-marrow. I think the notion is to use a drug-resistance gene to protect the marrow of patients who have solid tumors and where there is good evidence that dose intensification probably could cure more patients. And now whether or not one could use these kinds of approaches to treat leukemia, I would agree with you to be fairly pessimistic at the moment.

M. BOIRON : One should rather transfer drug-sensitivity genes which indeed have not been identified yet!

O.COHEN-HAGUENAUER : What about an antisense strategy ?

M. GOTTESMAN : The question comes up is to whether or not one could use antisense strategies, perhaps by introducing antisense genes. I think that is possible. A more direct approach is the pharmacologic one of trying to overcome the effects of these drug-resistance genes. I would take slight exception to the notion that there is no new treatment strategy available for leukemia. I think one big evidence that has appeared recently is that expression of the MDR-genes is quite common in relapse leukemia and therapy resistant leukemia. There are strategies beeing developed to overcome that drug resistance which might substantially affect cure rates in leukemia. We don't know that yet ; the clinical trials are just going to be started. But I think these are new approaches since 1970.

There are other chemotherapeutic modalities on the horizon which might potentially improve the treatment of leukemia. But the bottom line is that there will still be some drug resistant leukemias and we will need totally new ideas to treat them.

T.CASKEY : Any additional comments ?

P. LEHN : Yes, I would like to go back to general comment. I think that the most promising approach in a very far future is that of "vaccine". If you transfer cytokine genes into tumor cells it seems that you render them much more susceptible to destruction and induce a subsequent promotion of the immune system towards tumor destruction. The results of preliminary experiments look promising. It might be the most interesting approach considering cancer.

T.CASKEY : We are going to move on to inborn errors of metabolism. **Doctor MUNNICH**.

7. A. MUNNICH : Inborn errors of metabolism

I would like to remind you that inborn errors of metabolism are rare diseases ; each of them hardly reaching a frequency of 10 to the minus 4. But as a whole, they are numerous.

More than a hundred have been identified today. These diseases are usually expressed in the early neo-natal period and have a rapidly fatal outcome. For these diseases, we consider that mass-screening is too late and too expensive or even unreliable. A systematic neonatal screening is impossible according to our point of view : we thus screen for these patients according to clinical features and secondarily perform subsequent sophisticated biochemical investigations.

Inborn errors of intermediary metabolism can be split in two classes according to the pathophysiology. The first one would be intoxications and the second energy deficiencies.

Intoxications result of secondary accumulation of abnormal compounds. The primary genetic defect usually comes from liver cells, but the brain suffers from accumulation of metabolites. This situation corresponds to branched-chain-amino acid catabolism disorders and urea-cycle disorders. These diseases become apparent after two or three days of symptom-free period following birth. Babies require immediate toxin removal by blood exchange transfusion or peritoneal dialysis. Afterwards, low protein diets are set up.

A second class of diseases consists of energy deficiencies which are defects in either production or use of substrates. Enzymatic hypoglycemia, namely glycogenosis, neoglucogenesis disorders, inborn errors of pyruvate metabolism, of fatty acid oxidation and mitochondrial chain deficiencies and peroxisomal disorders belong to this class. In all these disorders, the problem is inside the cells ; there is no exported toxicity. As expected, no symptom-free period takes place ; these diseases sometimes have an antenatal onset. The clinical presentation consists of hypotonia, myopathia, cardiomyopathia, possible dysmorphia and rapidly progressive neurologic deterioration.

These energy deficiencies have no efficient therapy at the present time.

A third condition might also be considered, that is liver dysfunction in general; the main symptom beeing hepatomegalia with hypoglycemia. Hepatic failure is the major concern with these babies. These conditions are characterized by a dramatic response to glucose administration. The enzymatic defects included here are enzymatic hypoglycemia namely Glucose 6 phosphate and fructose diphosphatase deficiencies, tyrosinemia, fructose intolerance and galactosemia. In these last three disorders, milk withdrawal allows the baby to recover.

In the neonatal period, diagnosis can be made quickly on the basis of the status of the baby, namely acidosis, ketosis, blood lactate and amonemia level.

What are the present therapeutic possibilities in inborn errors of metabolism ? One has to consider two distinct groups of disorders. As for intoxications, vitamin therapy can be tried, together with drug administration and diet ; although vitamin responsive disorders are very rare, less than 1% in our experience ; drug administration helps to increase the urinary excretion of toxic metabolites in some cases, as for instance glycin which conjugates with iso-valeryl CoA with such efficiency that no additional dietary treatment is required in isovaleryl CoA dehydrogenase deficiency ; low protein diet is applied to most patients but it does not prevent them from acute episodes of coma-metabolic acidosis and even brain deterioration. Liver transplantation has been performed in OTC deficiency, citrullinemia and Mapple syrup urine disease. Unfortunately, expression from bone marrow would be too weak to allow clinical improvement.

As far as energy deficiencies are concerned, no diet, no effective treatment including toxin removal can be performed since the disorder is inside the cell.

Prospects for gene therapy in inborn errors of metabolism should be considered separately in intoxications and energy deficiencies. In the first class of diseases, no specific targeting of the organ in which the expression is missing is necessary. Whereas in energy deficiencies there is no alternative to the introduction of a functional transgene in the deficient cells.

I will finally emphasize on the fact that patients usually have profound enzymatic deficiencies. Restoring few percents of enzyme activity would probably allow normal phenotype recovery.

T.CASKEY : I would like to reinforce one point that you mentioned with regard to the insult of the central nervous system by inborn errors of metabolism. You can go into any inborn errors of metabolism clinic and you will see patients beautifully managed, all in very good metabolic balance, but it is basically a mental retardation clinic. I think that in spite the efforts of very good management by neonatologists and perinatologists and geneticists, the job is poorly done. I think it argues for as early an intervention as possible which in my opinion almost forces us to the point of newborn screening to identify the cases that would maximally benefit from the technology which will come in the future.

J.L.MANDEL : I will reemphasize the point I discussed yesterday with Pascale BRIAND about OTC deficiency. To my opinion in families where the defect has been identified, the use of prenatal dianosis renders gene therapy needness.

In contrast babies with sporadic cases can be born anywhere in a small hospital where the neurologic impairment will take place by the time the diagnosis is made.

T.CASKEY : Can I ask you a question about Europe ? Is newborn screening a requisite in virtually all countries in Europe ? Do you screen for metabolic defects ?

A.MUNNICH : As far as metabolic disorders are concerned, we only screen for Phenylketonuria (PKU) (The other systematic screening beeing hyopthyroidism).

T.CASKEY : But as long as the process is in place, you should convince the government to add tests to the list.

A.MUNNICH : But you have to consider the low frequency of the diseases and the time by which the disease becomes symptomatic and brain damages are irreversible.

T.CASKEY : A very large number of these diseases will be made DNA based diagnostics. You are not going to have to wait for a Guthrie. You will be able to do it on the basis of DNA. As for example you can screen for Duchenne Muscular Dystrophy now with 98% accuracy for duplication-deletion cases.

L.LUZZATTO : Do you mean that now in the States, rare metabolic disorders are screened for in every newborn ?

T.CASKEY : In the state of Texas we screen for six diseases and we include hemoglobinopathies.

L.LUZZATTO : But that is not a low frequency !

T.CASKEY : OK, but there are other errors of metabolism Mapple syrup urine disease, homocystinuria, hyperammonemia. They are tested by Guthrie. In the case of hemoglobinopathies it's CASKEY protein and DNA.

A.MUNNICH : But our opinion is that the clinical expression of these diseases is very early often before the reply of the screening test. The onset is so early!

T. CASKEY : This is just a technical problem!

M. GOTTESMAN : I just like to make one comment which may be broaden the discussion a bit. A point was made that some of these disorders of cellular metabolism need to be treated at the cellular level and in the specific cells involved. Obviously in terms of gene therapy one would need to be able to target the genes to those specific cells in an organism. I wonder whether anyone has any experience, this is not an issue that's been discussed in this meeting, but is there evidence or does anyone believes it is possible to design vectors which will be targeted with some efficiency to specific organs or tissue types.

S. GOFF : I think there are lots of efforts to target retroviruses with altering receptors. Those are very preliminary efforts so far as I know like targeting to the liver. I think it will be done but it will take time.

R. CRYSTAL : The other strategy that can be used is direct targeting. In the lung it is easy because of the air but in the other organs one could do it with the arterial system. Catheters are available to do that kind of things. An alternative strategy is to use cell-specific promoters in such a way that if the gene is elsewhere it should not be expressed except in the right tissues where it is desired.

G. SUTHERS : In energy-deficiencies where every cell is suffering from the defect, how would you hope to target your gene correction to every cell in the body ? What about crossing the boundary of somatic cell therapy to germline therapy for young male where you are trying to transfect every cell in the body?

P. LEHN : I think one should not mix up germline gene therapy and intentional modification of germ cells ! Let me remind you that modifications of germline cells follow radiation and chemotherapy. In some cases perhaps we will have to store away unmodified germ cells before conducting the treatment.

T. CASKEY : I heard a person I love very much make the following comments : "Yes, he would carry out germline therapy if he could do it **safely**, if he could do it **efficiently** and he would **improve the health** of the individual".

So I think we should not rule it out as long as you have those kinds of qualifies on it !

T. CASKEY : Let's move on to the next subject.

8. D. HOUSSIN : "Gene Transfer and liver cells".

The first thing I want to say is that each time I perform liver transplantation for children with Crigler-Najjar's syndrome, OTC deficiency or hyperoxaluria, I really feel that the treatment I am doing looks like an oversize treatment. This is the reason why I am very optimistic about the prospect of gene therapy.

Before going into my numerous slides, I want to thank Professor BOIRON and Odile for inviting a surgeon to this meeting though I am afraid to be the only one. And second I want to thank Odile for having acted as a middle woman between a group of liver surgery and a group of gene surgeons namely Jean-Michel HEARD, Olivier DANOS and Nicolas FERRY.

I would like to underline that the liver is a very interesting target organ (as you know) for gene therapy. It is a very large and very heavy organ. There are two main types of cells : hepatocytes which are very numerous and sinusoidal cells including Kupffer cells. Liver has a central role in human metabolism. It has something to do with some kind of a Japonese factory !

The first potential indication of liver gene therapy which is certainly utopian at present is the correction of susceptibility to alcohol toxicity. I don't know anything about genes but I suspect it might be possible. One should also include prevention of immune damage by modification of antigen expression which could avoid liver transplantation for viral or auto-immune diseases. There is also Alpha 1 antitrypsin deficiency because to me it is mainly a liver disease and I was very happy to hear yesterday that it was not restricted to the liver. The fourth one would be Wilson's disease. To get closer to potential developments of gene therapy let us now consider the treatment of liver-based enzyme abnormalities with extra-hepatic complications, mainly Crigler-Najjar's syndrome, and urea cycle deficiencies, together with hyperoxaluria, hypercholesterolemia, hemophilia, protein C deficiency and other metabolic storage diseases. But we also have to consider that liver could be used in the future as a factory manufacturing products which will then be excreted in blood-circulation. This would concern diseases which are not related to basic liver cell deficiency.

I will continue with a few words concerning technical matters. In terms of liver cells there are two possibilities. The first one is to take hepatocytes and isolate them from a piece of a resected liver. Then transfect cells in vitro and reimplant them in the same patient. It does not seem to be at present an efficient method, because transfected cells do not seem to be easily reimplantable.

That is the reason why we decided to test a second approach which is in vivo gene transfer using selective liver perfusion. You heard about this work yesterday (see FERRY et al, this issue) and I will not say anything about it. I just would like to emphasize that this probably is a field in which gene surgeons and surgeons meet. Surgeons are able to reach some of the specific requirements of gene therapy such as reimplantation of autologous cells at a proper site and mainly the specific targeting of a vector to an organ without infecting other organs ; the latter consisting in what we are trying to do with selective perfusion of the liver.

I will end in giving out a great concern of mine : one should keep in mind that if it happens that gene therapy fails, further liver transplantation might be necessary. The virus you will choose for the transfer should thus be compatible with the potential administration of immunosuppressive drugs further along. I was a bit worried by the use of adenoviruses since we have lost patients due to severe adenovirus infection following liver transplantation. That is all I wanted to say. Thank you.

T.CASKEY : I would like to ask a technical point on these new procedures of taking portions of liver and to do transplantations with portions of liver. And I wanted to ask what happens to the residual liver from the donor. Does it go into a rapid replication and expansion like the rat and the mouse where when you take out a lobe you suddenly see the liver expand ?

D.HOUSSIN : The process of liver regeneration is quite fast. Probably not as fast in man as it is in animals ; particularly in animals when you do a very large resection which you can't do in man because the risk of liver function impairment is too high. The regeneration rate is very fast. If you do a partial liver resection in a patient with a normal liver, a normal volume is restored within a few days or weeks.

T.CASKEY : Could I ask also ; there have been trophic factors isolated in Japan for stimulating hepatic growth. Are any of these growth factors in clinical trials at this point ?

D.HOUSSIN : Well. At the moment they are not used on patients but it is very promising since these factors could be added to some kind of minor liver resection in order to enhance regeneration and put the cells in the proper conditions to be targeted by a retrovirus vector.

T.CASKEY : We are going to move on to Cystic Fibrosis : **Ron Crystal**

9. R. CRYSTAL : Cystic Fibrosis

It is obvious for Cystic Fibrosis that all we need to do in the affected cells is to convert them to the heterozygote state since the heterozygotes do not have a significant disease. What I will outline here are some of the questions regarding gene therapy for Cystic Fibrosis and what are the hurdles that really have to be overcome. Is it feasible, yesterday we saw that it is feasible to transfer the genes, we also talked about safety. So what I would like to concentrate on are the other questions : 1°- which epithelial cells express the CFTR gene ; 2°- which of those epithelial cells require CFTR and how much do we have to get in ; 3°- and most importantly is modulation necessary ?

If you look at the tracheobronchial tree which is where CF manifests in its lethal form, what you see is a complex epithelium made up primarily of five cell types. The most common cell in the upper airway is the ciliated cell which is the terminally differenciated cell. There is the basal cell and there are serous cells and globlet cells which are mucus producing cells and then there is an undifferenciated cell which may in fact be the stem-cell for the other kind of ciliated cells.

The current evidence suggests that all these cells probably express CFTR. What is not known however is which cells require this chloride channel to revert the phenotype that we see clinically. We don't know whether it is all of these cells or a limited group of the cells. For example, the whole disease may be because these mucus producing cells, the serous cells and the goblet cells both on the surface and in the glands, may be critically dependent on CFTR, whereas these other cells may use it but not critically depend on it.

Having said all that, the initial strategies probably would be to try to put the gene in all of the cells. We have to keep this in mind. In addition, quantitative analysis of the amounts of CFTR show that there are only one or two copies average in these cells. So the job for gene therapy is not that difficult to overcome.

Most importantly, what I thought we would focus on in terms of discussion, because we haven't talked a lot about it in terms of gene therapy in general is will we have to allow the gene to be modulated in vivo ? For the strategies we have heard of mostly throughout this meeting, the genes are beeing put in with various kinds of viral promoters and other constitutive promoters so that we can see expression. But in fact, all these various genes are controlled and this may not be critically important for alpha-1-antitrypsin deficiency or ADA for example, but obviously it is critically important for the hemoglobins and may be important for CFTR.

If we look at the 5' region of CFTR, it turns out that it has the characteristics of a house-keeping like gene. It has no TATA box, it has a high G-C content, the very short fragments of a hundred base pairs will support transcription. We know from directly looking at transcription run-on in nuclei isolated from human bronchi, the transcription rate is very low compared to other genes. In addition, there is a variety of putative binding sites for all a variety of factors like SP1 sites, AP1, glucocorticoids, cyclic-AMP responsive elements. We know we can downregulate the gene either with phorbol-esters for example, or by mobilizing intra-cellular calcium. So the gene is modulatable. The question is "are we going to have to do gene therapy with a promoter that allows it to be modulated" ?

In summary, in terms of the various questions, I think that the most critical questions to consider for cystic fibrosis in addition to the safety question is going to be the question of modulation, is it necessary ? Putting together constructs with the cystic fibrosis promoter is not hard but the question is : Is it going to be necessary to do that ?

Thank you.

T.CASKEY : Open for discussion. Well the other hard question about this, Ron, is that it took quite some time for these regulatory elements in the hemoglobin locus to be discovered. We've had experience on the OTC locus finding an element another 1500 base pairs to 5' which is important. So to discover whether you have all the regulatory elements in your constructs is really a difficult issue. The gene may work ; but whether it really works properly is not easy.

R.CRYSTAL : There may be in the lung an advantage for gene therapy in that we could do it in a limited segment, such as one lobe for example and then see if there is any problem. Perhaps using transient systems rather than permanent, may be one stategy in case we do get into problems.

J.L. MANDEL : Is it still true that patients who carry null mutations are actually better off than patients with just the Δ F 508. Does this suggest things towards gene therapy or other therapies ?

R.CRYSTAL : This is a good question ! There has been two and maybe three cases of compound heterozygotes nulls in the field. Both have been caught in their twenties and they have both mild respiratory disease which has led to this concept that may be we could downregulate the gene, create the null state and may be the patients would be better off. But still two cases are anecdotal compared to the thousands of others and we don't know. What we can do is to shut down or at least markedly decrease transcription of the gene by at least two different methods : phorbol-esters probably through AP1 and by mobilization of intra-cellular calcium. So there might be pharmacologic ways to do it as well as gene therapy projects if that holds up.

O.COHEN-HAGUENAUER : I am afraid I will be a little provocative ! What do you think about alternative treatments of CF, speaking of drug-therapy rather than gene therapy itself ?

R.CRYSTAL : Well there are many strategies which have been used for cystic fibrosis. What has been the standard is to try to mobilize the secretions and antibiotics. What is coming along now is : recombinant aerosolized DNAases to cleave the DNA in sputtum and that helps the patient ; anti-proteases like alpha-1-antitrypsin to protect the epithelium ; antioxidants and also there is a study with amiloride which blocks sodium reabsorption which is suggested in short terms that it is a help ; it may be possible to try to modulate ion movements and do it pharmacologically. My guess is that it is going to be a lot harder than that ; and I think all these things should go on in parallel.

Another strategy has been considered which is basically to produce the protein in vitro and to aerosolize the protein so that it can be inserted in the membrane.

I think that this is so complex that we should go on along all these paths including gene therapy.

P. LEHN : What about RNAs into liposomes ?

R.CRYSTAL : Yes ; I think that trying to get the gene or something distal to that by any means is very rational.

O.COHEN-HAGUENAUER : When do you think that gene therapy should be done or be started in the course of the disease, or rather when that will be available, at what age should the treatment begin ?

R.CRYSTAL : I would think at a very early age. There has been now a variety of studies to see what is going on in the lung ; and it is certainly very early. It should probably be done around the age of one, before the age of three or four. I think a very early age would be ideal.

T.CASKEY : I would just like to make one point about the alpha 1. It is an acute reactive protein and one might imagine that it needs to be under regulation to be able to accomodate acute infectious disease of the lung.

R.CRYSTAL : That's been a concept in the field but there's been no clinical evidence that people with acute infections have any more lung damage. But you're right and perhaps the ideal way for that would be to be under an appropriate promoter.

T.CASKEY : We are making a switch here, we are going to move on to **Jean-Louis MANDEL** and he is going to discuss the latest developments out of his laboratory on the fragile X syndrome.

10. J.L.MANDEL : Fragile X syndrome

Some time ago, I guessed it was a joke to talk about fragile-X therapy. But I will present very shortly what we know about it and then try to think about what are the prospects for gene therapy.

Everybody used to consider fragile X syndrome as a favorite disease since it appeared to be one of the most frequent ones. This at least is the most frequent X-linked disease ; it affects one in 1500 male and there is one in about 2000 females with mild or moderate mental retardation due to fragile-X. So it is a very significant disease.

It appears as a chromosomal disease, and one would not have thought of gene therapy until now since the diagnosis is based on the presence of a fragile site on the X-chromosome ; the latter being induced by deoxynucleotides stress, like Fudr or, antifolates such as methotrexate.

A bizarre characteristic of this disease is that pedigree analyses have shown that a significant proportion of males carrying the mutation, at least 20%, have no clinical or even cytogenetic phenotype ; and these are called normal transmitting males.

So I will just shortly comment on recent results. I think that the most significant with respect to potential targets for gene therapy is that actually it might be a true monogenic disorder. The mutation might affect a single or at most two genes, according to our data.

The basis for this is that we and now others have observed that there is a single CpG-rich island which is methylated in affected males but is not methylated in normal transmitting males. Since it is known that methylation at a CpG-island, at least on the X-chromosome, is observed in the inactive X, it is most certain that the presence of such a methylation alters the expression of an adjacent gene, or maybe two adjacent genes at most. The region is now cloned. This fragile site which one could have thought as a very large segment, just because you can see it on a mitotic chromosome, is less than 100 kb long as shown by in situ hybridization. It might even be shorter than this.

So the target gene or couple of genes will certainly be identified very soon. Prospects for therapy will thus depend on the nature of the gene. If we are pessimistic we can think about a situation similar to that of Lesh Nyhan's disease, and it is going to be very difficult. On the other hand, we can be optimistic and speculate that it will ressemble phenylketonuria, and be easily accessible to therapy. But we have to wait for fragile-X gene identification.

Since there is a methylation problem, I will suggest as proposed several years ago for sickle-cell anemia and this is pretty much of a joke we could try azacytidine ; but I would in fact not push too strongly in favour of this !

T.CASKEY : What is the fragile site encoding for ?

J.L.MANDEL : I don't think that the fragile site is encoding a gene. The site is in a region where a gene might be located since CpG islands are associated to functional and expressed genes in general ; and in this particular case, the island is methylated on the inactive chromosome X, and not methylated on the active one.

D. GRAUSZ : What are the prospects for population screening ?

J.L.MANDEL : It probably looks pretty good in the near future. There might be ethical problems ; this should be discussed.

T.CASKEY : Actually, that is a good point, Jean-Louis. If you use DNA-based tests to identify diseases, you know that for this disorder you will be involved in some presymptomatic or in fact perhaps asymptomatic positives.

J.L.MANDEL : Yes, on the ethical point of view, there is just a problem ; there could be one very puzzling thought if you can detect non-transmitting males. The problem with these non transmitting males is their grand-children who have high risks of beeing affected ; so you will say to a kid : "when you will be grand father, you may have problems!"

T.CASKEY : This first of all is a very common disorder of extreme interest to quite a number of investigator groups ; undoubtedly this is going to be a complex disease to understand ; it will be a quite interesting story to follow.

11. T. CASKEY : I have been asked to make some comments on Duchenne Muscular Dystrophy.

I would like to make a few comments about what we should be targeting for gene transfer therapy for this disease.
The first point that I will make is fairly obvious with something like sixty or seventy percent of the body mass beeing represented by muscle tissue.
An effective means of gene transfer therapy that will be employed for this disease must have a very high efficiency delivery system. It is very clear in the case of Duchenne Muscular Dystrophy, the most severe phenotype of mutations in the Dystrophin locus, that one can have profound skeletal muscle disorder and then, at a later stage, profound cardiomyopathy with the disorder. So it is not just a matter of correcting just skeletal muscle ; one would, at some point have to deal with the cardiac failure problems of the disorder.
I guess, from a strategic point of view, we should be searching for high efficiency delivery systems. I think that means the virus ; I don't see how it is going to be possible to achieve that without a viral delivery system ; this is my opinion, there may be others that are different from that. I you look at the available viral delivery systems that were discussed at this conference, you heard discussion of use of the retrovirus, and the limitations of the retrovirus in its ability to package a wild type full-length dystrophin minigene.

But we have also heard of the possibility of truncating the dystrophin minigene such that less required components of the dystrophin sequence could be taken out and yet they would be an adequate phenotypic correction of the defect by such constructs. I think that it is a very interesting approach ; now there are some clinical evidence that would suggest that it might be done. But we should use caution in that strategy because we know that dystrophin is a very large molecule and does not have a singular function, since a number of associated proteins bind to dystrophin. So we are very early in the game of trying to understand structure-function relationships of dystrophin to be able to predict exactly what we could miss out and what we should include. It is early ; the strategy may work but it is one that I think needs to be monitored very carefully in terms of function.

I know of only one way to test that, and it is going to be in an intact animal and that will be transgenic since one can look only biochemical features in cultured cells. I think the ultimate test will be : "Can you correct the mouse ?".

I would make a single comment about the truncation approach : I put forward in my presentation the argument that the challenge should be to come up with a viral vector system that can accommodate full-length dystrophin and that is in the least hazardous or at least likely to fail approach for a therapeutic strategy. I will be quick to point out though that we now know that dystrophin is an extensively, alternatively spliced product. We do not understand at the present time the natural variants of dystrophin and how they influence specific cardiac functions ; and how they affect specific groups of skeletal muscle ; and so it is uncertain, even at this time, that we know exactly what type of full length wild type minigene is optimal ; the one that I talked about in my presentation is in fact the full length adult skeletal muscle but we know that there are alternative forms that operate in cardiac tissue ; so it is not certain at all that particular construct will in fact correct the phenotypic features of late onset cardiomyopathy for the disorder. So these are my comments on what we need in terms of understanding about have a truncated and alter the cDNAs for gene-transfer strategies.

Let me point out a few other features of Muscular Dystrophy which are confounding ; we should better pay attention to these, because in these confounding observations may be some very important new facts about this disease.

We discussed at some length, Lesh-Nyhan's syndrome and the knock-out of the HPRT gene not giving any phenotype for the disease. Well, you could exercise mdx-mice at a pretty hefty rate and not be very impressed that these animals were badly damaged.

They have a nonsense mutation which eliminates the production of the protein ; the latter is virtually non detectable by immunological techniques and yet, they are able to function rather well. How does that alternative functioning take place ? We do not have an understanding of why the mouse is protected from the loss of this particular expressed sequence. But in understanding that particular point, we may learn more about structure-function features of Duchenne Muscular Dystrophy. For those of you not in the field, there are possibilities of alternative froms of Dystrophin that might be having influence on this phenotype.

The other point that I would make is that I'm not sure that we really understand in man the correlation between clinical features and the actual mutations that exist within the gene. I think that have probably been some misleading papers in the litterature on this, going from deletion studies to predicting structural proteins. A number are probably going to be proven incorrect because you know from the case of beta-thalassemias, alternative splicing is a common event ; so you cannot just look at deletion pictures and predict what has been made by transcript. There was however new technology that was reported out of London last year which I thought was extremely interesting ; it is the ability to take lymphoblasts from patients that had these particular mutations and actually study the sequence of the messenger RNA made on the mutants.

Perhaps out of study of these unusual human examples of variants of the Dystrophin locus we will also come to understand the various structure-function features of the dystrophin molecule.

So there is a great deal to be learned out about this diseases. The challenge is fairly great for high efficiency delivery of the gene ; and we need to know what gene to deliver.

I will stop at that point. Any comments ?

G. SUTHERS : There is one other point too about delivery ; we got in the dis of another disease entity discussion at this meeting ; we talked about delivery are we going to deliver to the myofibrilla or are we going to deliver to the regenerating cells? And that of course is really an unanswered question at the present time ; do we know how to deliver to the regenerating cell ? the alive satellite or stem type.

L. LUZZATTO : I just thought that there is a very interesting developmental correlate there, because I think the evidence in the heterozygote is that because of fusion of myoblasts in normal muscle production, there is fusion of nuclei with either X chromosome beeing inactive. As a result, there are much fewer fibers affected in heterozygotes than you would have otherwise. I wonder if you could take that into account when thinking of gene therapy.

Dr. IOANNOU : Could you please comment on the possibilities of prevention through neonatal screening either by CK and then combination with multiplex.

T.CASKEY : In Germany and may be other places including France, there is a very cheap test that can be run which is CK, it is a fairly accurate screening test, it does not cost very much money ; you can separate out affected children from the wild type population pretty accurately.

You could cascade that with a DNA-based test very easily since a large proportion of the muscular dystrophy cases are either duplications or deletions; with the current multiplex PCR technology it should be possible for five or ten dollars of oligonucleotides and one PCR reaction to be able to confirm it at the genotype level. So I think it theoretically could be done ; but now what have you achieved by that ; you have achieved detection at the newborn phase for a disease that you do not have therapy for. So the hope is that some new technology comes forward which is useful.

For the family, there may be benefit in that a very high percentage of the mothers or even gonade mosaics are non-carriers for the defect. It would prevent perhaps the family carrying on with their family addition without knowledge that they already had one child with this disease. I can think of four families in which I have made the diagnosis of the affected child and the mother was pregnant in the room at the same time. We had the two things at once to ask. Perhaps we could have influence on that.

I guess if I were going to implement since it is a new mutation disease, if I were to have a very cheap and highly accurate testing method I would use it in utero. I would offer screening at the in utero phase since it is a new mutation event in many families and offer the mother the option in the prenatal diagnostic testing mode. That is fairly theoritical I guess.

Yes, go ahead Jean-Louis :

J.L. MANDEL : I would like to ask one question and to make one comment. Delivery of the DMD gene to a single muscle already seems very difficult but indeed what about aiming at every muscle and are there more important muscles that we should try to target first, like diaphragma for instance ?

T. CASKEY : I guess each muscular dystrophy patient if I ask this question might have different answers, but it would be my impression that the real bond state which comes on early for these children is the one that is most immediately disturbing so I would say skeletal muscle would be my first priority target based upon what I hear from patients. The cardiomyopathy disorder is a later onset disorder ; it is managed quite nicely by non invasive techniques for many years and now with very successful ability to do cardiac transplantation, one might envision that if you don't have a therapy for the heart, you might consider transplanting hearts in these individuals. There have been a couple of Duchenne patients that have received heart transplants.

M. BOIRON : Could we envisage direct transfusion of genes into the arteries for example ?

T. CASKEY : We certainly could envision that!!!

J.L. MANDEL : Another comment is related to one which has been made on CF and deals with when should the treatment be started ? It should certainly be performed at a stage where the child is still doing well ; since a recent paper (Cecilia Webster and Helen Blau. Somatic Cell Mol Genet 16 : 557-565, 1990) has demonstrated that in a 5 five years old normal child the myoblasts still have a potential of 56 doublings ; in Duchenne patients of the same age few myoblasts achieve more that 10 doublings. This will also be the problem with autologous transplantation since the potential for regeneration is already almost exhausted when the child is four or five.

T. CASKEY : That is a very interesting point. We have a clinical protocol which is active now at the Texas children's hospital. The protocol is as follows : children are brought in, they undergo open muscle biopsy ; muscle cells are taken out, shipped to Helen. Helen sorts for satellite which return to us for transfer. There is no proposal at this point to go back into the patient with the corrected myoblasts ; based on this paper and this experience, we have targeted on children less than one year of age with this disease.

She thinks that it is unlikely that there will be an adequate number of satellites just to make recovery from the muscle to do any experiments at all.

If you extrapolate that to let's not take satellite cells, but develop a gene replacement therapy which is going to use a vector ; I bet you that Helen's data is correct that the regenerating cell is at low count number; they are depleted in the patients with advancing disease.

If you follow this through, you might predict that Duchenne Muscular Dystrophy children are going to need to be treated prior to the age of one when the size of the child is small, the numbers of satellite cells are large or highest than in their life time and therefore have the highest likelihood of success. These are all uncertain issues, but I think that that paper of Helen's is an important one to pay attention to.

Let's move on to the next speaker : J. MALLET

12. J. MALLET : "CNS and Neurons"

Gene transfer experiments together with cell grafting can be envisaged in a number of neurological diseases such as Parkinson's disease, Alzheimer's, Huntington's together with spinal cord injury as well as epilepsy.

But most studies have focused on Parkinson's disease which is characterized by the disappearance of dopaminergic cells in the substantia nigra. Interestingly, the functional consequences are observed only when up to 80% of the cells have disappeared. This observation highlights the adaptive ability of the nervous system. Now remarkably, L. Dopa therapy has proven very effective in treating the disease; as if dopaminergic cells were only acting as mini-pumps to deliver Dopamine, since Dopa is locally transformed into Dopamine. This also raises the question as for the role of synapses in the functioning of this system. However Dopa-therapy is not as effective as time goes on ; besides this treatment has many side effects and is ineffective in particular patients. One aspect of Parkinson's disease is the availability of animal models ; for example, dopaminergic cells of substantia nigra can be locally destroyed by injection of the 6-hydroxy-dopamine toxin ; the degree of degenerescence of the substantia nigra pathway can be ascertained.

Functional recovery has been observed a few years ago, and more recently by A.Bjorklund using grafts of fetal cells originating from substantia nigra. However, a hierarchy in the degrees of recovery is observed ; it appears that it is correlated with the presence of functional synapses.

So synapses might be involved to some extent in the recovery. Graft experiments have also been done in human, with some success ; however, there are some problems with this therapy : 1st) there are very few dopaminergic cells.

2nd) the availability of such fetal tissue is problematic. 3rd) ethical issues also have to be considered.

So this is where engineered cells come into play. The strategy consists into taking particular types of cells and engineering them so that they produce L. Dopa or Dopamine, and to test functional recovery after grafting. In fact, this strategy will allow to define what is required for a full functional recovery ; the role of synapses could also be assessed.

A series of experiments have demonstrated the usefulness of genetically modified cells in animal models of Parkinson's disease.

In a first set of experiments, several cell lines (in Fred Gage's lab and Philippe Horellou in our lab), have shown the possibility of transfecting or infecting NIH 3T3 cells which then produce Dopa or AtT 20 cells or RIN cells which derive from pituitary gland and the pancreas respectively which not only produce Dopa but also Dopamine, since those cells express Dopa-decarboxylase. But most interestingly in those cells, we observe a regulated release of Dopamine, which means that this release is greatly increased following depolarization with potassium. We also observe in vivo release of Dopa and Dopamine from genetically engineered cells after grafting in denervated rat-striatum; the functional recovery interestingly, is more efficient with Dopa producing cells than with Dopamine producing cells. Thus Dopamine seems to be quickly degraded before it can reach its target whereas Dopa can be transported and locally transformed into Dopamine and therefore reach its target site. This is the first lesson we can draw from this first series of experiments.

Ongoing research is devoted to the immortalization of stem cells derived from the central nervous system with SV40 large antigen to avoid tumor formation when using cell lines ; this has been performed by several groups including Pierre Rouget's, who has immortalized mouse embryonic striatal cells; although they are immortalized, these cells have kept the capacity for cell contact inhibition, and do not grow tumors after grafting. R. Mc Kay's group has also immortalized cells from hippocampal and cerebellar origin using temperature sensitive oncogenes so that there is no way that tumors might be formed.

Recently R. Mc Kay has demonstrated that stem cells which are the precursors for neurons, can be stimulated to proliferate under the influence of specific growth factors, such as basic FGF (Fibroblast Growth Factor), and NGF (Nerve Growth Factor). A combination of these two factors is needed to stimulate the proliferation. So one possibility could be to grow cells in Petri-dishes with these factors, to infect them and finally graft these manipulated cells and allow them to differentiate.

In fact, if one withdraws the combination of FGF and NGF, the cells will differenciate to a neuronal phenotype. These procedures might lead to synapse formation which will be more adequate for optimal interactions between the graft and the host.

Although brain is a privileged tissue as far as immunological rejection is concerned, cyclosporine A still has to be administered in the experiments we have carried so far.

The next step would be to use autologous cells ; Fred Gage and coll have just published a paper showing primary cultures of fibroblasts followed by transfection whith an expression vector carrying Tyrosine-Hydroxylase. These cells survive after grafting, while they do express Dopa, at least during ten weeks.

An alternative method could consist in the use of hepatocytes since these cells express co-factors for Tyrosine-Hydroxylase which would then be convenient to express Dopa.

In our lab, with Philippe Horellou, we have chosen to grow astrocytes in vitro and modify them to produce Dopa and Dopamine. Grafting experiments are under ways to test the ability of those cells to survive and to compensate for the dopaminergic system cell deficit.

Another possibility which has also been addressed by Alfred Geller during this present meeting (see A. GELLER, this issue) is the use of viruses which infect non-dividing cells such as herpes-viruses ; we have also paid attention to adenovirus-derived vectors, which might be good candidates for these studies.

The next point to be addressed will be the regulation of neurotransmitter and release. Shall we be able in the long term to modulate in vivo the expression and the release ? If the grafting happened to turn wrong, a good point would be to be able to kill the cells in order to get rid of the burden of the graft if its effect happened to be deleterious.

One should also consider growth factors and we know about NGF and Alzheimer's disease. Recently, brain derived nerved growth factors have been shown to play an important role in dopaminergic cells survival.

So, an alternative strategy would be to provide BDNF to the striatum ; the problem in human would be to identify the proper type for BDNF injection, since 80% of the cells are destroyed when symptoms appear.

The next point to consider is how shall we also extend this therapy to other diseases such as Alzheimer's ? This also is under way using NGF producing cells.

Could we thus also help in case of Huntington, spinal cord injuries which in most cases lack the innervation from serotoninergic cells of the brain ? Finally, one should also consider the use of GABA producing cells in case of severe epilepsy.

P. LEHN : What would happen if you provoke an ectopic production of Dopa ?

J.MALLET : That's an interesting question ; at the present time, we just don't know ! It will depend on the development stage. If you have an ectopic production of Dopa or Dopamine during development you might ruin the organization of the nervous system. Such an ectopic production could be tried using transgenic technology. In adults, the synapses are more stabilized and there should be limited and less deleterious effects than in the young animal.

O.COHEN-HAGUENAUER : I would like to know how you will manage to infect CNS cells with adeno or herpes derived vectors ; in vivo, ex vivo ? Could you comment on this ?

J.MALLET : One possibility is to inject the viruses locally using stereotaxic pinpointing of the striatum ; and see whether the virus will be taken up by striatal cells and whether Dopa and/or Dopamine production will follow. We will know indeed whether some recovery could be achieved that way.

O.COHEN-HAGUENAUER : Sure, but CNS cells have already involuted at the time of clinical appearance of the disease.

J.MALLET : Yes, but if Dopamine is produced ectopically, it might still provide functional recovery of some behavioural disorders, in particular. There is a hierarchy in functional recovery ; some improvement is observed when Dopa or Dopamine are secreted locally ; the next step could be achieved through the reconstitution of part of the circuits, of some synapses. To me this could only be achieved using the stem cells and allow them to differenciate following grafting.

L.LUZZATTO : So there seems to be an important distinction between those conditions where you could really restore the production of neurotransmitters as opposed to conditions where there is an abnormality in the cell function in a more subtle way which has to do with each cell doing its job. It does not seem that you would consider this successful at the moment.

J.MALLET : Yes, right now we can address the question of Dopa or Dopamine production. The next step will be to try to build the circuitry and to have each cell do its own work.

L.LUZZATTO : Thank you. We will move on to the last presentation concerning ethical questions.

13. P. LEHN : "Scientific and ethical points to consider for the design of clinical trials of human gene therapy".

Until now, we heard a lot about the different methods of gene transfer and also about the potential applications of gene therapy in clinical medicine. I would now like to address the following question : "when and how to go from the laboratory to the clinic ?"

In the United States, a document entitled "Points to consider in the design and submission of human somatic cell gene therapy protocols" was developped by the Human Gene Therapy Subcommitte (HGTS) of the NIH Recombinant DNA Advisory Committee (RAC). It is intended to provide guidance for investigators preparing proposals for clinical trials. Also in Europe, both the European Parliamentary Assembly in Strasbourg and the European Medical Research Councils made statements about the guidelines for the conduct of research on gene therapy in man.

In a few minutes, I cannot discuss all the different points addressed in these documents but I would like to highlight some specific points and also raise a few questions, especially when looking at gene therapy in a very large perspective.

First, I would like to emphasize that, in the US, the meetings of the review committees are open to the public. Thus, the public can get direct information not only on the technical aspects of the proposals but also on the meaning and the long-range effects of the research.

Indeed, the broad membership of these review boards ensures a comprehensive approach to the full range of scientific, ethical and social issues raised by gene therapy.

Somatic-cell gene therapy for genetic diseases has the same goal as all other forms of treatment : the treatment of a single patient without risks to other persons or to the environment.

Thus, ethical issues are here very much identical to those raised by other new therapeutic approaches. As usual the review committee will have to seek evidence that the potential benefits to the patient outweigh the potential risks.

When considering the rationale of a proposal, one has to compare the proposed gene therapy with the existing alternative therapies. Thus, one can wonder how much information about gene therapy will be required, will be necessary when there is no alternative treatment. For example, for the treatment of muscular diseases, is it acceptable to use an in vivo transfection technique (like liposomes) knowing that the fate of the transferred DNA is then highly unpredictable, as integration is rare and leads to an unpredictable and even unstable structure ? Direct in vivo gene transfer (by a viral vector or a physical method) could also have an unintentional and undesirable consequence : the genetic modification of germline cells. Thus, in order to avoid the vertical transmission of these unwanted genetic changes, should one require the storage of unmodified germ cells before beginning the gene therapy treatment ? This situation appears to be somehow similar to the present situation in cancer patients undergoing radiation or chemotherapy.

The document "Points to consider" also deals with public-health considerations. It is in general expected that the recombinant DNA will be confined to the patient. Thus, a major question is the following : "is there a significant likelihood that the recombinant DNA will spread from the patient to other persons or to the environment ? Thus, for example, can one consider the use of a replication-defective viral vector possibly rescued and propagated (eventually from the patient to healthy persons) during a natural infection by the corresponding wild-type virus, as it could be the case for adenovirus vectors (in particular when used in the treatment of lung diseases) ?

In addition to its "correction" objective, gene therapy can also allow to transfer a new gene into a genetically normal cell to provide it with new properties. Indeed, gene transfer can also be considered as a very sophisticated pharmacologic method. For example, one could use genetically modified endothelial cells to secrete anti-clotting factors to inhibit local thrombosis.

Gene therapy can also be used as a tool for increasing the efficacy of other forms of treatment, as it is the case with immunotherapy, when TIL cells are engineered to express proteins (such as tumor necrosis factor) that contribute to the destruction of tumor masses.

I would like to stress that it seems to me that this kind of gene therapy can best be described as "enhancement somatic-cell gene therapy". However, it should be noted that it is still very different from the enhancement of a "general" human characteristic like intelligence, which appears technically unrealistic and would raise many new ethical problems. The previous considerations lead to emphasize that gene transfer is intrinsically different from transplantation.

Indeed, transplantation can only transplant natural cells and therefore remains limited to the correction of a defect. Only genetic engineering can allow to modify a somatic cell in order to enhance a specific function.

Finally, I would like to point out that diverse regulation authorities in the US and in Europe have concluded that it would be unethical to withhold somatic-cell gene therapy solely because it could lead to the development of techniques for germ line gene therapy or for enhancement genetic engineering. Although genetic modification of germ cells is at present still unrealistic, it will raise new ethical issues in the future, issues for which there is at present no consensus. Some, like T. FRIEDMANN, ask : "ought we to consider enhancing some particularly useful traits ?" Others, like Jean DAUSSET (who is the president of the Universal Movement for Scientific Responsability), see a darker side and suggest that : "Human genetic inheritance, given our present level of knowledge, should not be modified".

Obviously, the field of gene therapy still needs ethical exploration. However, it remains the responsibility of the regulation authorities to ensure the application of the agreed guidelines.

L.LUZZATTO : Thank you Doctor LEHN for highlighting a check-list. I like especially the point you made that new form of therapy should be no less stringent than of any other form of therapy but still it should be kept in perspective. Are there any questions or comments ?

M. PERRICAUDET : Indeed, I would like to comment on the possibility of recovering a recombinant adeno-virus which would be able to propagate by itself. We have to know that there is an upper limit for packaging viral DNA into an adenovirus capsid. Most of our recombinants reach this upper limit. Which means that if you want to recover essential genes for propagation, i.e.

E1a and E1b genes, the virus has to choose between either the foreign genes or other genes which are also essential for the virus to propagate. So, it is strictly impossible to recover a recombinant adenovirus which will be able to propagate itself.

The other point to consider is the situation where a patient who carries a recombinant adenovirus and is later superinfected by a wild type adenovirus. Will trans-complementation by the wild-type occur ? To me this is a more serious question. In order to eliminate this possibility mutated packaging sequences will be used and allow the counterselection of the defective virus versus the wild-type which co-infects the cell.

P.LEHN : Obviously what I said only addressed the second situation where you get infected by a wild type virus ; and even more restricted to the treatment of lung diseases since the lung is the natural tropism of adenoviruses. You could indeed get a copackaging of the recombinant by the wild-type. I am not speaking here of a recombination event.

M. BOIRON : I am surprised that we have not raised at all the question of potential side effects of retroviruses such as insertional mutagenesis. Is it a pure theoretical danger ?

O. DANOS : I think that if we use helper-free virus, retro-viral insertion will not be more deleterious than any other piece of DNA that you would insert in the genome by any means. So of course, the probability for oncogenic insertion is not null, but I would say that in the absence of propagation and subsequent reinfection it is very low. As a matter of fact, in animals receiving cells transduced with retroviruses, no insertional mutants have been observed in the absence of replication-competent virus. On a one hit event, this has not been detected yet.

L.LUZZATTO : But the frequency could be of the order of ten to the minus five and there might not have been enough events studied yet.

M. BOIRON : Especially when you deal with young children.

P. LEHN : We can not quantify this risk at present ; nevertheless it probably is extremely low. In addition, retroviruses are supposed to be used in severe diseases.

O. DANOS : We could state on the fact that according to this weak probability, the risk could be acceptable.

L.LUZZATTO : I think we are where the debate should be. I think it would be dangerous for us to say that there is no risk. Claudine JUNIEN has reminded us of the multistep nature of carcinogenesis. Transduced mice might not have been followed up long enough to observe all these steps. So I think it is better to admit that there is a very low final risk and that is part of the side-effects that we may or may not be willing to accept depending on the severity of the condition being treated.

O.DANOS : We should clearly distinguish between two orders of risk : the first one concerning the patient, and the second addressing his environment.

D. HOUSSIN : If the risk is for cancer, I think we should compare the risk of cancer with retrovirus for gene therapy to the one following organ transplantation and immunosuppression which is not low.

L.LUZZATTO : Very good point.

D. LOWY : I think that there is a question about the risk to the environment, without getting into issues of whether there might be an infectious retrovirus which would come out. I just would point out that acute transforming retroviruses do not propagate epidemiologically under natural conditions ; for example in felines where there is often an activation and transduction of oncogenes that is a problem for the individual cat but the acute transforming retrovirus does not propagate. The same thing is true in avian species where transduction of the retrovirus src gene occurs with some frequency.

O.COHEN-HAGUENAUER : I just would have liked to ask Michael BLAESE to make some comments about the steps he had to overcome before performing his first trial in man.

M. BLAESE : In the United States, there is a formal process that involved for us presentations before seven different formal regulatory agencies with fourteen of fifteen presentations over a span of three years. It was a very painful process personally to go through. But I think it was very important for the Society to have their representatives hear the discussion of these experiments.

They were discussed widely with lots of controversy and lots of people taking shots. But I think they are all appropriate things because in the United States, the experiments have been accepted as beeing an appropriate use of medical technology and we really had a lot of support.

So it continues to be painful for people who have followed on; there are now five protocols working in their way through for marker gene studies. Each of them has undergone the same level of review that our original protocols went through. I hope it becomes simpler in the future.

P. LEHN : I have an additional question for Michael BLAESE. This treatment is so highly publicized that one might wonder how you can take care of both private matters and the confidentiality of the whole thing ?

M. BLAESE : That has been a major concern of ours over the years of trying to keep the confidentiality and the privacy of the patients involved. The press generally in the United States has respected our wish, according to each patient's family.

Dr. IOANNOU : One thing that has not been discussed is the attempt of transgenic animals. It seems alright as long as you apply it to mice and to some lower mammals. But as the work progresses in the next decade, I think we might see transgenic chimpanzees potentially carrying human genes giving a few human characteristics. Where should we put the limit to this work ?

L. LUZZATTO : Well, evolution and reverse. Unfortunately hemoglobin of gorilla already is only a single amino-acid difference from the human. Transgenic primates, that may be a problem !

D. HOUSSIN : I don't really see any problem ! We are in this situation since "Lucy" that means a million years before !

P. LEHN : I will add that we are far more concerned by human ES cells. This is a great question.

O. DANOS : The point is that you probably don't need to wait for human ES cells to manipulate the human germ line. I mean all the technology is already available. You said it would not be possible yet but I am sure that there is nothing easier than taking a human oocyte and inject DNA in it.

L.LUZZATTO : Since you mention that do you agree that we don't want to do that ?

M. BOIRON : Yes !

L.LUZZATTO to P. LEHN : I think you left out germline gene therapy out of your discussion. It may be that you don't want to make it explicit what you think about !

P.LEHN : I did not say that I would leave it out, I just said that I leave it open !

L.LUZZATTO : Oh ! You leave it open ?

P.LEHN : Yes ; at the end you have to follow the regulation authorities. They have to follows the ensure that it follows the guidelines.

L.LUZZATTO : But you are making a legal issue, whereas I would like to know your view on the ethics, not the legality of the bureaucracy. We are talking of the ethics.

O. DANOS : But it is the bureaucracy which is important !

P.LEHN : The ethics might be different for each one, you know ! That is the reason why I cited both Theodore FRIEDMANN and Jean DAUSSET.

L.LUZZATTO : I for instance think that we should not do it !

P.LEHN : At the present time ! But who knows ?

J.L.MANDEL : Well. I really don't see the point of doing it at least with the aim of treating genetic diseases. If we know that the early embryo is affected, we should merely choose another embryo which is normal ; since in vitro fertilization and embryo selection is essential for going to germline cells. This would just consist of a mere selection without adding any modification to the genome. There is no point, I guess, of improving a normal embryo by germline gene transfer ; I would very much like to know what character Theodore FRIEDMANN is thinking about ! May be the gene for Nobel Prize ? The nature of which has not been localized yet !

M. BOIRON : If you transfer the gene for Nobel Prize, I think there simply will be no more Nobel Prizes ! It really makes nonsense ! It is not interesting at all.

14. L. LUZZATTO : Concluding remarks

If there are no other points, then next topic on the Agenda has been made easy by the fact that we were supposed to finish at eleven and since it is already eleven past eleven I think that I actually have achieved one of the purposes of this session that is that there will be no time for the concluding remarks !

Your might have noticed that Tom CASKEY said he was nervous, now I don't know what his concept of nervousness is ; perhaps he has already gone back to report to his lab what is going on !

My concept of nervousness is that I felt very nervous when Professor BOIRON asked me to make the "Concluding Remarks". In fact I wrote him a note which said : "I would rather not, but if you insist !" and of course I got no reply !

So here I am. And who am I to tell you the concluding remarks when you've heard an excellent summary of what is going on ! I thought therefore I would take the opportunity to just first of all thank all the organizers and particularly Michel BOIRON and Odile COHEN-HAGUENAUER because they have invited us here and have given us the opportunity to discuss matters that are really exciting ; and also given us most gracious hospitality with a characteristic sophistication that we have all very much appreciated.

Now, as I was saying, what can I stand here and tell you ? I went back to the humanistic tradition of the organizers and I thought : "let me really understand if we got guidance from the past as to what we should do in terms of gene therapy" ? (If I can have the first slide please) :

> "C'est une folie à nulle autre seconde
> de vouloir se mêler à corriger le monde"
> Molière,
> Le Misanthrope.

In fact I found some inspiration in the French humanistic tradition that "there is no greater madness than to interfere and try to correct the world". (Applauses)

So from that point of view, it is a good start ; it is a good warning I think, that if we want to do it we should do it properly. That is what the end of the discussion has brought us about. I thought of the questions of gene transfer as opposed to gene therapy and I think that it is very important.

This meeting has illustrated that in a very interesting way ; namely that there are a variety of uses and possible applications of gene transfer. I thought that the most advanced are not necessarily those which have to do with the last bit.

New definition of the gene : Indeed gene transfer has been at the center of trying to understand gene function in a new way ; and this I think is beeing extremely important. In fact to the extent that it has made a new thinking of the very definition of the gene. The traditional concept of gene that we teach to the students is that it is the unit of recombination - the unit of mutation - and the functional unit. We have learned of course that these three units are not the same. But the functional unit can now be operationally defined because we can transfer the gene and test what happens ! It has given us some considerable difficulty in equating with any of the traditional concepts ; for instance, when we came to molecular genetics then the gene became the transcription unit. But now, it turns out that there are regulatory elements which may be quite distant from the transcription unit. So I would define the gene as that piece of DNA which is required for the encoding of a particular product and its appropriate regulation. By that definition, that is highly relevant to what we need for gene therapy in the end.

The first use of gene transfer has been the gene cloning itself. That has enabled us to know of the structural changes in a great variety of different conditions which are now understood at the molecular level.

New developments and homologous recombination : Certainly what I found to be an especially interesting development in the last couple of years, and we've had some beautiful examples here is homologous recombination. Didier HOUSSIN has already reminded us of the parallelism between surgery and genetic engeneering. I thought of the idea of specifically knocking off a gene, which has been around now for some years, is certainly the ultimate in surgery ; that is traditional physiology to find out the function of an organ you just remove the organ ; that sounded a bit crude. Now, when you want to know the function of a gene, you just remove the gene ! You come to observe phenotypes which are sometimes what yo expect and sometimes quite different from what you expect ; I found it rather endearing to hear that molecular biologists now describe clinical phenotypes just like clinicians ;

they get caught into the variable expression and must develop some kinds of affection for their patients whatever their species. Certainly, the ultimate is the question of variable penetrance which has always bewildered us ; we thought that it was due to the rest of the genome and to the environment. Now we find that in isogenic animals with the same gene ablated, you still have variability of clinical expression. I Think that it is a very good lesson !

The other thing that I found rather touching is the reporter gene bêta galactosidase ; there are enough young people in the audience who probably would not remember that it is the system which led MONOD and JACOB in this country to develop the whole concept of gene regulation in the operon and the concept of the messenger RNA. So I think it is very nice that the blue colour is still coming useful in modern gene transfer.

As for gene expression we've heard some very telling examples of regulation. The beta-globin locus remains the kind of leading example, almost the reference point for every other system. In terms of the question of models of disease ; I have already mentioned that this is a complete new development whether it is by knocking off a gene or by introducing a gene from another species ; but the creation of these new models is also been preeminent in this meeting and that is now to me an almost awesome prospect because the potential is practically limitless. Practically for every gene and every disease there is the technology to do this ; we will have to be quite carefull in writing grants and persuading the granting agencies to what should be done because there is almost a bewildering possible variety of combinations.

Means of gene transfer : Well, the question of how to do gene transfer is also actually quite interesting from many points of view. The words that are used, the phraseology is also a very important point. There are different ways of operating gene transfer. One is called the calcium phosphate precipitate method ; it is very much like presenting to the cell something that looks quite nice which they take up ; it contains something that they did not quite expect, just like nitrogen-gas ? Phraseology is quite important. For instance electroporation seems just like there is quite a passion to give some "short sharp shock" and then something good will happen ; actually, it has been used in man very extensively and I am not sure very appropriately. It is thus better to do it to cells than human beings ! The next one is DNA coated gold particle and let us call it "bombardment". I am sure that people don't project their own views or tendancies ; but it is very interesting that you find these words cropping up in the field of gene transfer.

Of course, retroviral vectors unfortunately are quite reminiscent of "biological warfare"; but in fact, we've been told and I would share that view which is that it is the most realistic possibility at the moment. The fact that we've been able to disable the bullets of the biological warfare is quite important; we should extend that outside the strictly field of gene transfer. But compared to all that, Homologous Recombination could only be described as "a labour of love"; I would think that it probably stands as the way to go, in this age where we need love.

Gene transfer and gene therapy : The question of how to actually achieve the last objective namely gene transfer for the purpose of gene therapy is a very difficult one. I have tried to summarize but there is hardly any need because you've heard the examples. If we go from the very numerous in vitro experiments to the in vivo experiments, especially with emphasis on the long-term expression, that is quite difficult. I have just summarized a few of the systems where that has been actually achieved. This is not a complete list but I have not heard much else that has come out in this particular meeting. We have heard the progress done in the human case which are not listed here because it is not yet clear whether it is a permanent phenomenon, but we've heard the very encouraging results obtained by Michael BLAESE's group. I am sure there are other groups that are coming up even if they have not yet reached that stage.

One thing that I thought is encouraging in that respect is that while certain systems seem to be the most popular there are probably quite a variety of systems that can be utilized, there is indeed an increasing interest in diversification. So we've heard about a variety of vectors and a point was made today as "can we target vectors to individual tissues which are particularly appropriate" ? The use of Herpes Viruses we've heard from Doctor GELLER seems particularly relevant. We have heard things about every one of these organs namely : hemopoietic tissue, central nervous system, lymphoid cells, muscle, liver, lung and skin. It certainly seems that a combination of very sophisticated biological targeting together with the more kind of down-to-earth mechanical or topographical approach seems to be quite an important way to go.

G6PDH gene cloning characterization and transfer : Finally one thing that worries me a great deal, is to avoid speaking of gene therapy without actually having any data. I would not like to do that. I would like to rescue that because I thought of a different approach altogether.

Can I show you how a particular system that can be used to look at gene transfer in a variety of ways.

I thought if I had such a captive audience like this, it could not escape to hearing about glucose-6-phosphate-dehydrogenase which is an enzyme of the housekeeping type. One should emphasize on its importance in NADPH production and therefore cell-defense against oxidative damages. It is ubiquitous and it is crucial ; I am sure that any living deficient individual should have some residual activity since I am sure that total deficiency would be lethal. All patients that have been reported with complete deficiency, upon proper testings proved to have some residual activity.

I will not try to tell you that it the most common genetic disease because it isn't ! It is a relatively rare genetic disease but it is the most common genetic abnormality. There are more than four hundred million people that have the abnormal gene. The reason why they have no disease is because this is a conditional gene where the people are asymptomatic unless there are challenged by a variety of agents such as fava beans, drugs or infection. So it is a conditional mutant which is a very good way of extrapolating from what has been learned from conditional mutants in the prokaryotic systems.

There is a very striking genetic polymorphism and heterogeneity of the defect. There are an estimated 272 variants involved. One can argue about this number but I won't. I personally think that it may still be underestimated. Many variants interestingly are polymorphic and the reason for that is because they confer resistance against malaria ; so it is a case of biological selection.

Some years ago I was lucky to persuade Grazziela PERSICO to join our group and she obtained full length cDNA clones (the complete sequence in 1986) and then Giuseppe MARTINI worked out the genomic structure. In the last few years we have been able to characterize the mutations of about 20 different mutants ; I will not bore you with the details ; each one of these has an interesting story to tell. I would just like to point out two things. One is that so far, they are all individual point mutations. They are scattered all over the twelve coding exons ; we still have no mutant unfortunately on exon thirteenth, but it is coming. Except for one particular mutation which is a triplet deletion with subsequent disappearing of a single amino-acid. So the first point is that they seem to take place all over the gene.

The second point is that this is giving us a handle to understand why some have a mild disease and others a severe disease namely chronic non-spherocytic hemolytic anemia which may be life-crippling and require blood-transfusions. We thus are currenly trying to find out the reason for these distinct clinical phenotypic features.

This is hampered by the fact that the three dimensional structure of the protein has not yet been worked out. By gene transfer, we are now producing in E-coli, about 15 mg for one liter of culture which is about twenty times more than what you can get from human blood ; this enzyme has been cristallized and Margaret ADAMS at the moment is trying to work out the X-ray diffraction patterns.

Gene-transfer has also been used in a purpose which has not yet been mentioned here. When you find a mutation how do you know that this mutation is actually responsible for the phenotype that you observe ?

Philip MASON in our lab has placed the gene under the CMV promoter ; driven by this promoter the gene is expressed at high level in COS-cells ; the enzyme recovered from the COS-cells shows differences in its physico-chemical properties that you would expect in comparison with the enzyme which is recovered after transfection of a normal-native gene. This leads to conclude that physico-chemical differences are probably responsible for the severe clinical phenotype (G6PD mutant called Santiago de Cuba).

The last point is : "can we use this to investigate the significance of the structure of the gene" ? What Giuseppe MARTINI and his colleagues have done is a deletion analysis of the promoter that they can go into. They have also constructed a minigene which is genomic - then c-DNA - and then genomic and also a hybrid G6PD beta-globin construct. The results are very interesting ; namely, both in transfected cells and in transgenic mice, this genomic gene GD15 is expressed ; but the minigene is not. By contrast the hybrid G6PD-beta globin is expressed. That, I think, strongly implicates the function of a particular intron which is junk but shouldn't be all that junk because it is required for expression !

We were quite intrigued when we saw that in mice there were both a human and a mouse G6PD band and a third heterodimeric band as expected. Out of the two mice that have integrated DNA both show expression of the gene which seems to be copy-dependant : a single copy corresponding to low expression and two copies beeing associated to a level of expression comparable to the mouse endogenous gene. We hope that this is going to be a house-keeping gene which is going to tell us how to get that expressed and possibly driven by its own promoter it could be useful for other gene transfer systems when you want the genes expressed in all cells.

Conclusion : Just to finish, I thought that what everybody wants is to go home and know exactly what to do ! Again, who am I to tell you exactly what to do ? Let me however point out two aspects which seem to me very important. I think everybody would like to do that ; there is absolutely nothing original in this. In many cases, the gene is available and in some cases with the appropriate control regions. Now you have to get stem cells and purify them ; some progress is being made in that direction. Make retroviral constructs, we heard some of the difficulties of that ; and there must be a reason why retroviruses tend to be so small and only accomodate a small genome. That might have something to do with evolution. There might be reasons but it does not mean that you cannot help nature. So I am sure that human ingenuity will make it possible to obtain larger vectors or else to combine the "biological warfare" with the "labour of love" and obtain retroviruses that can effect homologous recombination. Now you have to infect and that does not seem to be too difficult by any of the methods which I have mentioned. But now what I would like to do is to simply say : "Ok, let us culture the stem cells", that was what Mario CAPECCHI indicated ; let us culture the stem cells decently just for a few weeks and if possible select for those which have been transfected. I mean I don't think at the moment anybody can actually do that. At the present time it is the kind of crucial bottleneck ; if anybody has got a good idea about that, don't tell anybody ! Just go and do it quickly !

Of course you finally want to autograft the transfected cells ; that is where we can capitilize on this excellent experience obtained with bone marrow transplantation ; and that is certainly going to be the logical way. I am sorry if I have introduced a bias in this ; that is that I assume that the first example will be hemopoietic cells ; I am not assuming that at all as a hematologist ; that would be a very presumptuous thing to do. I am just giving one example ; I am not saying at all : "it will be the first" ; because in fact I have not made any predictions at all.

The last thing I always like to tell to the patients is : "I can tell you what little I understand of your problem ; one thing I will not do is to predict what will happen because then we only make fools of ourselves".

I don't want to make any longer a fool of myself so I would just like to link up with what I said at the beginning :

"It may be madness, but yet, there is a method in it".
                                    Shakespeare.

Thank you very much.

Conclusion : M. BOIRON

Thank you Lucio for concluding so beautifully.

I would like to express my deep thanks and those of Odile to the participants who made this meeting a success.

The idea to bring together geneticists, physicians, virologists and even surgeons, proved a good one ; and we've had an excellent and productive meeting.

Thomas CASKEY told me that he was enthousiastic about this formula. He will be organizing, let's say on a two-years basis, an exchange between America and Europe, one meeting in America and each following one in Europe. the next one could take place in 1993 in the context of "Gordon Conference" with the same spirit of mixing people together.

As a general hematologist I learned a lot from this meeting and I suppose that I am not the only one !

Author index
Index des auteurs

Acsadi G. 263
Afanassieff M. 275
Antoniou M. 121
Arabian A. 287
Belmont J.W. 283
Beuzard Y. 295
Blaese R.M. 137
Boiron M. 3, 347
Bolhuis R.L.H. 113
Bonifer C. 267
Bordignon C. 103
Braakman E. 113
Brandenburger A. 285
Briand P. 159
Brody S.L. 147
Broxmeyer H.E. 95
Buckingham M. 271
Calise D. 169
Capecchi M. 209
Carillo S. 177
Carow C. 95
Caskey C.T. 17, 283, 293, 324
Cavard C. 159
Charbit A. 237
Chasse J.F. 159
Chebloune Y. 275
Chong W. 263
Clément J.M. 237
Cohen-Haguenauer O. 3
Collins M.K.L. 285
Cooper S. 95
Cosset F.L. 275
Cournoyer D. 283
Crystal R.G. 147, 319
Danos O. 169
Dillon N. 121
Drynda A. 275
Duke D. 263
Duplessis O. 169
Einerhand M.P.W. 85
Eloit M. 249
Etienne-Julan M. 177
Faure C. 275
Federoff H.J. 63
Feldman R.A. 273
Ferrari G. 103

Ferry N. 169
Fischer A. 113, 298
Fraser P. 121
Fung-Leung W.P. 287
Geller A.I. 63
Giavazzi R. 103
Gilboa E. 103
Girard M. 33
Gluckman E. 302
Goff S.P. 217
Gottesman M.M. 185
Grimber G. 159
Grosveld F. 121, 267
Guénet J.L. 195
Hangoc G. 95
Hanscombe O. 121
Heard J.M. 169
Hendrie P.C. 95
Hofnung M. 237
Houssin D. 169, 317
Jani A. 263
Jeanteur P. 177
Jiao S. 263
Johnson G.R. 279
Junien C. 307
Leclerc C. 237
Legras C. 275
Lehn P. 333
Leserman L. 75
Levrero M. 159
Lévy J.P. 27
Lindenbaum M. 121
Lowy D.R. 273
Luzzatto L. 340
Mak T.W. 287
Makeh I. 159
Mallet J. 329
Mandel J.L. 271, 322
Martineau P. 237
Mavilio F. 103
Metcalf D. 279
Mitani K. 283
Molina R.M. 275
Moore K.A. 283
Muir S. 237
Munnich A. 312

Nigon V.M. 275
O'Callaghan D. 237
Pastan I. 185
Perricaudet M. 51, 159, 249, 271
Philipsen S. 121
Piechaczyk M. 177
Pruzina S. 121
Quantin B. 271
Ragot T. 249
Rahemtulla A. 287
Robertson E.J. 217
Rommelaere J. 285
Ronfort C. 275
Rossini S. 103
Roux P. 177
Russell S.J. 285
Scarpa M. 283
Schaison G. 310
Schilham M. 287
Schwartzberg P.L. 217
Sippel A.E. 267
Stratford-Perricaudet L.D. 51, 159
Szmelcman S. 237
Tajbakhsh S. 271
Talbot D. 121
Tambourin P.E. 273
Thomas J.L. 275
Valerio D. 85, 113
Valsésia S. 275
Valverius E.M. 273
Van Beusechem V.W. 113
Van Krimpen B.A. 113
Velu T.J. 273
Verdier G. 275
Villeval J.L. 279
Visser J.W.M. 85
Wagner E.F. 227
Wakeham A. 287
Williams P. 263
Wolff J.A. 263
Yannoutsis N. 267

List and address of participants
Liste et adresse des participants

Akhurst Rosemary J., Department of Genetics, Glasgow University, Yorkhill, G3 8SJ Glasgow, UK

Alizon Marc, Rétrovirus et Transfert Génétique, Institut Pasteur, 25, rue du Docteur Roux, 75724 Paris Cedex 15, France

Auffray Charles, Groupe de Génétique Moléculaire, Institut d'Embryologie du CNRS et du Collège de France, 49 bis, avenue de la Belle Gabrielle, 94736 Nogent-sur-Marne Cedex, France

Auriol (d') Luc, Genset, 1, passage E. Delaunay, 75011 Paris, France

Bach Jean-François, INSERM U 25, Centre de l'Association C. Bernard, Immunologie Clinique, Hôpital Necker, 161, rue de Sèvres, 75743 Paris Cedex 15, France

Behr Jean-Paul, Laboratoire de Chimie Génétique, URA 1386 CNRS/Université Louis Pasteur, 74, route du Rhin, BP 24, 67401, Illkirch Cedex, France

Berger Roland, INSERM U 301, Institut de Génétique Moléculaire, Hôpital Saint-Louis, 27, rue Juliette Dodu, 75010 Paris, France

Bernard Bruno A., Département de Biologie Cellulaire, CIRD Galderma, Sophia Antipolis, 06565 Valbonne, France

Bernardi Alberto, Laboratoire d'Enzymologie, CNRS – Bâtiment 34, avenue de la Terrasse, 91198 Gif-sur-Yvette Cedex, France

Birg Françoise, INSERM U 119, Institut Paoli Calmettes, 27, boulevard Lei Roure, 13009 Marseille, France

Bohnlein Ernst, Sandoz Forschungsinstitut, PO Box 80, Brunner Strasse 59, A 1235 Wien, Autriche

Bonifer Constanze, Institut für Biologie III, Universität Freiburg, Schaenzle Strasse 1, D7800 Freiburg, Allemagne

Bories Dominique, INSERM U 91, Hôpital Henri Mondor, 51, avenue du Maréchal de Lattre de Tassigny, 94010 Créteil, France

Bosselut Rémy, CNRS URA 532, Institut Curie, Bâtiment 110, Centre Universitaire, 91405 Orsay Cedex, France

Boué André, INSERM U 73, Château de Longchamp, 75016 Paris, France

Brady Hugh J.M., Laboratory of Gene Structure and Expression, National Institute for Medical Research, The Ridgeway, Mill Hill, London NW7 1AA, UK

Brandenburger Annick, Laboratoire de Biophysique et de Radiologie, Faculté des Sciences, ULB, rue des Chevaux, 67, 1640 Rhode-St-Genèse, Belgique

Brulet Philippe, Service de Génétique Cellulaire, Institut Pasteur, 28, rue du Docteur Roux, 75274 Paris Cedex 15, France

Bréchot Christian, INSERM U.75 et Unité d'Hépatologie, Hôpital Laennec, 42, rue de Sèvres, 75340 Paris Cedex 07, France

Brice Pauline, Polyclinique d'Hématologie, Hôpital Saint-Louis, 1, avenue Claude Vellefaux, 75010 Paris, France

Brison Olivier, Laboratoire d'Oncologie Moléculaire, Pavillon de recherche 1, Institut Gustave Roussy, 39, rue Camille Desmoulins, 94805 Villejuif Cedex, France

Burger H., TNO Division of Health Research, Institute of Applied Radiobiology and Immunology, PO Box 5815, 2280 HV, Rijswijk, Pays-Bas

Buttin Gérard, Unité de Génétique Somatique, Institut Pasteur, 25, rue du Docteur Roux, 75724 Paris Cedex 15, France

Calvo Fabien, Laboratoire de Pharmacologie Expérimentale, Institut de Génétique Moléculaire, Hôpital Saint-Louis, 1, avenue Claude Vellefaux, 75010 Paris, France

Casadevall Nicole, INSERM U.152 et Service d'Hématologie, Hôpital Cochin, 27, rue du Faubourg Saint-Jacques, 75014 Paris, France

Cazillis Michèle, Institut Jacques Monod, 2, place Jussieu, Tour 43, 75251 Paris Cedex 05, France

Cesbron Jean-Yves, Centre d'Immunologie et de Biologie Parasitaire, Institut Pasteur, 1, rue du Pr. A. Calmette, BP 245, 59019 Lille, France

Chamberlain Sue, Department of Biochemistry and Molecular Genetics, St Mary's Hospital Medical School, Norkolk Place, London W2 1PG, Royaume-Uni

Chebloune Yahia, Laboratoire de Biologie Cellulaire et Moléculaire/CNRS UMR 106, Université Claude Bernard Lyon I, 43, boulevard du 11 Novembre 1918, 69622 Villeurbanne Cedex, France

Chrétien Stany, INSERM U 76, Centre National de Transfusion Sanguine, 6, rue Alexandre Cabanel, 75739 Paris Cedex 15, France

Cohen Daniel, CEPH, Hôpital Saint-Louis, 27, rue Juliette Dodu, 75010 Paris, France

Coppey Jacques, Section de Biologie, Institut Curie, 25, rue d'Ulm, 75231 Paris Cedex 05, France

Cosset François-Loïc, Laboratoire de Biologie Cellulaire, INRA, CNRS UMR 106, Université Claude Bernard Lyon I, 43, boulevard du 11 Novembre 1918, 69622 Villeurbanne Cedex, France

Cotten Matthew, Forschungs Institute für Molekulare Pathologie, Research Institute of Molekulare Pathologie, Geschaftsfuhrender, Dr. Bohr-Gasse 7, A1030 Wien, Autriche

Coulombel Laure, Pavillon de Recherches 1, Institut Gustave Roussy, 39, rue Camille Desmoulins, 94805 Villejuif, France

Cournoyer Denis, Department of Medicine, Mac Gill University, Montreal, Quebec, Canada

Courvalin Pierre, Unité des Agents Antibactériens, Institut Pasteur, 25, rue du Docteur Roux, 75724 Paris Cedex 15, France

Coze Carole, Service d'Oncologie Pédiatrique, Hôpital d'Enfants de la Timone, 13385 Marseille Cedex 5, France

Cramer Philippe, Transgène, 16, rue Henri Regnault, 92411 Courbevoie Cedex, France

Darmon Michel, Département de Biologie Cellulaire, CIRD Galderma, Sophia Antipolis, 06565 Valbonne, France

Dautry François, Laboratoire d'Oncologie Moléculaire, Institut Gustave Roussy, 39, rue Camille Desmoulins, 94805 Villejuif Cedex, France

Dubart Anne, Institut Gustave Roussy, 39, rue Camille Desmoulins, 94805 Villejuif Cedex, France

Dubreuil Patrice, INSERM U 119, Institut Paoli Calmettes, 27, boulevard Lei Roure, 13009 Marseille, France

Dumenil Dominique, Institut Gustave Roussy, 39, rue Camille Desmoulins, 94805 Villejuif Cedex, France

Dupressoir Thierry, INSERM U.186 Institut Pasteur, 1, rue Calmette, BP 245, 59019 Lille Cedex, France

Dzierzak Helen, Medical Research Council, National Institute for Medical Research, The Ridgeway, Mill Hill, London NW7 1AA, UK

Eloit Marc, Génétique des Virus Oncogènes, Institut Gustave Roussy, 39, rue Camille Desmoulins, 94805 Villejuif Cedex, France

Favrot Marie, Laboratoire d'Immunologie, Centre Léon Bérard, 28, rue Laënnec, 69373 Lyon Cedex 08, France

Fellous Marc, INSERM U 276, Immunogénétique Humaine, Institut Pasteur, 25, rue du Docteur Roux, 75724 Paris Cedex 15, France

Ferry Nicolas, Institut Pasteur, 28, rue du Docteur Roux, 75015 Paris, France

Feugeas Olivier, INSERM U 184, LGME Institut de Chimie Biologique, Faculté de Médecine, 11, rue Humann, 67085 Strasbourg Cedex, France

Forestier François, Service de Biologie Fœtale, Institut de Puériculture de Paris, 26, boulevard Brune, 75014 Paris, France

Galibert Francis, Laboratoire d'Hématologie Expérimentale, Centre Hayem, Hôpital Saint-Louis, 1, avenue Claude Vellefaux, 75010 Paris, France

Garel Marie-Claude, INSERM U 91/CNRS UA 607, Hôpital Henri Mondor, 51, avenue du Maréchal de Lattre de Tassigny, 94010 Créteil, France

Gazzolo Louis, CNRS UMR 30, Immuno-Virologie Moléculaire et Cellulaire, Faculté de Médecine A. Carrel, rue Guillaume Paradin, 69372 Lyon Cedex 08, France

Gérard Catherine, Institut de Recherche Interdisciplinaire en Biologie Humaine et Nucléaire, ULB, Faculté de Médecine, Hôpital Erasme, route de Lennik 808, 1070 Bruxelles, Belgique

Gerrard Ann, Sir William Dunn School of Pathology, Chemical Pathology Unit, University of Oxford, South Parks Road, Oxford OX1 3RE, UK

Gespach Christian, INSERM U 55, 184, rue du Faubourg Saint-Antoine, 75571 Paris Cedex 12, France

Ghysdael Jacques, Section de Biologie, Institut Curie, Bâtiment 110, 91405 Orsay Cedex, France

Gilgenkrantz Hélène, INSERM U 129, ICGM, 24, rue du Faubourg Saint-Jacques, 75014 Paris, France

Gisselbrecht Christian, Coquelicot 6, Hôpital Saint-Louis, 1, avenue Claude-Vellefaux, 75010 Paris, France

Gisselbrecht Sylvie, INSERM U 152, Hôpital Cochin, 27, rue du Faubourg Saint-Jacques, 75014 Paris, France

Goossens Michel, INSERM U.91, Laboratoire de Biochimie, Hôpital Henri Mondor, 51, avenue du Maréchal de Lattre de Tassigny, 94010 Créteil Cedex, France

Grausz David, INSERM U 301, IGM, Hôpital Saint-Louis, 27, rue Juliette Dodu, 75010 Paris, France

Guillouzo Christiane, INSERM U 49, Recherches Hépatologiques, Hôpital Pontchaillou, 35033 Rennes Cedex, France

Haddad Patrick, INSERM U 93, Centre Hayem, Hôpital Saint-Louis, 2, place du Docteur Fournier, 75010 Paris, France

Hardouin Sylvie, Unité de Recherche sur la Régulation de la Croissance, INSERM U 142, Hôpital Saint-Antoine, 184, rue du Faubourg Saint-Antoine, 75571 Paris Cedex 12, France

Heard Jean-Michel, Laboratoire de Rétrovirus et Transfert Génétique, Institut Pasteur, 28, rue du Docteur Roux, 75724 Paris Cedex 15, France

Heidmann Thierry, INSERM U 140, Institut Gustave Roussy, 39, rue Camille Desmoulins, 94805 Villejuif, France

Houge Gunnar, INSERM U. 301, Institut de Génétique Moléculaire, 27, rue Juliette Dodu, 75010 Paris, France

Huet Thierry, CEPH, Hôpital Saint-Louis, 27, rue Juliette Dodu, 75010 Paris, France

Ioannou Panayiotis, The Cyprus Institute of Neurology and Genetics, PO Box 3462, Nicosia, Chypre

James Michael, CEPH, Hôpital Saint-Louis, 27, rue Juliette Dodu, 75010 Paris, France

Jones Richard, Merrell Dow Research Institute, 16, rue d'Ankara, BP 447 R9, 67009 Strasbourg Cedex, France

Jordan Bertrand, INSERM-CNRS Marseille Luminy, 70, route Léon Lachamp, 13288 Marseille Cedex 9, France

Kahn Axel, INSERM U.129, Institut Cochin de Génétique Moléculaire, 24, rue du Faubourg Saint-Jacques, 75014 Paris, France

Kaplan Jean-Claude, INSERM U.129, Biochimie Génétique, ICGM, 24, rue du Faubourg Saint-Jacques, 75014 Paris, France

Klatzmann David, CERVI, Groupe Hospitalier Pitié-Salpétrière, 47-83, boulevard de l'Hôpital, 75651 Paris Cedex 13, France

Koering Catherine, Unité d'Oncologie Moléculaire, Institut Pasteur, 1, rue Calmette, BP 245, 59019 Lille Cedex, France

Korman Alan, Immunogénétique, Institut Pasteur, 28, rue du Docteur Roux, 75724 Paris Cedex 15, France

Lacombe Catherine, INSERM U 152, ICGM, Hôpital Cochin, 27, rue du Faubourg Saint-Jacques, 75014 Paris, France

Larsen Christian, INSERM U.301, IGM, Hôpital Saint-Louis, 1, avenue Claude-Vellefaux, 75010 Paris, France

Lavau Catherine, INSERM U 163/CNRS URA 271, Institut Pasteur, 28, rue du Docteur Roux, 75724 Paris Cedex 15, France

Le Gall Isabelle, CEPH, Hôpital Saint-Louis, 27 rue Juliette Dodu, 75010 Paris, France

Léger Jean-Jacques, INSERM U 300, Faculté de Pharmacie, Bâtiment K, avenue Charles Flahaut, 34100 Montpellier, France

London Jacqueline, Laboratoire de Biochimie Génétique, Université René Descartes, Hôpital Necker-Enfants Malades, 149, rue de Sèvres, 75743 Paris Cedex 15, France

Lopez Bernard, Institut Curie, Section de Biologie, 26, rue d'Ulm, 75231 Paris Cedex 05, France

Mamoun R.Z., INSERM U 328, Fondation Bergonie, 229, cours de l'Argonne, 33076 Bordeaux Cedex, France

Mannoni Patrice, INSERM U.119 et Service de Biologie Cellulaire et Moléculaire, Institut Paoli Calmette, 232, boulevard de Ste-Marguerite, BP 156, 13273 Marseille Cedex 9, France

Marty Michel, Sevice d'Oncologie, Hôpital Saint-Louis, 1, avenue Claude-Vellefaux, 75010 Paris, France

Mathieu-Mahul Danièle, INSERM U 301, IGM, Hôpital Saint-Louis, 27, rue Juliette Dodu, 75010 Paris, France

Meneguzzi Gerrino, Laboratoire de Virologie, UER Médecine, avenue de Vallombrose, 06000 Nice, France

Middleton L.T., The Cyprus Institute of Neurology and Genetics, PO Box 3462, Nicosia, Chypre

Monier Roger, Laboratoire d'Oncologie Moléculaire, Institut Gustave Roussy, 39, rue Camille Desmoulins, 94805 Villejuif Cedex, France

Montplaisir Nicole, Genset, 1, passage E. Delaunay, 75011 Paris France

Moraine Claire, Unité de Génétique, Laboratoire Gen-DEP, CHRU de Tours, Hôpital Bretonneau, 2, boulevard Tonnelé, 37044 Tours Cedex, France

Morinet Frédéric, Service de Bactério-Virologie, Hôpital Saint-Louis, 1, avenue Claude-Vellefaux, 75010, Paris, France

Mornex Jean-François, INSERM U.80 et Hôpital Cardiovasculaire et Pneumologique Louis Pradel, 28, avenue du Doyen Lépine, 69500 Bron, France

Mouliet Philippe, Rétrovirus et transfert génétique, Institut Pasteur, 28, rue du Docteur Roux, 75015 Paris, France

Naffak Nadia, Institut Pasteur, 28, rue du Docteur Roux, 75015 Paris, France

Najean Yves, Service Central de Médecine Nucléaire, Hôpital Saint-Louis, 1, avenue Claude-Vellefaux, 75010 Paris, France

Nandi Pradip, Laboratoire de Pathologie Infectieuse et Immunologie, INRA, Centre de Recherches de Tours, 37380 Nouzilly, France

Nemani Mona, Service de Médecine Nucléaire, Hôpital Saint-Louis, 1, avenue Claude-Vellefaux, 75010 Paris, France

Nicolas Jean-François, Biologie Moléculaire du Développement, Institut Pasteur, 25, rue du Docteur Roux, 75015 Paris, France

Ouazana Roland, Centre de Génétique Moléculaire et Cellulaire, Bâtiment 741, Université C. Bernard Lyon I, 43, boulevard du 11 Novembre 1918, 69622 Villeurbanne Cedex, France

Palmer Mark S., Department of Biochemistry and Molecular Genetics, St Mary's Hospital Medicine School, Norfolk Place, London W2 1PG, UK

Péault Bruno, Systemix, 3400 West Bayshore Road, Palo Alto, CA 94303, États-Unis

Perbal Bernard, Laboratoire d'Oncologie Virale et Moléculaire, Institut Curie, Bâtiment 110, Centre Universitaire, 94405 Orsay Cedex, France

Ploemacher Rob E., Department of Cell Biology and Genetics, Erasmus University, PO Box 1738, 3000 Dr, Rotterdam, Pays-Bas

Poenaru Livia, Institut Cochin de Génétique Moléculaire, INSERM U 129, 24, rue du Faubourg Saint-Jacques, 75014 Paris, France

Pontoglio Marco, Institut Pasteur, 28, rue du Docteur Roux, 75724 Paris Cedex 15, France

Quantin Béatrice, LGME/CNRS, INSERM U 184, Institut de Chimie Biologique, Faculté de Médecine, 11, rue Humann, 67085 Strasbourg Cedex, France

Rabourdin-Combe Chantal, Immuno-Biologie Moléculaire, ENSL CNRS UMR 13, 46, allée d'Italie, 69364 Lyon Cedex 07, France

Radman Minoslav, Laboratoire de Mutagénèse, Institut Jacques Monod, Tour 43, 2, place Jussieu, 75251 Paris Cedex 05, France

Rahemtulla Amin, Ontario Cancer Institute, Princess Margaret Hospital, 500 Sherbourne Street, Toronto, Ontario, M4X 1K9, Canada

Rain Jean-Didier, Service de Médecine Nucléaire, Hôpital Saint-Louis, 1, avenue Claude-Vellefaux, 75010 Paris, France

Richard Patrice, Biologie de la Moelle Osseuse, Institut d'Hématologie, Hôpital Saint-Louis, 2, place du Docteur Fournier, 75010 Paris, France

Romeo Paul-Henri, INSERM U 91, Hôpital Henri Mondor, 51, avenue du Maréchal de Lattre de Tassigny, 94010 Créteil, France

Rommelaere Jean, ULB, Faculté des Sciences, Laboratoire de Biophysique et Radiobiologie, rue des Chevaux, 67, 1640 Rhode-St-Genèse, Belgique

Rosa Jean, INSERM U 91, Hôpital Henri Mondor, 51, avenue du Maréchal de Lattre de Tassigny, 94010 Créteil, France

Salvetti Anna, Immuno-Virologie Moléculaire et Cellulaire, UMR 30 CNRS, Faculté de Médecine Alexis Carrel, rue Guillaume Paradin, 69372 Lyon Cedex 08, France

Sarda Laure, Service de Médecine Nucléaire, Hôpital Saint-Louis, 1, avenue Claude-Vellefaux, 75010 Paris, France

Scarpa Maurizio, Department of Pediatrics, University of Padova, Padova, Italie

Schneider-Maunoury Sylvie, Laboratoire de Génétique Moléculaire, École Normale Supérieure, 46, rue d'Ulm, 75230 Paris Cedex 05, France

Scholte Bob J., Cell Biology I, Erasmus University, PO Box 1738, 3000 Dr., Rotterdam, Pays-Bas

Schwartz Olivier, Institut Pasteur, 28, rue du docteur Roux, 75015 Paris, France

Sigaux François, Laboratoire de Biologie Moléculaire, Centre Hayem, Hôpital Saint-Louis, 1, avenue Claude-Vellfaux, 75010 Paris, France

Silverman Paul H., Beckman Instruments Inc, 2500 Harbour Bld, Fullerton, CA 92634, États-Unis

Sonigo Pierre, Laboratoire de Génétique des Virus, Institut Cochin de Génétique Moléculaire, 22, rue Méchain, 75014 Paris, France

Stoll Claude, Institut de Puériculture, Hôpital Central, Hospices Civils, 23, rue de la Porte de l'Hôpital, BP 426, 67091 Strasbourg Cedex, France

Stratford-Perricaudet Leslie, Laboratoire des Virus Oncogènes, CNRS URA-1301, Institut Gustave Roussy, PR2, 39, rue Camille Desmoulins, 94805 Villejuif, France

Suthers Graeme, Institute of Molecular Medicine, John Radcliffe Hospital, Headington, Oxford, OX 39 DU, UK

Sylla B.S., Unité des Mécanismes de la Cancérogenèse, Centre International de Recherche sur le Cancer, 150, cours Albert Thomas, 69372 Lyon Cedex 08, France

Tanzer Joseph, CHRU de Poitiers, Centre de Transfusion Sanguine, rue Guillaume Le Troubadour, 86021 Poitiers, France

Tata Frederick, Department of Biochemistry and Molecular Genetics, St-Mary's Hospital Medical School, Norfolk Place, London W2 1 PG, UK

Tavitian Armand, INSERM U 248, Faculté de Médecine Lariboisière-Saint-Louis, 10, avenue de Verdun, 75010 Paris, France

Teissie Justin, CRBGC-CNRS, 118, route de Narbonne, 31062 Toulouse Cedex, France

Thierry Dominique, Biologie de la Moelle Osseuse, Institut d'Hématologie, Hôpital Saint-Louis, 1, avenue Claude Vellefaux, 75010 Paris, France

Tiraby Gérard, Laboratoire de Microbiologie et de Génétique Appliquées du CNRS CRBGC, Université P. Sabatier, 118, route de Narbonne, 31062 Toulouse Cedex, France

Tosi Mario, INSERM U 276, Immunogénétique, Institut Pasteur, 28, rue du Docteur Roux, 75724 Paris Cedex 15, France

Touraine Jean-Louis, INSERM U 80, Hôpital Édouard Herriot, Pavillon P5, place d'Arsonval, 69374 Lyon Cedex 08, France

Tremp Gunter, Centre de Technologie de Vitry-Alfortville, Rhône-Poulenc Rorer SA, 13, quai Jules Guesde, BP 14, 94403 Vitry-sur-Seine Cedex, France

Vainchenker William, INSERM U 91, Hôpital Henri Mondor, 51, avenue du Maréchal de Lattre de Tassigny, 94010 Créteil, France

Valere Thomas, Laboratoire de Génétique des Virus, ICGM, 22, rue Méchain, 75014 Paris, France

Vasseur Marc, Genset, 1, passage E. Delaunay, 75011 Paris, France

Velu Thierry, Département de Génétique Médicale, Institut de Recherche Interdisciplinaire en Biologie Humaine et Nucléaire, ULB, Campus Hôpital Erasme, route de Lennik 808, 1070 Bruxelles, Belgique

Vermeulen R.J., Institute of Applied Radiobiology and Immunology, TNO Lange Kleiweg 151, PO Box 5815, 2280 HV Rijswijk, Pays-Bas

Verneuil (de) Hubert, Faculté de Médecine Xavier Bichat, Laboratoire de Génétique Moléculaire, 16, rue Henri Huchard, 75018 Paris, France

Vidaud Michel, INSERM U.91 et Laboratoire de Biologie Moléculaire, Institut de Puériculture, 26, boulevard Brune, 75014 Paris, France

Villeval Jean-Luc, INSERM U 91, Hôpital Henri Mondor, 51, avenue du Maréchal de Lattre de Tassigny, 94010 Créteil, France

Vilmer Etienne, Unité d'Hémato-Immunologie, Hôpital Robert Debré, 48, boulevard Serrurier, 75019 Paris, France

Viville Stéphane, Unité de Biologie Moléculaire et de Génie Génétique, INSERM U.184, Institut de Chimie Biologique, 11, rue Humann, 67085 Strasbourg Cedex, France

Wagemaker Gérard, Institute of Applied Radiobiology and Immunology, TNO Lange Kleiweg 151, PO Box 5815, 2280 HV Rijswijk, Pays-Bas

Weber Anne, INSERM U 129, CHU Cochin-Port-Royal, 24, rue du Faubourg Saint-Jacques, 75014 Paris, France

Whalen Robert, Département de Biologie Moléculaire, Institut Pasteur, 25, rue du Docteur Roux, 75724 Paris, France

Wolff Jon A., Departments of Pediatrics and Genetics, Waisman Center, University of Wisconsin, Madison WI53706, États-Unis

Zillhardt Katy, Direction Scientifique, Rhône-Poulenc, 25, quai Paul Doumer, 92408 Courbevoie, France

Zouali M., Immunogénétique Cellulaire, Institut Pasteur, 28, rue du Docteur Roux, 75724 Paris Cedex 15, France

We thank Dr Nadia Blumenfeld-Charbit for her help with english reviewing of the manuscript.

Colloques **INSERM**
ISSN 0768-3154

Other *Colloques* published as co-editions by John Libbey Eurotext and INSERM

153 Hormones and Cell Regulation (11th European Symposium). *Hormones et Régulation Cellulaire (11ᵉ Symposium Européen).*
Edited by J. Nunez and J.E. Dumont.
ISBN : John Libbey Eurotext 0 86196 104 8
INSERM 2 85598 324 X

158 Biochemistry and Physiopathology of Platelet Membrane. *Biochimie et Physiopathologie de la Membrane Plaquettaire.*
Edited by G. Marguerie and R.F.A. Zwaal.
ISBN : John Libbey Eurotext 0 86196 114 5
INSERM 2 85598 345 2

162 The Inhibitors of Hematopoiesis. *Les Inhibiteurs de l'Hématopoïèse.*
Edited by A. Najman, M. Guignon, N.C. Gorin and J.Y. Mary.
ISBN : John Libbey Eurotext 0 86196 125 0
INSERM 2 85598 340 1

164 Liver Cells and Drugs. *Cellules Hépatiques et Médicaments.*
Edited by A. Guillouzo.
ISBN : John Libbey Eurotext 0 86196 128 5
INSERM 2 85598 341 X

165 Hormones and Cell Regulation (12th European Symposium). *Hormones et Régulation Cellulaire (12ᵉ Symposium Européen).*
Edited by J. Nunez, J.E. Dumont and E. Carafoli.
ISBN : John Libbey Eurotext 0 86196 133 1
INSERM 2 85598 347 9

167 Sleep Disorders and Respiration. *Les Evénements Respiratoires du Sommeil.*
Edited by P. Lévi-Valensi and D. Duron.
ISBN : John Libbey Eurotext 0 86196 127 7
INSERM 2 85598 344 4

169 Neo-Adjuvant Chemotherapy. *Chimiothérapie Néo-Adjuvante.*
Edited by C. Jacquillat, M. Weil, D. Khayat.
ISBN : John Libbey Eurotext 0 86196 150 1
INSERM 2 85598 349 5

171 Structure and Functions of the Cytoskeleton. *La Structure et les Fonctions du Cytosquelette.*
Edited by B.A.F. Rousset.
ISBN : John Libbey Eurotext 0 86196 149 8
INSERM 2 85598 351 7

Colloques INSERM
ISSN 0768-3154

172 The Langerhans Cell. *La Cellule de Langerhans.*
Edited by J. Thivolet, D. Schmitt.
ISBN : John Libbey Eurotext 0 86196 181 1
INSERM 2 85598 352 5

173 Cellular and Molecular Aspects of Glucuronidation. *Aspects Cellulaires et Moléculaires de la Glucuronoconjugaison.*
Edited by G. Siest, J. Magdalou, B. Burchell
ISBN : John Libbey Eurotext 0 86196 182 X
INSERM 2 85598 353 3

174 Second Forum on Peptides. *Deuxième Forum Peptides.*
Edited by A. Aubry, M. Marraud, B. Vitoux
ISBN : John Libbey Eurotext 0 86196 151 X
INSERM 2 85598 354 1

176 Hormones and Cell Regulation (13th European Symposium). *Hormones et Régulation Cellulaire (13ᵉ Symposium Européen).*
Edited by J. Nunez, J.E. Dumont, R. Denton
ISBN : John Libbey Eurotext 0 86196 183 8
INSERM 2 85598 356 8

179 Lymphokine Receptors Interactions. *Interactions Lymphokines-récepteurs.*
Edited by D. Fradelizi, J. Bertoglio
ISBN : John Libbey Eurotext 0 86196 148 X
INSERM 2 85598 359 2

191 Anticancer Drugs (1st International Interface of Clinical and Laboratory responses to anticancer drugs). *Médicaments anticancéreux (1ʳᵉ Confrontation internationale des réponses cliniques et expérimentales aux médicaments anticancéreux).*
Edited by H. Tapiero, J. Robert, T.J. Lampidis
ISBN : John Libbey Eurotext 0 86196 223 0
INSERM 2 85598 393 2

193 Living in the Cold (2nd International Symposium). *La Vie au Froid (2ᵉ Symposium International).*
Edited by A. Malan, B. Canguilhem
ISBN : John Libbey Eurotext 0 86196 234 9
INSERM 2 85598 395 9

Colloques INSERM
ISSN 0768-3154

194 Progress in Hepatitis B Immunization. *La Vaccination contre l'épatite B.*
Edited by P. Coursaget, M.J. Tong
ISBN : John Libbey Eurotext 0 86196 2494
INSERM 2 85598 396 7

196 Treatment Strategy in Hodgkin's Disease. *Stratégie dans la maladie de Hodgkin.*
Edited by P. Sommers, M. Henry-Amar,
J.H. Meezwaldt, P. Carde
ISBN : John Libbey Eurotext 0 86196 226 5
INSERM 2 85598 398 3

198 Hormones and Cell Regulation (14th European Symposium). *Hormones et Régulation Cellulaire (14e Symposium Européen).*
Edited by J. Nunez, J.E. Dumont
ISBN : John Libbey Eurotext 0 86196 229 X
INSERM 2 85598 400 9

199 Placental Communications : Biochemical, Morphological and Cellular Aspects. *Communications placentaires : aspects biochimique, morphologique et cellulaire.*
Edited by L. Cedard, E. Alsat, J.C. Challier,
G. Chaouat, A. Malassiné
ISBN : John Libbey Eurotext 0 86196 227 3
INSERM 2 85598 401 7

204 Pharmacologie Clinique : Actualités et Perspectives. (6e Rencontres Nationales de Pharmacologie clinique).
Edited by J.P. Boissel, C. Caulin, M. Teule
ISBN : John Libbey Eurotext 0 86196 225 7
INSERM 2 85598 454 8

205 Recent Trends in Clinical Pharmacology (6th National Meeting of Clinical Pharmacology).
Edited by J.P. Boissel, C. Caulin, M. Teule
ISBN : John Libbey Eurotext 0 86196 256 7
INSERM 2 85598 455 6

206 Platelet Immunology : Fundamental and Clinical Aspects. *Immunologie plaquettaire : aspects fondamentaux et cliniques.*
Edited by C. Kaplan-Gouet, N. Schlegel,
Ch. Salmon, J. McGregor
ISBN : John Libbey Eurotext 0 86196 285 0
INSERM 2 85598 439 4

Colloques INSERM
ISSN 0768-3154

207 Thyroperoxidase and Thyroid Autoimmunity. *Thyroperoxydase et auto-immunité thyroïdienne.*
Edited by P. Carayon, T. Ruf
ISBN : John Libbey Eurotext 0 86196 277 X
INSERM 2 85598 440 8

208 Vasopressin. *Vasopressine.*
Edited by S. Jard, R. Jamison
ISBN : John Libbey Eurotext 0 86196 288 5
INSERM 2 85598 441 6

210 Hormones and Cell Regulation (15th European Symposium). *Hormones et Régulation Cellulaire (15ᵉ Symposium Européen).*
Edited by J.E. Dumont, J. Nunez, R.J.B. King
ISBN : John Libbey Eurotext 0 86196 279 6
INSERM 2 85598 443 2

211 Medullary Thyroid Carcinoma. *Cancer Médullaire de la Thyroïde.*
Edited by C. Calmettes, J.M. Guliana
ISBN : John Libbey Eurotext 0 86196 287 7
INSERM 2 85598 440 0

212 Cellular and Molecular Biology of the Materno-Fetal Relationship. *Biologie cellulaire et moléculaire de la relation materno-fœtale.*
Edited by G. Chaouat, J. Mowbray
ISBN : John Libbey Eurotext 0 86196 909 1
INSERM 2 85598 445 9

215 Aldosterone. Fundamental Aspects. *Aspects fondamentaux.*
Edited by J.P. Bonvalet, N. Farman, M. Lombes, M.E. Rafestin-Oblin
ISBN : John Libbey Eurotext 0 86196 302 4
INSERM 2 85598 482 3

217 Sleep and Cardiorespiratory Control. *Sommeil et contrôle cardio-respiratoire.*
Edited by C. Gaultier, P. Escourrou, L. Curzi-Dascalora
ISBN : John Libbey Eurotext 0 86196 307 5
INSERM 2 85598 484 X

LOUIS-JEAN
avenue d'Embrun, 05003 GAP cedex
Tél. : 92.53.17.00
Dépôt légal : 739 — Septembre 1991
Imprimé en France